Biochemistry and Molecular Biology in the Post Genomic Era

Medicine & Health
New York

Biochemistry and Molecular Biology in the Post Genomic Era

Structure and Function of Cytochromes
Elaine J. Mathis (Editor)
2022. ISBN: 979-8-88697-102-6 (Hardcover)
2022. ISBN: 979-8-88697-122-4 (eBook)

Laboratory Guide: Concepts and Protocols for Practical Courses in Biochemistry and Molecular Biology
Shafat Ahmad Latoo, M.S., PhD (Editor)
Mohammad Asif Shah, M.S., PhD (Editor)
2022. ISBN: 978-1-68507-862-1 (Hardcover)
2022. ISBN: 979-8-88697-028-9 (eBook)

Omics for Animal Sciences: Principles and Approaches
Asif Nadeem (Author)
Maryam Javed (Author)
2022. ISBN: 978-1-68507-722-8 (Hardcover)
2022. ISBN: 978-1-68507-901-7 (eBook)

The Future of Metabolic Engineering
Abhishek Sharma, PhD (Editor)
Dhruti Amin, PhD (Editor)
2022. ISBN: 978-1-68507-362-6 (Hardcover)
2022. ISBN: 978-1-68507-464-7 (eBook)

Recent Advances in Computer Aided Drug Designing
Akhil Varshney, PhD, Ashutosh Mani, PhD (Editors)
2021. ISBN: 978-1-53619-739-6 (Hardcover)
2021. ISBN: 978-1-53619-904-8 (eBook)

More information about this series can be found at
https://novapublishers.com/product-category/series/biochemistry-and-molecular-biology-in-the-post-genomic-era/

Sevgi Durna Daştan
and Taner Daştan
Editors

Metabolomics and Clinical Approach

nova
Medicine & Health
New York

NOTICE TO THE READER

Library of Congress Cataloging-in-Publication Data

ISBN: 979-8-89113-095-1

Published by Nova Science Publishers, Inc. † New York

Contents

Preface

Metabolomics is the scientific study of chemical processes involving metabolites, substrates, intermediates, and namely all reagents and products of cell metabolism. Metabolomics and Clinical Approach will contribute to the the large-scale scientific study of small molecules within cells, biofluids, tissues or organisms and their interactions within a biological system. Also this book gives a perspective about study steps of metabolomics, the relationship of different diseases and metabolites, and the use of metabolomics in the treatment processes of different clinical pictures and diseases in the light of current information obtained from the literature. This book aims to describe all types of contents, effects, and kinetics of metabolite production related with metabolomics, as well as to summarize from the beginning to the end. Because the significance of metabolomics science and clinical trials increases day by day. Some diseases like cancer are an important cause of mortality for which no definitive treatment has yet been found. Further investigation of the relationship between metabolomics and diseases will open new horizons for diagnosis and treatment of many kind of diseases. This book presents all about metabolomics from the beginning to the end, as many kind of studies, potential mechanisms, diagnosis techniques, the metabolomics technologies like GC-MS, LC-MS, and software programmes about metabolomics analysis.

Chapter 1 - Responses provided by living beings to environmental stimuli and other effects can exhibit variation. Sufficiently convincing explanations for the physiological reasons for such variation could not be obtained from studies utilizing transcriptomics or proteomics. The final part of the physiological cascade of a given mechanism is open to environmental effects. Metabolites can be used to evaluate such changes. Detailed investigations and categorizing metabolites are now possible due to the development of analytical techniques, which pave the way for metabolomic studies. Metabolomics is a sub-branch in the field of systems biology. Metabolomics defines the comprehensive categorization of metabolites that are formed by genomic mechanisms and interactions with environmental stimuli. In recent years, novel tools and databases have been developed to enable the confident analysis, identification, and quantification of metabolites from various sources (e.g., plants, animals, humans, foods, and environment) and to process large-scale data sets for easier access. The core of systems biology includes blending data provided by omics (e.g., transcriptomics, proteomics, nutrigenomics, lipidomics, glycomics, interactomics, and fluxomics) with bioinformatic processing. Today, metabolomics is extensively used in various research areas, including diagnostics, biomarker identification, cancer research, genetic disorders, metabolic pathway research, pharmaceutical research, toxicity determination, animal science, and agricultural and nutritional research.

Chapter 2 - Obesity is one of the non-infectious public health problems that is constantly increasing worldwide. With the results of cardiovascular, cerebrovascular, and metabolic diseases due to obesity, it is an important health problem. In the prediction of obesity and its causes of health problems, it is possible to take measures with the help of metabolomic methods, which benefit from small molecular markers. A large number of metabolites have been used in the calculation of personal metabolic BMI, and the most important of these will be considered. In this chapter, information about the relationship between metabolomics and BMI and their possible uses is given.

Chapter 3 - Aging is a multifactorial and inexpugnable period of biological organisms. By age, many biological and metabolic events occur to destroy organs in the human body. With age, muscle mass starts to decrease, chronic and neurodegenerative disease diagnoses increase, and response to infections become weaker. Diet, physical activities, infections, and genetic factors are the components of how aging will be. The research can be carried out in both non-mammalian and mammalians subjects and with a sample of body fluids easily. Investigations with metabolomics will be the future of many treatment modalities, end of the diseases, and may be the key to a long-life span.

Chapter 4 - The integrative science of metabolites, metabolomics, today encompasses life sciences in every aspect, ranging from the discovery of metabolic pathways in species to the identification of significant biomarkers for various physiological and pathological conditions. Metabolism is the foundation of living systems that contains small and low molecular weight substances called metabolites in its entirety, which is an intricate network of numerous molecular pathways working seamlessly. As a discipline, metabolomics studies the metabolome, which is the integrative whole of all the steps of metabolism and its interactions in a living system. The entire DNA existence of a living system is called the genome, which contains all the genes responsible for functional units of transcripts and proteins. The genome also has its own set of modifications primarily on genes called the epigenome, which adds to its complexity. Metabolites as substances differ from gene-encoded products of transcripts and proteins by their intermediary and transitive natures, which are not well-defined as the gene-encoded products. In this chapter, the genetic basis of metabolomics and its possible applications in the research are reviewed.

Chapter 5 - The development and advancements in technology, artificial intelligence, and fields of bioinformatics, enabled the use of enormous data coming from genes, transcripts, and proteins processed by the omics in medicine as biomarkers. Scientists are improving different methods, such as stem-cell therapies, applications of regenerative medicine, and enhanced drug interactions in personalized medicine, using omics technologies in a broad scope of biology. Thus, the omics can discern functions of individual genes, proteins, and metabolites; to evaluate drug effects of drugs made or derived from such substances; and analyze differences in cellular pathways that occur from these drugs. The combined use of omics with system biology in regenerative medicine research, and pharmacology fields increases the information regarding concealed molecular mechanisms of diseases, their potential therapies, and personalized applications of stem-cell applications. Improved characterization of living systems along with a detailed evaluation of clinical and pharmacological data are required aspects for the further development of studies containing multiple omics methodologies. The application of data mining on the present data from the literature would enable to obtain experimental evidence in a cost-effective manner by reducing the prior experimental research. Metabolomics in pharmacology serves to attain personalization in medicinal treatments to preserve health and prevent diseases. Different branches of omics, such as metabolomics, transcriptomics, proteomics, and toxicogenomics, would lead to improved and easier use of pharmacometabolites in treatment protocols.

Chapter 6 - Metabolomics detects, identifies, and quantifies small molecule-containing metabolites in cells, tissues, and physiological fluids through high-performance yielding technologies. Metabolomics is an integral part of biotechnology, which includes drug activity investigations, enzyme-to-substrate interactions, biomarker identifications, and metabolomic pathway analyses. Metabolite profiling can be achieved cost-effectively in a short time with high precision and specificity through High-Performance Liquid Chromatography (HPLC), one of the analytical methods. Metabolomics research is seen in different fields, including nutrition, toxicology, environmental pollution, drug research and development, and a broad spectrum of biochemical and industrial analyses. Here in this chapter, fundamental basics about HPLC will be given, and the use and importance of HPLC in metabolomics will be highlighted.

Chapter 7 - The field of metabolomics is becoming an indispensable part of clinical research with its potential for the discovery of biomarkers and diagnostic molecules along with its potential for revealing concealed aspaects of pathophysiological conditions. Basically, metabolomics aims to objectively identify and quantify all metabolites present in a living system at a particular state or point of time. In summary, all metabolomics research contains steps of sample collection and processing, detection, and analysis of raw data, and evaluation of the results. A frame of the metabolic state of a eukaryotic living system can be understood by using various biological samples ranging from cerebospinal fluid to tissues to blood plasma. Each biological sample contains a large set of endogenous compounds that are classified under various compounds, e.g., organic acids, amino acids, peptides, carbohydrates, etc. Both internal (gender, age, health, physiological state, etc.) and external (diet, lifestyle, pollution, environment, etc.) stimuli affect the metabolite composition, sometimes quite strikingly. A large number of variables are effective in the composition of metabolites, which requires a careful design of the research and the use of standardized experimental procedures encompassing all the steps. There are conventional standardized methods for the individual identification of particular metabolites based on their compound classes. Metabolomics methods, however, aim to detect and profile the global metabolite context by applying pattern recognition and profiling on complex sets of metabolite data. Currently, there is no single approach to achieve such a daunting task. Therefore, different analytical approaches are used according to the intended metabolomics study. An analytical method should be both sensitive and comprehensive to cover large data series of metabolites in a robust and specific manner. Of the available methods, nuclear magnetic resonance (NMR) and mass spectrometry are the best instrumental and analytical methods frequently used for metabolomics research. The high sensitivity and wide dynamic range provided by mass spectrometry (MS) can be coupled with chromatography methods to achieve large-scale analysis of metabolites from biological samples. Mass spectrometry can be coupled with liquid chromatography (LC) for the metabolite profiling of thermolabile or involatile compounds. The LC-MS-based metabolomics research that used the liquid chromatography-mass spectrometry (LC-MS) approach was reviewed in this chapter.

Chapter 8 - All biochemical elements that are part of the metabolism are represented in their entirety as the metabolome. It enables researchers to link the phenotype to the function provided as a whole from the genome and environmental variables. Cellular investigations of different components, e.g., DNA, mRNA, proteins, and their interactions, are now largely complemented with metabolomic research for revealing the function and interactions of individual metabolites. Different repositories for various molecules and molecular pathways are present for researchers. The metabolism itself is a vast network of intricate biochemical interactions, and mathematical models are required for a detailed analysis of particular pathways. Such a complex network of interactions can be better assessed using computational algorithms employing precise mathematical models. Metabolomics is already a noteworthy field in discovering novel therapeutic agents. In response to the increased demand for metabolomics research in various fields, different in silico tools were developed for the integrative analysis of metabolic systems, which have their own algorithms and pipelines for data simulation and evaluation. Some of the noteworthy metabolomic databases and associated software are introduced in this chapter.

Chapter 9 - Metabolomics is a field of omics that developed after genomics, transcriptomics, and proteomics as an important study area of systems biology. Metabolomic studies have gained an important place in various research areas, especially in the early diagnosis and treatment of diseases. For this purpose, metabolites are identified through software databanks using various separation and detection methods. Thanks to the development of software and computer and analytical device technology, new ones are added to what we know about the metabolome and metabolites every day. This chapter aims to guide researchers in a sequential manner on the past, present, and future goals of metabolomics studies.

Chapter 10 - Traumatic brain injury (TBI) is an important pathology that can cause severe disability and unexpected sudden death. In the pathogenesis of TBI, many biochemical reactions develop at the cellular level and these mechanisms can cause significant changes in some of the body's metabolites. Clinical, radiological, and biochemical data are used in the evaluation of traumatic brain injuries due to the complex physiology of the brain. For the classification of trauma, clinicians often use the Glasgow Coma Scale (GCS). In addition, radiologically taken MR Spectroscopy evaluations and biochemical markers made from samples such as blood and cerebrospinal fluid provide enlightening information about TBI. Metabolomics can be biochemically detected in body fluids such as blood, cerebrospinal fluid, etc., in sudden traumatic brain injury and can give important information about the course of the disease and the severity of the trauma and the mortality and morbidity of the patient.

Chapter 11 - Diabetes mellitus is a chronic metabolic disease in which hyperglycemia results from insulin resistance and reduced insulin, as in type 2 diabetes (T2D), or destruction of insulin-producing pancreatic β-cells as in type 1 diabetes (T1D). The mortality rate is higher in the diabetes population than in the general population, largely owing to cardiovascular and renal complications. Recent studies have shown that the only essential factor is the patient, not the disease. The genomic structure of each patient shapes the disease in its unique way. In this determination, an -omic identity emerges. The application of metabolomics in diabetes has simplified the identification of metabolites that can serve as screening and prognostic biomarkers. Metabolomic studies on diabetic subjects demonstrated many altered metabolic pathways and variations. Identifying predictive biomarkers involved in the pathogenesis of diabetes is essential, and avoiding complications related to personalized phenotyping and individualized drug response are recent study subjects. So, it is aimed to review the use of metabolomics and its impacts on diabetes research in this chapter.

Chapter 12 - Metabolomics is the process of detecting, quantifying, and recognizing metabolites present in the whole organism over a period of time as biomarkers or by using technologies to study disease pathogenesis. Many platforms are used for these procedures, including NMR and several MS technologies. Recently, metabolites have been used in many areas of orthopedics. Metabolite markers have been identified in many orthopedic diseases. An understanding of the pathogenesis of diseases was achieved. First, a metabolomic study of osteoarthritis was conducted. Additionally, metabolites show us an important way in many cases such as the diagnosis of diseases, treatment, fusion of bone fractures, and biomaterials used in orthopedics.

Chapter 13 - It is essential to select the best embryos to transfer in any in vitro fertilization (IVF) treatment. Human embryos could only be assessed morphologically in the clinical setting until recent times. However, since this assessment is observation-based, it is open to both interpersonal and variability between observations made by the same person at different times. Preimplantation embryo metabolism demonstrates distinctive features associated with the developmental potential of embryos. On this basis, it has been assumed that the metabolite content of the culture medium reflects the implantation potential of individual embryos. The need for a non-invasive, reliable, and rapid embryo assessment strategy has promoted IVF metabolomic studies to increase the success rates of single embryo transfers. It is crucial to assess glucose, protein, or oxygen utilization according to the metabolism of human embryos.

Metabolomic profiling is an analysis of cell-free DNA released by the embryo into the culture medium. Although it is the most promising technologies developed to date for embryo selection, it is currently not suitable for clinical use.

Chapter 14 - The pregnancy process is an intricate and unique period that requires control examinations to ensure the continuity of the well-being of the mother and the baby. The accompanying changes are also evident biologically, physiologically, psychologically, and socially. Several factors must be considered to determine when a woman's pregnancy is at risk and when unfavorable pregnancy outcomes will occur. Biomedical indicators are critical in medicine. Studies show that the variables in these indicators are vital in determining the risk status. Once the metabolic pathways are understood clearly in healthy and diseased conditions, we can gain more applicable information on disease mechanisms and precise treatment approaches. The prenatal medicine practices require the development of novel non-invasive approaches that cover diverse categories of diseases with lower rates of false-positives. Metabolomics for this purpose has the potential of great advantage. Metabolomic studies measure and analyze the biochemistry products of cells. As a biomarker, metabolomics may uncover new diagnostic and therapeutic approaches. This chapter reviews the idea and utilization of metabolomics for maternal health and perinatal medicine, emphasizing the latest developments in metabolomics studies and the research agenda. In addition, the existence of studies that will increase our knowledge about the etiopathogenesis of maternal complications is exciting and promising.

Chapter 15 - Metabolomics has presented specific findings about metabolite variations in multi-biofluids and tissues and has provided countless potential biomarkers and therapeutic targets. Metabolomics is significant when considering the need for diagnostic biopsies of the central neural system tissues in neurological diseases and difficulties in clinical practice.

Additional metabolic pathways that show involvement in different disease steps are demonstrated despite the genetic and pathophysiological heterogeneity of neurological diseases. Metabolic pathways are variable dynamic systems that are controlled by endogenous circadian mechanisms. Experimental models on metabolic reprogramming are significantly informative about the molecular mechanisms underlying metabolic changes.

These mechanisms and steps are essential in terms of defining the therapeutic window. Additionally, knowing the next step in the disease progress enables critical practices for treatment to be applied.

Chapter 16 - Metabolomics is the large-scale study of small molecules produced from the metabolic activities of the organism, and these molecules are generally called metabolites. The relationships of these metabolites with each other and with the biological system are called the metabolome. Unlike genomics, proteomics and transcriptomics, metabolomics is a field of study that examines in a broad spectrum of all metabolic activities in organisms. These metabolites are commonly divided into two groups, targeted and untargeted: targeted metabolites are based on quantitative methods that allow the metabolite concentration to be measured; and untargeted metabolites are those that envisage the simultaneous evaluation of large-scale metabolites without any prior sample information to form hypotheses. It is also suitable for describing changes in different pathophysiological conditions. There are many considerations about the functions of metabolic processes and individual metabolites, and important information has been recorded. They have important roles in immune cells. To identify metabolites that explain how the immune system works, the use of mass spectrometry and NMR spectroscopy-based platforms provides important biomarkers of how the immune system functions. This section gives important clues about how metabolomics is used in the immunology field. In particular, future roles of metabolomics in the immune system will be discussed.

Chapter 17 - Neurological and psychiatric diseases and disorders remain great public health hazards. There is a need for research for their early diagnosis and for developing more effective treatment approaches. In neurological and psychiatric diseases, which are multifactorial conditions without a single gene mutation, metabolomics is important for a holistic assessment. Nuclear magnetic resonance (NMR)-based and chromatography/mass spectrometry-based approaches can be clinically applied to assess the metabolome. MS has become significantly important in biological and biomedical research in the last 20 years. Ionization sources, matrix-assisted laser desorption/ionization (MALDI), secondary ion mass spectrometry (SIMS), and desorption electrospray ionization (DESI), are now included in the most important mass spectrometry imaging (IMS) studies. The ability to identify the spatial distribution of hundreds of analytes in a single imaging study without needing a label or preliminary information is one of the main advantages of MALDI-IMS over other imaging methods. Studies using MALDI-IMS have been conducted to better understand the cellular pathology and/or severity of the disease in neurology and psychiatry. Moreover, MALDI-IMS has enabled the matching of specific classes of analytes with brain regions that may have been lost using more traditional methods. The clinical uses of mass spectrometry-based approaches in neurology and psychiatry will be addressed in this section.

Chapter 18 - Metabolomics deals with small molecule metabolites, and one of their main purposes is to identify those small molecules that make differences in the metabolic effects of different diets. Thus, deepening our knowledge of the interactive and regulatory roles of human health and nutrition. Metabolomics, pharmacology, and toxicology have also been widely adopted, but they are relatively new to human nutrition. Today, scientists play an important role in the health status of people by finding new bioactive food components that prevent cancer, obesity, diabetes, cardiovascular and chronic diseases, as well as prolong life and improve physical and mental health. In this context, the use of high-throughput metabolomics techniques contributes to the development of nutritional models, the benefits of a diet to metabolism, and the improvement of physiological responses to this diet. That is, it provides a better understanding of the effects of genes, enzymes, proteins, metabolites, and microenvironments at the cellular level. Metabolomics can assist in the design of nutritional programs and improve our understanding of nutrition and the role of nutrients in promoting and maintaining cellular functions and overall health. The purpose of this section is to make a general assessment of nutritional metabolomics, to emphasize the effects of nutritional metabolomics on clinical studies, and to contribute to the scientific literature on these issues.

Chapter 19 - Comparing the vast variation in biochemical processes seen in tumor cells with normal cells can be considered the initiation of metabolomics research, which is now used in different medical fields. Currently, there is an undisputed need for clinically relevant biomarkers that can be used for the diagnosis and prognosis of urologic cancer types, e.g., prostate, bladder, and metabolomics can be considered promising at this stage. Novel and relevant biomarkers are required for specialized diagnosis, monitoring, and treatment of a particular disease, which would also contribute to the improvement, enhancement, and personalization of a designed therapy. While considerable progress has been made in determining important biomarkers, more challenges remain to be solved for the further integration of metabolomics into clinical practices. This chapter reviews relevant metabolomics research conducted in the field urology.

Chapter 20 - The definition of metabolomics encloses an efficient description of small molecule metabolites present in different biological matrices. Metabolomics has shown up as a prominent tool for various areas including health diseases, drug research, plant science, food science, and nutrition. The metabolomics has recently been used to investigate some parameters in particular for food quality, processing, and the safety of both raw materials and final products. Food metabolomics has also a position in human nutrition research. This book chapter focuses on the novel and potential applications of metabolomics in food science and nutrition by summarizing some metabolomic analysis of food components, metabolomics from the preferential, presumable, and informative approaches in food processing, food microbiology, food safety, food quality, and benefits of foodomics in human nutrition and related health diseases.

Chapter 21 - Recently, many articles and reviews on metabolomics have been published in the fields of perinatology, obstetrics, and pediatrics. Metabolomics, which lies at the end point of the "omics cascade," allows for the detection of alterations in systems-level metabolites within biological pathways, thus providing insights into the mechanisms that underlie various physiological conditions and pathologies. Metabolomics, along with transcriptomics, has an essential role in discovering connections between genetic regulation, metabolite phenotyping, and biomarker identification. Biomarkers discovered through metabolomics may shed some light on the etiology of certain newborn pathological conditions (such as preterm birth, intrauterine growth retardation, asphyxia, metabolic diseases, neurological disorders, organ pathologies, sepsis, nutritional problems) and their adverse effects on infant development and improve current clinical conditions.

Chapter 22 - Preterm birth is a multi-sided condition affecting more than 15 billion infants and women per year around the world. In the challenges of dealing with preterm birth and its accompanying morbidities, including respiratory and neurological disorders, increase the medical and pecuniary burden due to the increased survival of very preterm infants. Therefore, prevention and early detection of preterm birth associated mortality and/or morbidity is crucial to deal with these challenges. Metabolomics are promising 'clue' molecules of human metabolism. Maternal, fetal, and neonatal body fluids include many metabolomics that can be used as either early biomarkers or targeted therapeutic molecules of major preterm birth-related morbidities, including respiratory distress syndrome, pulmonary hypertension, and bronchopulmonary dysplasia. Given the wide range of prematurity associated disorders and human body fluid bioenvironment, more metabolomics are expected to be identified to improve quality of care. Thus, future research on body fluid metabolomics is expected to bring today's individualized medicine closer to predict PTB by providing a better understanding of its underlying mechanisms.

Chapter 23 - Metabolites are small molecules that are the end products of enzymatic processes in the human body. Inborn errors of metabolism (IEM) are inherited, known to have a poor prognosis, generally and luckily rarely diseases. More than 1000 diseases were defined about metabolite deficiency, enzymatic dysfunction, or absence (Ferreira & van Karnebeek, 2019). The first studies on inborn errors of metabolism started in the 1900s with most popular diseases including albinisim, cystinuria, and alkaptonuria (Vangala & Tonelli, 2007). From those years, with the help of new technology, new studies are performed with a few drops of blood and provided to check more than 20 metabolic diseases with one sample. More than 100 years before, diagnosed metabolic diseases numbers were smaller, but for now the diagnostic ratio of IEM increased 5 times much more than those years. Thus, an early diagnosis can be possible with screening all newborns, not only probable patients or newborns with a family history. So, in many countries it becomes a part of the routine neonatal screening programme to diagnose in early newborn period before symptoms occur. By the help of technological systems, the new study area of the point is metabolomics and the analysing of the metabolite profiles of the biological system to understand genes' effects in many metabolic inherited diseases.

Chapter 24 - Metabolomics is the systematic analysis of the particular chemical fingerprints of small molecules or metabolite profiles which are associated with a different cellular metabolic process in a cell, organ, or organism. Events in a cell are not described completely by messenger RNA gene expression data and proteomic analyses, but metabolic profiling supplies direct and indirect physiological insights, which can possibly be measurable in a broad range of biospecimens. Even though not specific to cardiac conditions, identification, confirmation, clinical validation, and bedside tests are a biomarker exploration path to translate metabolomics into cardiovascular biomarkers. Technological progress in metabolomic tools (such as nuclear magnetic resonance spectroscopy and mass spectrometry) and more complicated bioinformatics and analytical techniques help to evaluate low-molecular-weight metabolites in biospecimens and ultimately supply a unique insight into determined and novel metabolic pathways. Systematic metabolomics can provide physiological knowledge of cardiovascular disease states in addition to traditional profiling and can include the definition of metabolic reactions of an individual or population to therapeutic interventions or environmental exposures.

Chapter 1

The Concept of Metabolomics

Sinan Vıcıl[1,*], PhD
and Tünay Karan[2], PhD
[1]Department of Biochemistry, Tekirdag Namık Kemal University, Tekirdag, Turkey
[2]Department of Genetics, Yozgat Bozok University, Yozgat, Turkey

Abstract

Responses provided by living beings to environmental stimuli and other effects can exhibit variation. Sufficiently convincing explanations for the physiological reasons for such variation could not be obtained from studies utilizing transcriptomics or proteomics. The final part of the physiological cascade of a given mechanism is open to environmental effects. Metabolites can be used to evaluate such changes. Detailed investigations and categorizing metabolites are now possible due to the development of analytical techniques, which pave the way for metabolomic studies. Metabolomics is a sub-branch in the field of systems biology. Metabolomics defines the comprehensive categorization of metabolites that are formed by genomic mechanisms and interactions with environmental stimuli. In recent years, novel tools and databases have been developed to enable the confident analysis, identification, and quantification of metabolites from various sources (e.g., plants, animals, humans, foods, and environment) and to process large-scale data sets for easier access. The core of systems biology includes blending data provided by omics (e.g., transcriptomics, proteomics, nutrigenomics, lipidomics, glycomics, interactomics, and fluxomics) with bioinformatic processing. Today, metabolomics is extensively used in various research areas, including diagnostics,

* Corresponding Author's Email: sinanvicil@hotmail.com.

In: Metabolomics and Clinical Approach
Editors: Sevgi Durna Daştan and Taner Daştan
ISBN: 979-8-89113-095-1

biomarker identification, cancer research, genetic disorders, metabolic pathway research, pharmaceutical research, toxicity determination, animal science, and agricultural and nutritional research.

Keywords: metabolites, metabolomics, omics, systems biology

Introduction

Living beings display differences in the answers according to the situations they encounter while continuing their lives, e.g., the prognosis of a given disease or reactions to a given drug provide differences between organisms. The Human Genome Project (HGP) was considered effective in interpreting the individual variations in such responses. In short, the HGP is an international scientific project to reveal and identify the genomic sequence, structure, and functions of human genes and map these genes, which was initiated in 1990 and declared complete in 2003. The project enabled the deciphering of the entire human genome. The project revealed the existence of approximately 30k genes with 99.9% sequential similarity with 0.1% individual variation. Translating these variations to physiology using transcriptomics and proteomics did not reveal convincing results. Under physiological conditions, the final parts of any mechanism are susceptible to environmental stimuli. Metabolites are the biological variables in such conditions, termed the "clinical phenotype" (Venter, 2003; Bren, 2005).

Metabolites

Metabolites are small chemical compounds with low molecular weights, such as signal transducers, hormones, intermediaries, or final products, resulting from biochemical reactions. These compounds are the result of cellular synthesis and enzymatic processing. They would not aggregate in tissues and transform into other products. They generally have lower than 1500 Da molecular weights. Biomolecules of carbohydrates, lipids, proteins, peptides, amino acids, amines, steroids, nucleosides, oligonucleotides, aldehydes, ketones, and alkaloids are metabolites. The amount of metabolites in a given living system is variable. It can amount to several hundred in lower eukaryotes, several thousand in higher eukaryotes (i.e., mammals), and several hundreds of thousands in plants due to their complex sets of metabolic cascades (Van der Werf et al., 2007; Kaplan & Celebier, 2020).

Plant metabolites are called primary and secondary metabolites according to how they are synthesized and their functions. The synthesis of primary metabolites is similar among living systems, and they have essential functions in maintaining life, reproduction, growth, development, and metabolism. Secondary metabolites do not have a role in fundamental life functions but are functional in environmental interactions and adaptiveness. They are structurally more complex compared to primary metabolites. They are the biologically active parts of the plant metabolome that would be effective in pharmaceutical applications. Secondary metabolites have different chemical groups that are divided into alkaloids, phenolics, terpenes, and steroids (Topcu & Çölgeçen, 2015).

The determination and quantification of metabolites have been used for diagnostics and treatment for years. However, the concept of the metabolite profile has arisen due to omics integration into systems biology. Metabolite profiling aims to reveal physiological cascades and their association with various pathologies by the determination and analysis of metabolites present in the cellular milieu and bodily fluids. Metabolite profiling has a beneficial prospect in diagnosing and prognostics of various diseases with their providence of biomarkers.

Systems Biology

The Concepts of Systems Biology and the Omics

While Systems Biology is an already established field of study, it has been more pronounced in the scientific community since 2000. Some attribute this increased visibility to the HGP completed in 2003. Nevertheless, the insufficient contribution of the data revealed by the HGP to existing problems leads the scientific community to different approaches. At this point, the field of systems biology has come into the scene as a discipline of integrative research on structure, form, and interactions of mechanisms of organisms (Kasap et al., 2010). The conventional approach to studying cells, tissues, and organs includes investigations independent of each other, whereas systems biology includes an integrative approach to all mechanisms of living systems. There are some agreed-upon definitions for systems biology; (1) it is a scientific discipline that aims to understand biological systems as a whole instead of at the molecular level (Kitano, 2002); and (2) it is a multidisciplinary novel scientific division that investigates genes, proteins, and biochemical pathways as a whole with their inter-relations (Institute for Systems Biology) (Vailati-Riboni et al., 2017).

Researchers embracing this novel concept aim to investigate integratively system-wide genes, proteins, and all other parts with their relationships and dependencies instead of at the individual level. It is known that parts that constitute the organisms are not genuinely functional by themselves but truly gain their functions together with others. This integrative composition includes the parts and the biochemical pathways that regulate the interactions between these parts. Back in 1940, Bertalanffy proposed the idea of integrative investigations of biological systems instead of investigating separately, but this idea could not proceed past postulation and remained dormant (Kasap et al., 2010). Systems biology accumulated more interest starting in 2000 due to the astonishing developments in genomics and associated technologies. The developed tools contributed to understanding the flow of information from genes to proteins and their associated mechanisms of action. In parallel to these developments, improvements in biochemical techniques have accelerated the identification of protein-to-enzyme relationships in a biochemical pathway. The conventional understanding of the investigation of biological systems, including humans, provided limited data about the functions of operations and failed to provide convincingly adequate explanations for various conditions and diseases. The drive behind systems biology was the idea of an impairment in the primary mechanism in the case where an integral part becomes hampered (Kitano, 2002).

With the development of imaging methods, a more objective approach could be put forward by considering the three-dimensional structures of molecules. It has started to be used in software development, and technologies that can make experimental models elucidate mechanisms have been used. The addition of software to systems biology studies contributed to being multidisciplinary and paved the way for the virtual modeling of living beings. Such models have started to be used in areas of the formation of disease mechanisms and the preliminary trials of drugs. In addition, the elucidation of the mechanisms for the reflection of the information at the gene level by changing with the environmental conditions has also taken its place among the objectives of the modeling studies (Kasap et al., 2010).

In systems biology studies, data from sub-disciplines of genomics, transcriptomics, and metabolomics should be identified with bioinformatics.

The –omics suffix in the names of the sub-disciplines in question adds the meaning of "all-to-whole" to the term. The –omics suffix has started to appear more frequently with the prominence of integrative approaches. Its first use dates back to the 1920s. Hans Winkler used the word genome on this date. By the 1980s, the term genomics entered the literature, and after the developments in the field of genomics, other -omics technologies were encountered following the 2000s. These technologies are transcriptomics, proteomics, metabolomics, nutrigenomics, lipidomics, glycomics, interactomics, and fluxomics. Systems biology is the blending of -omics technologies and bioinformatics. The non-targeted detection of genes, proteins, and metabolites in a biological sample is a fundamental issue of systems biology (Budak & Donmez, 2012).

The main feature of the approach, in which the -omics technologies are used, is to better understand a complex system by considering it as a whole. In integrative approaches, all available data are carefully collected and analyzed with appropriate methods. This approach is practical when the hypothesis is unknown, unpredictable, and suitable for hypothesis-generating experiments. When applied to well-constructed models, the -omics approaches help reveal the connections and interactions between parts of a complex mechanism (Levin et al., 2016).

The Omics Technologies

Genomics

The gene is an inheritable fundamental element that carries the codes of enzymes and similar molecules, especially protein structures, controls the functioning of all biochemical and physiological mechanisms required for the continuation of life, and ensures the transfer of hereditary characteristics to the next generations. Genes consist of nucleotide sequences located at a certain point on the chromosomes. The genome represents all the genetic information carried by the chromosomes. Regarding the genome, the studies carried out to identify all genes in a living being, solve their structures and functions, and understand the mechanisms are called genomics. It is one of the first developing fields of omics. The Human Genome Project is a vital step in genomics (Basaran et al., 2010). All data obtained in the project were processed into a common database with the developed software. In this way, a detailed source of information about all genes' locations, structures, and functions has been created. With the Human Genome Project, the genetic risk distribution of various chronic diseases has been determined, and essential data have been provided to investigate many genetic diseases' diagnoses and treatment possibilities. Today, it is known that it is impossible to prevent, diagnose, or treat diseases with only genomic studies, and other omic techniques are needed to determine specific individual strategies in the health field. Genomics is divided into two sub-disciplines: (1) structural genomics, which aims to discover and comprehend genetic information using gene mapping and nucleotide sequencing, and (2) transcriptomics, which aims to discover and elucidate gene functions and relations using genome-wide analysis of gene expressions, modes and periods of gene expressions, and their functional reflection to the organism (Horgan & Kenny, 2011; Basaran et al., 2010; Recber, 2019).

Transcriptomics

All mRNA (messenger RNA) transcripts in a cell for a specific period are called the transcriptome. An mRNA is responsible for transmitting the genetic code of the amino acid combination of the protein to be synthesized, which is formed as a result of the transcription of DNA, to the ribosomes. One of the mechanisms sought to be elucidated in living beings is understanding how the same genome can give rise to different cell types and how gene expression is regulated. Comparing mRNAs at different times in cells and tissues with transcriptomic analyses is influential in determining how gene expression changes in different organisms and the emergence of diseases. With these studies, it is possible to obtain information about which genes are active during a given disease, but it is not yet possible to know at what rate these genes are used (Recber, 2019). This situation occurs because an mRNA is not always translated into a protein; therefore, mRNA levels do not fully reflect the encoded protein activity. It is known that proteins are much more effective than genes and transcripts in regulating cell functions (Tyers & Mann, 2003).

Proteomics

Proteins are structures of amino acids linked by peptide bonds. They have essential functions in many cellular mechanisms, including being structurally present in cells, catalyzing their metabolic reactions, DNA replication, responsiveness to stimuli, and transporting molecules from one location to another. All proteins encoded by the genome in an organism or system, which can differentiate between cells and change over time, constitute the proteome. Proteomics, on the other hand, is the process of determining the structures, locations, amounts, modifications, functions, and interactions of all proteins with other proteins and molecules under certain conditions in a particular biological system or organism. The proteome is a more dynamic structure compared to the genome and transcriptome. Therefore, proteomic studies are much more complex in analysis and data evaluation than genomics (Bren, 2005). Genomic studies have determined that there are approximately 30k genes in the human genome, and there is a 0.1% difference between individuals in this gene structure. Many transcriptomic and proteomic studies have been carried out to understand the functions of the genes that cause this genetic difference and to gain more information about the diseases. However, the results obtained were insufficient to explain the phenotypes clinically. Therefore, the information carried by the metabolites in the cell is needed to explain the clinical phenotypes (Madsen et al., 2010; Recber, 2019). While genomic, transcriptomic, and proteomic studies can only provide information about what can happen in the organism, metabolomic studies can directly and accurately reflect the current state of the organism and provide information about what exactly is happening in the organism (Madsen et al., 2010).

Bioinformatics

The data obtained as a result of studies in the field of omics are quite large and complex. Working with large-scale data requires significant resources and investments in time, finance, and the workforce. There is a need to develop computational and analytical technologies to deal with large-scale data and ensure that the data can circulate freely and openly and be used to the maximum effect by the broader research community. For this purpose, bioinformatics techniques have been shaped by integrating specially developed software, algorithms, databases, and statistical techniques with information from biology databases. Bioinformatics facilitates integration in the fields of omics and acts as a bridge with other disciplines (Blekherman et al., 2011). In recent years, with the increasing impact of basic biological research on medical sciences and clinical fields, it has pioneered the development of modern epidemiological, diagnostic, diagnostic, and therapeutic modules. It is thought that the importance of bioinformatics studies for clinical sciences will increase even more, and it is suggested that applications such as including DNA sequence information in patients' medical files will be started (Kasap et al., 2010; Levin et al., 2016).

Others

The glycome is the name of all the carbohydrate structures in a cell or tissue. The sub-discipline that tries to define the locations, amounts and relationships of carbohydrates is called glycomics. Since carbohydrates are functional in the receptor structures of cells and the mechanisms of glycosylation that affect the function of many proteins are crucial considerations in an integrative approach to the system. In this respect, systems biology draws on the field of glycomics. Interactomics examines the interactions between cellular molecules, their effects, and results, especially in terms of proteins, while fluxomics examines local changes in molecules within the cell over time (Kasap et al., 2010).

Metabolomics

The term "Metabolome" is used to describe all of the metabolites found in the organism. Metabole roughly means change, and the -om suffix means roughly total in Greek. The metabolome as a field can be defined as metabolites within the biological system and their interactions under certain genetic, nutritional, and environmental conditions. As the metabolome is the end product downstream, changes and interactions between gene expression, protein expression, and the environment are directly reflected in the metabolome, making it physically and chemically more complex than others (Guijas et al., 2018a; Nalbantoglu, 2019). According to the species, intracellular metabolites are called the endometabolome, and metabolites secreted into the extracellular fluid or the external environment are called the exometabolome. The term metabolome was first defined in 1998 during yeast metabolism studies as a complete complement of small molecules in a biological system or fluid (Stephen et al., 1998).

Metabolomics is the detection, quantification, identification, and comparison of small molecule metabolites from carbohydrates, lipids, hormones, vitamins, and other cell components in tissues, cells, and physiological fluids over a specified period, using high-throughput technologies. Metabolomics is the closest to the phenotype among other omic approaches and best modulates the molecular phenotype of health and disease. Genotype-to-genomics and phenotype-to-metabolomics relationships have been shown to refer to specific gene variations and metabolite relationships that inform about genetic, epigenetic, and phenotypic changes. In this sense, metabolomics is an intriguing resource for biomarker discovery, which has advantages over other omics approaches. Metabolomic analyses can usually be performed on body fluids such as serum, urine, cerebrospinal fluid, plasma, saliva, or tissues (Tsoukalas et al., 2017; Nalbantoglu, 2019).

Different living beings, from single-celled microorganisms to higher biological systems such as mammals, are investigated using the metabolomics approach. The number of metabolites is less than the number of proteins, transcriptomes, and genomes found in humans. Despite this less quantity, the number of external factors affecting metabolites is high. The metabolome is dynamic and easily affected by environmental factors and can change. This variability gives particular clues in the follow-up of an organism's disease or health status. Changes in metabolite levels can be considered as the final response of the organism to genetic modifications, environmental factors, changes in intestinal microflora, and changes in the kinetic activity of enzymes. Therefore, this new research platform is considered to be most closely related to the phenotype among other omic technologies (Klupczyńska et al., 2015).

While genomics, transcriptomics, and proteomics, which are the fields of omics, give clues about what will happen, metabolomics gives information about what happens. This aspect comes to the fore, especially in clinical phenotype studies. There is increasing interest in metabolomics research since genomics, transcriptomics, and proteomics cannot fully explain the response of organisms to physiological and pathophysiological stimuli. Metabolomics defines the comprehensive characterization of small molecules derived from the genome (endogenous metabolites) and their interaction with the environment (exogenous metabolites). In recent years, advanced methods have been developed that allow the reliable identification, detection, and quantification of new metabolites in food, plant, environmental, animal, and human research. The combined use of untargeted and targeted metabolomics has demonstrated many advantages beyond analytical chemistry. Advances in omics approaches have provided important insights into novel biomarkers and their potential to generate hypotheses. Advanced data processing systems have greatly helped characterize metabolic pathways in different biological systems (Di Minno et al., 2022).

Metabolomics is a multidisciplinary field that includes biology, chemistry, mathematics, and biostatistics with its diversity and integrative approach. Unlike classical biochemical approaches that focus on single metabolites, single metabolic reactions, their kinetic properties, and defined linked (i.e., precursor/product, intermediate metabolism) reactions and cycles, metabolomics collects quantitative data on a more extensive series. It creates a dynamic picture in which changing environmental conditions are also reflected in the result (Kristal et al., 2007).

The concept of metabonomics is the term used to describe analyzing and evaluating metabolites in response to various biological stimuli or genetic modifications (Nicholson & Lindon, 1999). "Metabonomics" broadly considers metabolic profiling by examining non-genomic environmental effects in metabolic disorders. However, while there are scientists who argue that there are no defining differences in the way both terms are used, there are also scientists who argue that metabolomics studies should be associated with metabolite analysis of plants and microorganisms. According to this group, using the term metabonomics in human studies would be adequate (Robertson, 2005; Lindon & Nicholson, 2008).

The main reason for recent developments in metabolomics studies compared to other omic fields is that technologically necessary opportunities were more limited in previous years. It is thought that there are between 3k to 20k metabolites in the human body (Nalbantoğlu, 2019). The diversity in the chemical structures of metabolites also affects the analysis methods. In addition, the mechanisms associated with these metabolites and other components in these mechanisms may differ in the disease state. These reasons affect the dependency on technological developments in metabolite detection and biomarker discovery studies. Despite this, current developments are progressing in a promising way. Therefore, with the samples to be produced from physiological fluids or the breath of living beings, issues such as whether there is a pathological condition, which diseases the individual has encountered before, and the effectiveness of the ongoing treatment process will gradually increase (Kaplan & Celebier, 2020).

Historical Process

Although metabolomics studies within the scope of systems biology are considered relatively new, the origins of studies on metabolomes date back to ancient civilizations. It is the first example to be noticed that ants attracted in the urine of people with diabetes in ancient China in 2000 BC (Van der Greef & Smilde, 2005). In the 4th century BC, Hippocrates associated the sweet-fruity smell in human breath with diabetes. In 1506, Ullrich Pinder worked on diagnosing some diseases with the color spectrum modeling known as the "urea wheel" (Klupczyńska et al., 2015).

However, Williams's idea in the late 1940s can be cited as the beginning of modern metabolomics studies, with the idea that individuals can have a metabolic profile that can be reflected in the structure of their physiological fluids. For this purpose, Williams et al., collected more than 200,000 urine and saliva samples from mental disorders, alcoholics, schizophrenic patients, and many different disease groups. They analyzed the samples by paper chromography and categorized the results according to disease groups, revealing the first metabolite profiling studies (Kaplan & Celebier, 2020). Subsequent progress has been made thanks to technological advances. In 1971, Hornings & Horning studied metabolites found in human tissues and urine by gas chromatography (GC-MS). They were the first to use the term "metabolic profiling" in the literature (Horning & Horning, 1971). In addition, Horning & Horning contributed to developing GC-MS methods for analyzing urinary metabolites. NMR spectroscopy, which was first discovered in the 1940s, started to be used in the field in 1974 with the studies of Seeley et al., Accessing the information that 90% of ATP in the muscle cell forms a complex with Mg using NMR has given the idea that a new analytical tool can be used in metabolite studies. In 1989, Bell et al., used NMR spectroscopy in metabolite profiling from physiological fluids (Kaplan & Celebier, 2020). After Games et al.'s studies of black pepper components with an LC-MS device, LC-MS started participating in metabolomic studies with NMR in the 1990s. In a study conducted in 1995, CSF analysis was performed in sleep-deprived mice with GC-MS and LC-MS, and as a result, a component called oleamide was found. This component was determined to act as a sleep inducer (Cravatt et al., 2015). This study was recorded as the first study in which GC-MS and LC-MS were used together. During this period, capillary electrophoresis and HPLC began in metabolomics studies (Plumb et al., 2004). Fiehn first mentioned the metabolome in 2002 (Kaplan & Celebier, 2020).

The acceleration of metabolomics studies and the developing technologies have created a need for a common database in this field. In 2005, METLIN, the first metabolomic tandem mass spectrometry database, was launched at the Siuzdak Laboratory of the Scripps Research Institute. METLIN is a mass spectrometry database repository to aid in metabolite identification. This pool contains distinctive data such as peak lists and mass ranges of endogenous metabolites, pharmaceutical drugs, and some organic compounds. The first issue of the field-specific journal "Metabolomics" was published in the year METLIN was launched (Guijas et al., 2018b).

In 2005, which was a busy year in terms of studies in the field, studies were started by the Canadian Alberta University, Canadian Innovation Agency, and Genome Canada for the Human Metabolome Project (HMP) to reveal the unknowns about the human metabolome. This project aimed to establish a relationship between the metabolome and the disease through metabolic pathways, to evaluate drug metabolism and toxicology, to establish a link between human metabolism and the human genome, to develop software for metabolomics studies in examining the identification, diagnosis, and treatment of diseases and the response to the treatment process. This purpose aims to create a freely accessible electronic database containing detailed information about metabolites that can be used for general applications and biomarker discovery from physiological fluids and tissues in the human body (Kaplan & Celebier, 2020). Thus, a database (Human Metabolome Data Base-HMDB) in which all metabolites found in blood plasma, urine, cerebrospinal fluid, and leukocytes are defined, their measurement results and reference value ranges are determined, and an electronic library (Human Metabolome Library-HML) that will make these data freely accessible in the electronic environment has emerged. The data is constantly updated within the project scope and made available to everyone at the web address "www.hmdb.ca."

The first version of HMDB was released in January 2007, and the last version, 5.0, was released on January 17, 2022. Chemical data, clinical data, and metabolite molecular biology/biochemical data are linked in the database. The database contains data on 220,945 water and fat-soluble metabolites. In addition, 8,610 protein sequences (enzymes and transporters) depend on these metabolite entries. Many data domains are linked to other databases (KEGG, PubChem, MetaCyc, ChEBI, PDB, UniProt, and GenBank) and structure and pathway imaging applications. The HMDB database supports extensive text, sequence, chemical structure, and MS and NMR spectral query searches. Four additional databases, DrugBank, T3DB, SMPDB, and FooDB, are all part of the HMDB database suite. DrugBank contains equivalent information on ~2832 drugs and 800 drug metabolites, T3DB contains information on ~3670 common toxins and environmental pollutants, and SMPDB contains ~132,335 pathway diagrams for human metabolic drug and disease pathways and ~60,628 pathways for other organisms. The FooDB database also contains ~70,000 food ingredients and additives information (Human Metabolome Database, 2022).

Metabolomics in Different Fields of Study

As a result of the standardization and widespread use of metabolomics techniques, their use in many different fields is increasing. The main ones are medicine, biology, veterinary medicine, food, plant sciences, drug research, and toxicology studies.

Diagnostics and Biomarker Identification

Especially in the field of health sciences, metabolomics is used intensively and is progressing rapidly. Looking at the sub-headings in the field of health, one of the areas of focus is biomarker studies. The only aim of biomarker studies is not to find pathways and metabolites that will provide an early diagnosis. The selection of the therapeutic method, the follow-up of the prognosis, and the evaluation of the efficacy of the treatment are also among the aims of the biomarker studies. Obtaining samples with ease in metabolomics and, generally, non-invasiveness encourages its further use in routine practice. Again, the possibility of working with many metabolites at once is an essential factor in preference (Klupczyńska et al., 2015).

Cancer Research

One of the areas where metabolomics studies are concentrated in medicine is cancer research. In cancer cases where early diagnosis is critical, biomarker research is one of the priority and desired topics. In this way, it will be possible to detect the disease in advance and reveal the pathophysiological changes that occur in the biochemical pathways. Different research groups continue their studies for these purposes by conducting metabolic profiling. In profiling studies, an effort is made to obtain results by comparing healthy and diseased groups (Klupczyńska et al., 2015). For this purpose, in a study conducted on kidney cancer patients, both groups were compared regarding urinary metabolites. It was found that the excretion of α-ketoglutarate, acylcarnitine, and quinoline differed in the urine samples of the cancer group (Ganti et al., 2012). Again, metabolite findings affecting metastasis in cancer patients or metabolome information that can be used in the phase-staging of tumors continue to be investigated (Vermeersch & Styczynski, 2013).

Hereditary Diseases

Another goal of the studies that are expected to benefit from the metabolomic approach is to provide the diagnosis of inherited metabolic disorders with different methods. It is expected that the methods to be developed will serve the purpose of early diagnosis and thus enable rapid treatment procedures. The diagnosis of phenylketonuria with high levels of the phenylalanine metabolite in newborns is the most typical example in this field (Chace et al., 2002; Raghuveer et al., 2006).

Metabolic Pathway Investigations

Thousands of chemical reactions occur every second to sustain life in living organisms. These reactions are constantly connected with the pathways they belong to and with each other. Even though some of the pathways have been uncovered as a result of scientific studies, there are still some waiting to be discovered. The elucidation of these mechanisms is vital as a biological discovery and to treat the reflection of disorders in the mechanism as a disease. At this point, metabolomic studies are essential considering environmental and genetic factors. For these reasons, studies are carried out with sensitive analytical techniques (Yang et al., 2019).

Pharmaceutical and Toxicology Research

The discovery of biochemical pathways in living beings, which have not yet been fully elucidated, will both provide an understanding of the structure and contribute to the emergence of new targets for drugs in terms of disease treatment. Again, metabolomic methods have been used in drug development studies to measure efficacy or evaluate toxicity. These directional studies are called pharmacometabolomics. Metabolomic methods are also used in research on toxic substances, and biomarker studies are continued for early diagnosis (Zhang et al., 2012).

Research in Veterinary Medicine

Veterinary physicians prefer more accessible methods that will not harm animal health and welfare while screening for diseases or taking samples from pets and farm animals for diagnostic purposes. Metabolomics is being used more and more every day with the advantage it provides in this sense. For example, degenerative mitral valve disease, one of the common cardiopathies in some breeds of dogs, is being investigated through metabolomic analysis to improve the early detection of the disease (Li et al., 2015; Ophoff, 2019). With the increased obesity in pets, non-targeted metabolomics is used for diabetes (O'Kell et al., 2019). Metabolic methods identify metabolites that differ as body condition scores increase in obesity in cats. Metabolomics has gained tremendous popularity in equine diseases, especially since it concerns the racing industry. Diseases such as equine joint injuries and osteoarthritis are studied by metabolomics using articular cartilage biopsy samples, joint fluid, blood, and urine. Metabolomics has highlighted the advantage of biomarker identification over standard imaging procedures for osteoarthritis cases. The effects of exercise on muscle health in racing thoroughbreds were examined by metabolomic methods in muscle, urine, and plasma samples, contributing to the field. In terms of veterinary medicine, it is a fact that there are many subjects to be researched in the field of metabolomic methods, which are considered at the beginning of the road (Ophoff, 2019).

Food and Nutrition Research

Bioactive food studies are one of the pillars of the studies carried out to reduce the incidence of diabetes, obesity, and the metabolic and cardiovascular diseases that develop due to these, which are becoming more and more problems in people with lifestyle changes. Metabolomic methods are used in studies such as better elucidating the effects of foods on the body according to their content, creating consumption patterns, and examining the effect of the applied diet on physiological parameters (Yang et al., 2019). As a result of the development and practice of metabolomic techniques, composition analysis in foods can be performed quickly and with more accurate results. Again, analyzes of food quality and studies on fraudulent product detection also benefit from metabolomic technologies (Budak & Donmez, 2012).

Agricultural and Crops Research

Metabolomics-based studies are increasingly used in different scientific fields, especially agronomy and plant biology, to understand the behavior of plants under different stress conditions (Do Prado et al., 2018). Plants are affected by many environmental factors during their development period. Element composition and amount in the environment are one of them. In the metabolomics study conducted in plants with regular and excessive molybdenum exposure, it has been revealed that organic compounds such as gluconic acid, 2-oxoarginine, D-gluconic acid, L-nicotine, and citric acid are effective in eliminating the toxic effect of excess molybdenum. This conclusion was reached by revealing the metabolic status of the roots and leaves of the plant seedling by UPLC-MS/MS (Xu et al., 2018). Similar studies can be found frequently in the field. Metabolomics technology is widely used in agricultural product value measurement and disease diagnosis fields and contributes to increasing agricultural income (Yang et al., 2019).

Conclusion

The metabolomics approach, which started with the sensory observations of scientists in ancient times, entered scientific practice in the real sense with the development of chromatographic methods from the beginning of the 21st century. Cancer research and biomarker discovery studies, especially in medicine, continue to gain momentum with each passing day. In terms of other life sciences, metabolomics approaches have begun to be accepted as more robust alternatives. Considering that analytical technologies are developing daily, it can be said that more practical applications will become standardized soon. One of the most striking factors in these developments is the integration of bioinformatics and scientific data. The resulting metabolomics databases and online libraries are very functional in providing ease of access to users. Through guiding technologies, radical breakthroughs will likely emerge in the coming period, such as elucidating the processes of fundamental mechanisms in life sciences, making progress in personalized medicine, creating virtual models of organisms, and developing biotechnological production methods.

References

Basaran, E., Aras S., Cansaran Duman D. (2010). General Outlook and Applications of Genomics, Proteomics and Metabolomics. *Turkish Bulletin of Hygiene and Experimental Biology,* 67(2): 85-96.

Bell, J. D., Brown, J. C., Sadler P. J., (1989). NMR studies of body fluids. *NMR In Biomedicine*, 2(5-6), 246-56. https://doi.org/10.1002/nbm.1940020513.

Bertalanffy, V. L. (1940). Der Organismus als physikalisches System betrachtet. *Die Naturwissenschaften*, 28, 521–531.

Blekherman, G., Laubenbacher, R., Cortes, D. F., Mendes, P., Torti, F. M., Akman, S., Torti, S. V., Shulaev, V. (2011). Bioinformatics tools for cancer metabolomics. Metabolomics: *Official Journal of The Metabolomic Society*, 7(3), 329–343. https://doi.org/10.1007/s11306-010-0270-3.

Bren, L. (2005). Metabolomics: working toward personalized medicine. *FDA Consumer*, 39(6), 28-33. https://doi.org/10.1002/mas.21548.

Budak, Ş. Ö., Donmez, S. (2012). Gıda Biliminde Yeni Omik Teknolojileri (Novel Omics Technologies in Food Science). *The Journal of Food*, 37(3), 173-179.

Chace, D. H., Kalas, T. A., & Naylor, E. W. (2002). The application of tandem mass spectrometry to neonatal screening for inherited disorders of intermediary metabolism. *Annual Review of Genomics and Human Genetics*, 3, 17–45. https://doi.org/10.1146/annurev.genom.3.022502.103213.

Cravatt B. F., Prospero-Garcia, O., Siuzdak, G., Gilula, N. B., Henriksen, S. J., Boger, D. L., Lerner, R. A. (1995). Chemical characterization of a family of brain lipids that induce sleep. *Science*, 268 (5216), 1506–9. https://doi.org/10.1126/science.7770779.

Di Minno, A., Gelzo, M., Caterino, M., Costanzo, M., Ruoppolo, M., Castaldo, G. (2022). Challenges in Metabolomics-Based Tests, Biomarkers Revealed by Metabolomic Analysis, and the Promise of the Application of Metabolomics in Precision Medicine. *International Journal of Molecular Sciences*, 23(9), 5213. https://doi.org/10.3390/ijms23095213.

Do Prado, R. M., Porto, C., Nunes, E., de Aguiar, C. L., Jorge, P. E. (2018). Metabolomics and Agriculture: What Can Be Done? *mSystems*, 3(2), 156-17. https://doi.org/10.1128/mSystems.00156-17.

Fiehn, O. (2002). Metabolomics--the link between genotypes and phenotypes. *Plant Molecular Biology*, 48(1-2), 155–171. https://doi.org/10.1023/A:1013713905833.

Games D. E., Alcock N. J., van der Greef J., Nyssen L.M., Maarse H, Ten MC, Brauw D. N. (1984). Analysis of pepper and capsicum oleoresins by high-performance liquid chromatography--mass spectrometry and field desorption mass spectrometry. *Journal of Chromatography A*, 294, 269-79. https://doi.org/10.1016/S0021-9673(01)96133-3.

Ganti, S., Taylor, S. L., Kim, K., Hoppel, C. L., Guo, L., Yang, J., Evans, C., & Weiss, R. H. (2012). Urinary acylcarnitines are altered in human kidney cancer. *International Journal of Cancer*, 130(12), 2791–2800. https://doi.org/10.1002/ijc.26274

Guijas C., Montenegro-Burke J. R., Warth B., Spilker M. E., Siuzdak G. (2018a). Metabolomics activity screening for identifying metabolites that modulate phenotype. *Nature Biotechnology*, 36(4), 316-320. https://doi.org/10.1038/nbt.4101.

Guijas, C., Montenegro-Burke, J. R., Domingo-Almenara, X., Palermo, A., Warth, B., Hermann, G., Koellensperger, G., Huan, T., Uritboonthai, W., Aisporna, A. E., Wolan, D. W., Spilker, M. E., Benton, H. P., & Siuzdak, G. (2018). METLIN: a technology platform for identifying knowns and unknowns. *Analytical chemistry*, *90*(5), 3156-3164. https://doi.org/10.1021/acs.analchem.7b04424.

Horgan, R. P., Kenny L. C. (2011). Omic'technologies: genomics, transcriptomics, proteomics and metabolomics. *The Obstetrician Gynaecologist*, 13(3), 189-95. https://doi.org/10.1576/toag.13.3.189.27672.

Horning, E. C., Horning, M. G., (1971). Metabolic profiles: Gas-Phase methods for analysis of metabolites. *Clinical Chemistry*, 17(8), 802-9. https://doi.org/10.1093/clinchem/17.8.802.

Human Metabolome Database. (2022, Oct 01) *"About the Human Metabolome Database,"* https://hmdb.ca/about .

Kaplan O., Celebier M. (2020). Past, present and future of metabolomic studies. *Turkiye Klinikleri Journal of Medical Sciences*, 40(3), 366-374. https://doi.org/10.5336/medsci.2020-75489.

Kasap H., Pazarcı P., Erkoç M. A. (2010). Sistem Biyolojisi [Systems Biology]. *Archives Medical Review Journal,* 19, 25-35.

Kitano, H. (2002). Systems biology: a brief overview. *Science*, 295(5560), 1662–1664. https://doi.org/10.1126/science.1069492.

Klupczyńska, A., Dereziński, P., Kokot, Z. J. (2015). Metabolomıcs in Medıcal Scıences-Trends, Challenges and Perspectıves. *Acta Poloniae Pharmaceutica*, 72(4), 629–641.

Kristal B. S., Kaddurah-Daouk R., Beal M. F., Matson W. R. (2007). Metabolomics: concept and potential neuroscience application. In: Handbook of Neurochemistry and Molecular Neurobiology: Brain Energetics. In A. Lajtha (Eds.), *Integration of Molecular and Cellular Processes.* Springer: New York, 889–912. https://doi.org/10.1007/978-0-387-30411-3_33.

Levin, N., Salek, R. M., Steinbeck, C. (2016). Chapter 11 - From Databases to Big Data. In E. Holmes, J. K. Nicholson, A. W. Darzi, J. C. Lindon (Eds.), *Metabolic Phenotyping in Personalized and Public Healthcare,* 317–331, Academic Press.

Li, Q., Freeman, L. M., Rush, J. E., Huggins, G. S., Kennedy, A. D., Labuda, J. A., Hannah, S. S. (2015). Veterinary Medicine and Multi-Omics Research for Future Nutrition Targets: Metabolomics and Transcriptomics of the Common Degenerative Mitral Valve Disease in Dogs, OMICS: *A Journal of Integrative Biology*, 19(8), 461-470. https://doi.org/10.1089/omi.2015.0057.

Lindon, J. C., Nicholson, J. K. (2008). Analytical technologies for metabonomics and metabolomics, and multi-omic information recovery. *TrAC Trends in Analytical Chemistry*, 27, 194–204. https://doi.org/10.1016/j.trac.2007.08.009.

Madsen, R., Lundstedt, T., Trygg, J. (2010). Chemometrics in metabolomics-a review in human disease diagnosis. *Analytica Chimica Acta*, 659 (1-2), 23-33. https://doi.org/10.1016/j.aca.2009.11.042.

Nalbantoglu, S. (2019). Metabolomics: Basic Principles and Strategies. In S. Nalbantoglu, & H. Amri (Eds.), *Molecular Medicine. IntechOpen.* https://doi.org/10.5772/intechopen.88563.

Nicholson, J. K., Lindon J. C., Holmes E. (1999). Metabonomics: understanding the metabolic responses of living systems to pathophysiological stimuli via multivariate statistical analysis of biological NMR spectroscopic data. *Xenobiotica; the Fate of Foreign Compounds in Biological Systems*, 29(11), 1181–9. https://doi.org/10.1080/004982599238047.

O'Kell, A. L., Garrett, T. J., Wasserfall, C., & Atkinson, M. A. (2019). Untargeted metabolomic analysis in non-fasted diabetic dogs by UHPLC–HRMS. *Metabolomics*, 15(2). https://doi.org/10.1007/s11306-019-1477-6.

Ophoff A. (2019). Metabolomics in veterinary medicine: Untargeted metabolomic analysis of porcine reproductive and respiratory syndrome virus and targeted metabolomic analysis of Salmonella Enteritidis. Iowa State University *Veterinary Microbiology and Preventive Medicine Program*, MSc Thesis, Ames, Iowa.

Plumb, R., Castro-Perez, J., Granger, J., Beattie, I., Joncour, K., & Wright, A. (2004). Ultra-performance liquid chromatography coupled to quadrupole-orthogonal time-of-flight mass spectrometry. *Rapid communications in mass spectrometry, RCM*, 18(19), 2331–2337. https://doi.org/10.1002/rcm.1627.

Raghuveer, T. S., Garg, U., Graf, W. D. (2006). Inborn errors of metabolism in infancy and early childhood: An update. *American Family Physician*, 73, 1981–90.

Recber, T. (2019). Determination of Targeted Metabolites in Breast Cancer by LCMS/ MS Method. Hacettepe University Graduate School Health Sciences, *Analytical Chemistry Program*, Ph.D. Thesis, Ankara.

Robertson, D. G. (2005). Metabonomics in toxicology: a review. *Toxicological Sciences*, 85(2), 809–22. https://doi.org/10.1093/toxsci/kfi102.

Stephen, G., Oliver, Michael K. Winson, Douglas B. Kell, Baganz, F. (1998). Systematic functional analysis of the yeast genome. *Trends in Biotechnology*, 16(9), 373-378, https://doi.org/10.1016/S0167-7799(98)01214-1.

Topcu, Ş., Çölgeçen, H. (2015). Bitki Sekonder Metabolitlerinin Biyoreaktörlerde Üretilmesi [The Production of Plant Secondary Metabolites Using Bioreactors]. *Turkish Journal of Scientific Reviews*, (2), 9-29.

Tsoukalas, D., Alegakis, A., Fragkiadaki, P., Papakonstantinou, E., Nikitovic, D., Karataraki, A., Nosyrev, A. E., Papadakis, E. G., Spandidos, D. A., Drakoulis, N., Tsatsakis, A. M. (2017). Application of metabolomics: Focus on the quantification of organic acids in healthy adults. *International Journal of Molecular Medicine*, 40(1), 112-120. https://doi.org/10.3892/ijmm.2017.2983.

Tyers M., Mann M. (2003). From genomics to proteomics. *Nature Protocols*, 422 (6928),193-7. https://doi.org/10.1038/nature01510.

Vailati-Riboni, M., Palombo, V., Loor, J. J. (2017). What Are Omics Sciences?. In: Ametaj, B. (eds) Periparturient Diseases of Dairy Cows. *Springer*, Cham. https://doi.org/10.1007/978-3-319-43033-1_1.

Van der Greef, J., Smilde, A. K. (2005). Symbiosis of chemometrics and metabolomics: past, present, and future. *Journal of Chemometrics*, 19: 376-386. https://doi.org/10.1002/cem.941.

Van der Werf, M. J., Overkamp, K. M., Muilwijk, B., Coulier L., Hankemeier T. (2007). Microbial metabolomics: Toward a platform with full metabolome coverage. *Analytical Biochemistry*, 370 (1), 17-25. https://doi.org/10.1016/j.ab.2007.07.022.

Venter J. C. (2003). A part of the human genome sequence, *Science*. 299(5610):1183-5. https://doi.org/10.1126/science.299.5610.1183.

Vermeersch, K. A., Styczynski, M. P. (2013). Applications of metabolomics in cancer research. *Journal of Carcinogenesis*, 12, 9. https://doi.org/10.4103/1477-3163.113622.

Xu, S., Hu, C., Hussain, S., Tan, Q., Wu, S., Sun, X. (2018) Metabolomics analysis reveals potential mechanisms of tolerance to excess molybdenum in soybean seedlings, *Ecotoxicology and Environmental Safety*, 164, 589–596. https://doi.org/10.1016/j.ecoenv.2018.08.062.

Yang, Q., Zhang, A.H., Miao, J.H., Sun, H., Han, Y., Yan, G.L., Wu, F.F., Wang, X.J. (2019). Metabolomics biotechnology, applications, and future trends: *A systematic review. RSC Advances*, 9, 37245–37257. https://doi.org/10.1039/C9RA06697G.

Zhang, A., Sun, H., Wang, P., Han, Y., & Wang, X. (2012). Metabonomics for discovering biomarkers of hepatotoxicity and nephrotoxicity. *Die Pharmazie-An International Journal of Pharmaceutical Sciences*, 67(2), 99-105.

Chapter 2

Metabolomics and BMI

Bade Ertürk Arik*, MD

Department of Family Physician, Istikbal Family Health Center, Kayseri, Turkey

Abstract

Obesity is one of the non-infectious public health problems that is constantly increasing worldwide. With the results of cardiovascular, cerebrovascular, and metabolic diseases due to obesity, it is an important health problem. In the prediction of obesity and its causes of health problems, it is possible to take measures with the help of metabolomic methods, which benefit from small molecular markers. A large number of metabolites have been used in the calculation of personal metabolic BMI, and the most important of these will be considered. In this chapter, information about the relationship between metabolomics and BMI and their possible uses is given.

Keywords: metabolomics, BMI, mBMI, food, obesity, amino acids, lipids, nucleic acids

Introduction

Obesity is one of the concerns affecting an increasing number of individuals each year and threatens public health (World Health Organization, 2021). Obesity is known to cause proven health problems such as cardiovascular disease or diabetes mellitus. Also, it has a close association with ischemic stroke and cancer (Hales et al., 2017). The incidence and prevalence of obesity

---

* Corresponding Author's Email: badeerturkarik@gmail.com.

In: Metabolomics and Clinical Approach
Editors: Sevgi Durna Daştan and Taner Daştan
ISBN: 979-8-89113-095-1

are increasing throughout the world. When the data from 2016 is evaluated, 39% of the world's population is considered in the overweight category (GBD 2015 Obesity Collaborators, 2017). According to WHO data, the increase in obesity nearly tripled between 1975 and 2016. Obesity has not only affected adults but also affected children, and it is estimated that 39 million children under 5 years of age are overweight or obese. 2.8 billion or more people die annually from obesity-related causes (World Health Organization, 2021). BMI (Body mass index) has usually been used to evaluate practically obesity and its caused risks. As regards the definition of WHO, overweight is ≥25, and obesity is over ≥30 (World Health Organization, 2021). Even though BMI is commonly used, it is affected by situations such as ethnicity, age, and gender and could not provide direct knowledge about body fat and muscle. Furthermore, it is unclear how morbidity progresses, although 20% of patients with metabolically healthy obesity (MHO) or type 2 diabetes have a normal BMI (Carnethon et al., 2012).

Various molecule measurements, such as lipid, glucose, and HbA1c measurements, were used before in research on obesity and its effects. However, all of these are insufficient to explain obesity or its effects on its own. Metabolomics involves the detection of carbohydrates, proteins, lipids, vitamins, or smaller sized metabolites using various advanced techniques and researching their effects in the organ, tissue, cell, or briefly the whole organism. Three different and advanced methods are used mainly in metabolite research, which are mass spectrometry, nuclear magnetic resonance, and high liquid chromatography. By using these methods, metabolites can be detected better and their effects can be investigated (Patti et al., 2012). With metabolomic, healthy individuals can be compared by analyzing metabolite changes related to obesity in the whole body. In this way, the metabolic profile of individuals can be created (Badoud et al., 2015), and the right prediction can be made on obesity and its caused effects with the created profiles through metabolomic methods (Vijay & Valdes, 2019).

Methods and Aims

In research on metabolomic and obesity (BMI), many biological samples are used, such as serum, plasma, urine, and exhaled breath. The most commonly used are serum and plasma samples (Payab et al., 2022). Research on obesity is still new although metabolomic has an essential role in the pharmacology field. The method by which the samples taken will be analyzed has not been standardized either. In current research, the most commonly used method is gas chromatography-mass spectrometry (GC-MS), a type of mass spectrometry. However, it is noticeable that the methods used are plurality (Table 1) and not standardized (Payab et al., 2022). In research on the relation between metabolomic and BMI, the researchers mostly researched carbohydrates, lipids, proteins, and nucleic acids, xenobiotics, and vitamins/cofactors, and they analyzed the correlation between metabolites and BMI (Payab et al., 2022). Thus, they tried to do a prediction of obesity, benefit from metabolomic profile in weight loss, or predict possible side effects of obesity. Besides that BMI with metabolomic BMI(mBMI) terms and slim but metabolically risky (mBMI) individuals with healthy and normal BMI individuals are compared with different points of view, and it is demonstrated that individuals with mBMI have twice more type 2 diabetes in the future (Ottosson et al., 2022). Individuals with mBMI have twice the cardiovascular risk, and they also have a significant increase in insulin resistance (Cirulli et al., 2019).

Table 1. Methods used in Metabolomic and BMI research

1	Gas chromatography mass spectrometry
2	Tandem mass spectrometry
3	Nuclear magnetic resonance
4	Liquid chromatography
5	Ultra-high performance liquid chromatography
6	Liquid chromatography- mass spectrometry
7	Ultra performance liquid chromatography coupled to a triple quadruple mass spectrometer
8	Liquid chromatography coupled with flow injection mass spectrometry
9	Exactive plus orbitrap mass spectrometry, capillary electrophoresis
10	UPLC liquid chromatography mass spectrometer
11	Flow injection analysis electrospray ionization- mass spectrometer
12	Nexera X2 U- High performance liquid chromatography

Nucleic acids and BMI

The closest relation between BMI and nucleic acid is demonstrated between the urate metabolites. In the obese, an increase in the urate level is detected

(Ali et al., 2018; Biradar et al., 2020; Cirulli et al., 2019; Li et al., 2021). Elizabeth T. Cirulli et al., show that the closest relation with obesity is the urate metabolite, and Menni C et al., also show a positive correlation between increased adipose tissue and urate (Cirulli et al., 2019; Menni et al., 2016). However, in other research, there is no relation between increased ureta acid and adipose tissue (Biradar et al., 2020). The increase in nucleic acid metabolites N2, N2-dimethylguanosine, and N6-carbamoylthreonyladenosine also has a weaker relationship with obesity (Cirulli et al., 2019).

Proteins and BMI

Until now, research has shown a close relation between some amino acids and BMI. Glutamate/glutamic acid is closely related to the waist circumference and obesity, and a glutamic increase is observed in the obese (Payab et al., 2022). In many research works, glutamate has the closest relation to obesity among the amino acids (Cirulli et al., 2019; Ottosson et al., 2022). In their research, Filip Ottosson et al., revealed that the most distinct amino acid negatively related to obesity is acylcarnitine (Ottosson et al., 2022). There is also a positive correlation between glutamic acid and increased fat mass. High glutamate is related to increased inflammation in visceral adipose tissue (Petrus et al., 2020).

Amino acids known to be closely related to the increase in BMI, isoleucine, valine, and leucine, were named branched-chain amino acids (BCAAs). BCAAs, which are essential amino acids that are not synthesized by the human body, are related to various metabolic pathways (Jennings et al., 2016; Siddik & Shin, 2019). Insulin secretion is essential in the relation between adipogenesis BCAAs and obesity (Siddik & Shin, 2019). It is thought that the amount of BCAAs increase by the reason of differentiation in amino acid catabolism in adipose tissue in overweight or obese individuals (Newgard, 2012).

There is significant research on the N-acetylglycine decrease in the obese. Also, glycine is inversely proportional with the increasing adipose tissue (Alves et al., 2019; Cirulli et al., 2019).

There are articles demonstrating that phenylalanine levels increase as well as decrease in the obese (Badoud et al., 2014; Cirulli et al., 2019; Pohle-Krauza et al., 2008).

The common features of valine, leucine, isoleucine, tyrosine, glutamate, phenylalanine, and lysine are their increase in adipose tissue increase and metabolic syndrome (Jourdan et al., 2012; Menni et al., 2016).

Lipids and BMI

Considering the relation between lipids and BMI, there are articles showinga decrease in the level of lysophosphatidylcholine in the obese (Rauschert et al., 2016; Tulipani et al., 2016).

In their research, Elizabeth T. Cirulli et al., analyzed more than 1000 metabolites and determined that 49 metabolites were closely related to obesity. 24 of them were lipid-derived metabolites, and the most important one was 1-(1-enil-palmitoil)-2-oleoil-GPC.

The decrease in the level of plasma has been found to be related to obesity (Cirulli et al., 2019).

There are articles that show an increase in the level of plasma choline (Kochhar et al., 2006) or a decrease in the obese (Ho et al., 2016). Similarly, there are also conflicting results on glycerophosphocholine, diacylphosphatidylcholines, and phosphatidylcholines (Ho et al., 2016; Rauschert et al., 2016).

In the obese, acylcarnitines (C14:2 and C18:2) show a negative alteration, and it has been used for determination mBMI in the research (Ottosson et al., 2022).

Carbohydrates and BMI

Research reveals that mannose and glucose have a positive relation with obesity. Furthermore, glycerin/glycerol is also known to be high in the obese in relation to lipids. Lactate has a role in gluconeogenesis and its increase is an essential indicator of increased oxidative stress in diabetes (Cirulli et al., 2019; Ottosson et al., 2022; Weisberg, 2015).

Conclusion

Metabolomic research on obesity has provided a different point of view from BMI. Metabolically healthy obesity (MHO) is a definition that has recently increased in importance. Even though there are no known accepted criteria, it defines the obese who has not impaired glucose tolerance, dyslipidemia, or metabolic syndrome (Denis & Obin, 2013; Stefan et al., 2013). It is estimated that the possible negative effects of obesity are less in individuals with MHO. The mBMI term, which is thought to better predict the negative effects of obesity, has emerged as a result of metabolomic research compared to the MHO definition created with the limited number of data.

There are no known and accepted direct criteria for mBMI. MBMI has been defined using different numbers of metabolites in research (Cirulli et al., 2019; Ottosson et al., 2022).

In their research, Filip Ottosson et al., have indicated that individuals (the difference between them is at least 5 kg/m2) with mBMI >BMI have two times greater development of type 2 diabetes. Also, the possibility of death increases considerably. mBMI can provide information about the possible negative effects of obesity up to about 20 years ago (Ottosson et al., 2022).

In the research by Elizabeth T. Cirulli et al., the important consequences of obesity, in cardiovascular events, there was no significant history in the mBMI < BMI group, while the mBMI > BMI group had a similar cardiovascular event frequency to the obese. Furthermore, the use of medication for blood pressure has been detected to be significantly higher in the mBMI > BMI group. During the 13-year follow-up period, a significant increase in cardiovascular and stroke risk was found in the obese mBMI group compared to normal mBMI. Additionally, cardiovascular events occur later in the normal mBMI group (Cirulli et al., 2019).

All findings allow us to understand obesity through metabolomic research and predict the possible health problems by taking precautions. However, the determination of standardized methods and markers has not yet depended on obtaining more research and results.

References

Ali, N., Perveen, R., Rahman, S., Mahmood, S., Rahman, S., Islam, S., Mohanto, N. C., Nurunnabi, S. M., Ahmed, S., & Rahman, M. (2018). Prevalence of hyperuricemia and the relationship between serum uric acid and obesity: A study on Bangladeshi adults. *PLoS One*, *13*(11), e0206850. https://doi.org/10.1371/journal.pone.0206850.

Alves, A., Bassot, A., Bulteau, A. L., Pirola, L., & Morio, B. (2019). Glycine Metabolism and Its Alterations in Obesity and Metabolic Diseases. *Nutrients*, *11*(6). https://doi.org/10.3390/nu11061356.

Badoud, F., Lam, K. P., DiBattista, A., Perreault, M., Zulyniak, M. A., Cattrysse, B., Stephenson, S., Britz-McKibbin, P., & Mutch, D. M. (2014). Serum and adipose tissue amino acid homeostasis in the metabolically healthy obese. *J Proteome Res*, *13*(7), 3455-3466. https://doi.org/10.1021/pr500416v.

Badoud, F., Perreault, M., Zulyniak, M. A., & Mutch, D. M. (2015). Molecular insights into the role of white adipose tissue in metabolically unhealthy normal weight and metabolically healthy obese individuals. *Faseb j*, *29*(3), 748-758. https://doi.org/10.1096/fj.14-263913.

Biradar, M. I., Chiang, K. M., Yang, H. C., Huang, Y. T., & Pan, W. H. (2020). The causal role of elevated uric acid and waist circumference on the risk of metabolic syndrome components. *Int J Obes (Lond)*, *44*(4), 865-874. https://doi.org/10.1038/s41366-019-0487-9.

Carnethon, M. R., De Chavez, P. J., Biggs, M. L., Lewis, C. E., Pankow, J. S., Bertoni, A. G., Bertoni, A. G., Golden, S. H., Liu, K., Mukamal, K. J., Campbell-Jenkins, B., & Dyer, A. R. (2012). Association of weight status with mortality in adults with incident diabetes. *JAMA*, *308*(6), 581-590. https://doi.org/10.1001/jama.2012.9282.

Cirulli, E. T., Guo, L., Leon Swisher, C., Shah, N., Huang, L., Napier, L. A., Kirkness, E. F., Spector, T. D., Caskey, C. T., Thorens, B., Venter, J. C., & Telenti, A. (2019). Profound Perturbation of the Metabolome in Obesity Is Associated with Health Risk. *Cell Metab*, *29*(2), 488-500.e482. https://doi.org/10.1016/j.cmet.2018.09.022.

Denis, G. V., & Obin, M. S. (2013). 'Metabolically healthy obesity': origins and implications. *Mol Aspects Med*, *34*(1), 59-70. https://doi.org/10.1016/j.mam.2012.10.004.

GBD 2015 Obesity Collaborators (2017). Health Effects of Overweight and Obesity in 195 Countries over 25 Years. *N Engl J Med*, *377*(1), 13-27. https://doi.org/10.1056/NEJMoa1614362.

Hales, C. M., Carroll, M. D., Fryar, C. D., & Ogden, C. L. (2017). Prevalence of Obesity Among Adults and Youth: United States, 2015-2016. *NCHS Data Brief*(288), 1-8.

Ho, J. E., Larson, M. G., Ghorbani, A., Cheng, S., Chen, M. H., Keyes, M., Rhee, E. P., Clish, C. B., Vasan, R. S., Gerszten, R. E., & Wang, T. J. (2016). Metabolomic Profiles of Body Mass Index in the Framingham Heart Study Reveal Distinct Cardiometabolic Phenotypes. *PLoS One*, *11*(2), e0148361. https://doi.org/10.1371/journal.pone.0148361.

Jennings, A., MacGregor, A., Pallister, T., Spector, T., & Cassidy, A. (2016). Associations between branched chain amino acid intake and biomarkers of adiposity and cardiometabolic health independent of genetic factors: A twin study. *Int J Cardiol*, *223*, 992-998. https://doi.org/10.1016/j.ijcard.2016.08.307.

Jourdan, C., Petersen, A. K., Gieger, C., Döring, A., Illig, T., Wang-Sattler, R., Meisinger, C., Peters, A., Adamski, J., Prehn, C., Suhre, K., Altmaier, E., Kastenmüller, G., Römisch-Margl, W., Theis, F. J., Krumsiek, J., Wichmann, H. E., & Linseisen, J.

(2012). Body fat free mass is associated with the serum metabolite profile in a population-based study. *PLoS One*, *7*(6), e40009. https://doi.org/10.1371/journal.pone.0040009.

Kochhar, S., Jacobs, D. M., Ramadan, Z., Berruex, F., Fuerholz, A., & Fay, L. B. (2006). Probing gender-specific metabolism differences in humans by nuclear magnetic resonance-based metabonomics. *Anal Biochem*, *352*(2), 274-281. https://doi.org/10.1016/j.ab.2006.02.033.

Li, F., Chen, S., Qiu, X., Wu, J., Tan, M., & Wang, M. (2021). Serum Uric Acid Levels and Metabolic Indices in an Obese Population: A Cross-Sectional Study. *Diabetes Metab Syndr Obes*, *14*, 627-635. https://doi.org/10.2147/dmso.S286299.

Menni, C., Migaud, M., Glastonbury, C. A., Beaumont, M., Nikolaou, A., Small, K. S., Brosnan, M. J., Mohney, R. P., Spector, T. D., & Valdes, A. M. (2016). Metabolomic profiling to dissect the role of visceral fat in cardiometabolic health. *Obesity (Silver Spring, Md.)*, *24*(6), 1380-1388. https://doi.org/10.1002/oby.21488.

Newgard, C. B. (2012). Interplay between lipids and branched-chain amino acids in development of insulin resistance. *Cell Metab*, *15*(5), 606-614. https://doi.org/10.1016/j.cmet.2012.01.024.

Ottosson, F., Smith, E., Ericson, U., Brunkwall, L., Orho-Melander, M., Di Somma, S., Antonini, P., Nilsson, P. M., Fernandez, C., & Melander, O. (2022). Metabolome-Defined Obesity and the Risk of Future Type 2 Diabetes and Mortality. *Diabetes Care*, *45*(5), 1260-1267. https://doi.org/10.2337/dc21-2402.

Patti, G. J., Yanes, O., & Siuzdak, G. (2012). Innovation: Metabolomics: the apogee of the omics trilogy. *Nat Rev Mol Cell Biol*, *13*(4), 263-269. https://doi.org/10.1038/nrm3314.

Payab, M., Tayanloo-Beik, A., Falahzadeh, K., Mousavi, M., Salehi, S., Djalalinia, S., Ebrahimpur, M., Rezaei, N., Rezaei-Tavirani, M., Larijani, B., Arjmand, B., & Gilany, K. (2022). Metabolomics prospect of obesity and metabolic syndrome; a systematic review. *J Diabetes Metab Disord*, *21*(1), 889-917. https://doi.org/10.1007/s40200-021-00917-w.

Petrus, P., Lecoutre, S., Dollet, L., Wiel, C., Sulen, A., Gao, H., Tavira, B., Laurencikiene, J., Rooyackers, O., Checa, A., Douagi, I., Wheelock, C. E., Arner, P., McCarthy, M., Bergo, M. O., Edgar, L., Choudhury, R. P., Aouadi, M., Krook, A., & Rydén, M. (2020). Glutamine Links Obesity to Inflammation in Human White Adipose Tissue. *Cell Metab*, *31*(2), 375-390.e311. https://doi.org/10.1016/j.cmet.2019.11.019 .

Pohle-Krauza, R. J., Navia, J. L., Madore, E. Y., Nyrop, J. E., & Pelkman, C. L. (2008). Effects of L-phenylalanine on energy intake in overweight and obese women: interactions with dietary restraint status. *Appetite*, *51*(1), 111-119. https://doi.org/10.1016/j.appet.2008.01.002.

Rauschert, S., Uhl, O., Koletzko, B., Kirchberg, F., Mori, T. A., Huang, R. C., Beilin, L. J,. Hellmuth, C., & Oddy, W. H. (2016). Lipidomics Reveals Associations of Phospholipids With Obesity and Insulin Resistance in Young Adults. *J Clin Endocrinol Metab*, *101*(3), 871-879. https://doi.org/10.1210/jc.2015-3525.

Siddik, M. A. B., & Shin, A. C. (2019). Recent Progress on Branched-Chain Amino Acids in Obesity, Diabetes, and Beyond. *Endocrinol Metab (Seoul)*, *34*(3), 234-246. https://doi.org/10.3803/EnM.2019.34.3.234.

Stefan, N., Häring, H. U., Hu, F. B., & Schulze, M. B. (2013). Metabolically healthy obesity: epidemiology, mechanisms, and clinical implications. *Lancet Diabetes Endocrinol*, *1*(2), 152-162. https://doi.org/10.1016/s2213-8587(13)70062-7.

Tulipani, S., Palau-Rodriguez, M., Miñarro Alonso, A., Cardona, F., Marco-Ramell, A., Zonja, B., Lopez de Alda, M., Muñoz-Garach, A., Sanchez-Pla, A., Tinahones, F. J., & Andres-Lacueva, C. (2016). Biomarkers of Morbid Obesity and Prediabetes by Metabolomic Profiling of Human Discordant Phenotypes. *Clin Chim Acta*, *463*, 53-61. https://doi.org/10.1016/j.cca.2016.10.005.

Vijay, A., & Valdes, A. M. (2019). The Metabolomic Signatures of Weight Change. *Metabolites*, *9*(4). https://doi.org/10.3390/metabo9040067.

Weisberg, L. S. (2015). Lactic Acidosis in a Patient with Type 2 Diabetes Mellitus. *Clin J Am Soc Nephrol*, *10*(8), 1476-1483. https://doi.org/10.2215/cjn.10871014.

World Health Organization (2021). *Obesity.* Retrieved from https://www.who.int/news-room/facts-in-pictures/detail/6-facts-on-obesity.

Chapter 3

Metabolites Associated with Age and Aging

Ali Sağlik*, MD

Department of Emergency Medicine, Faculty of Medicine, Istinye University, Istanbul, Turkey

Abstract

Aging is a multifactorial and inexpugnable period of biological organisms. By age, many biological and metabolic events occur to destroy organs in the human body. With age, muscle mass starts to decrease, chronic and neurodegenerative disease diagnoses increase, and response to infections become weaker. Diet, physical activities, infections, and genetic factors are the components of how aging will be. The research can be carried out in both non-mammalian and mammalians subjects and with a sample of body fluids easily. Investigations with metabolomics will be the future of many treatment modalities, end of the diseases, and may be the key to a long-life span.

Keywords: aging, biological process, life span, metabolites

Introduction

Aging is a biological process that is composed by decreased physiological and metabolic functions and an increased incidence of chronic diseases (López-Otín et al., 2013). Genomic instability and metabolite alterations are the primary disturbances in the aging process (Ke et al., 2017; López-Otín et al., 2013; Srivastava, 2017). Progressive molecular damage due to free oxygen

* Corresponding Author's Email: alisaglik83@hotmail.com.

In: Metabolomics and Clinical Approach
Editors: Sevgi Durna Daştan and Taner Daştan
ISBN: 979-8-89113-095-1

radicals, mistakes in biochemical and biological reactions, and programmed destruction in multisystems are the main sources of aging (Golubev et al., 2017; Jin, 2010). Factors such as diet, physical activity, and infections can also affect the aging process (Biagi et al., 2017; Wei et al., 2017). For many years, the first aim of researchers is to decrease the effects of years in living organisms and especially in humans.

Metabolites Usage in Aging Process

By age physical capacity, muscle strength, and flexibility, skin elasticity, visual acuity decrease, and some biomarkers, such as hormones, lipids, and amino acids, levels alter. There is a lot of research on the effects of aging on an organism, not only on human being. In a study with worms, they found that by aging trehalose sugar and branched chain amino acid levels (BCAA) increase (Fuchs et al., 2010). In another study, Avanesov et al. checked metabolites in flies by liquid chromatography mass spectrometry and found that by aging metabolites variety and metabolome remodelling increased whereas tolerance to damage decreased (Avanesov et al., 2014). In another study showed that suppressing age dependent S-adenosyl-homocysteine (SAH) metabolite accumulation results in methionine restriction and a longer lifespan (Parkhitko et al., 2019). In a study with bat feces, 41 metabolite differences were found between young and older bats, but the most important difference was in between tryptophan metabolism, and it shows that protein metabolism is important for a long-life span (Laye et al., 2015). In mice it is found that for metabolomics, biologic age is more important than chronological age (Tomás-Loba et al., 2013). Telomerase deficient mice have a metabolic profile like an older and telomerase overexpressed mice have like a younger age mice metabolic profile. This finding provides an anti-aging effect of telomerase (Tomás-Loba et al., 2013).

The metabolic differences in mammalian are categorized according to organs (de Guzman et al., 2013). For example, metabolites in the brain diverged less than other organs. Moreover, a long-life span was found in correlation with low levels of triacylglycerols, low tryptophan products, low amino acid account in the brain, high sphingomyelin, and high uric acid/allantoin ratio (de Guzman et al., 2013).

The last studies focus on omics, such as genomics, metabolomics, proteomics, lipidomics, in biologic organisms to understand metabolic changes by age (Valdes, Glass, & Spector, 2013). A human being is the result of genetics and non-genetic factors such as diet, lifestyle, and environmental factors. In many studies about metabolomics, it is shown that metabolic profiles are correlated with chronologic and biological age (Chaleckis et al., 2016; Chen et al., 2016; Jové et al., 2016a; Yu et al., 2012). Lawton et al. checked 269 people's metabolomic levels and found that more than 100 metabolites alter with age (Lawton et al., 2008). In another study with fasting serum, it is found that metabolomic profiles are age-dependent (Yu et al., 2012). In research performed with twins, it is found that 22 metabolites altered with age, and the most important one C-glycosyl tryptophan (C-glyTrp) was directly correlated with chronological age (Menni et al., 2013). Collino et al. reported that serum tryptophan concentration is reduced with aging, alteration of specific glycerophospholipids and sphingolipids related with long life span (Menni et al., 2013). In another research, it reveals that the structure and composition of gut microbiota is important for life span. Levels of phenylacetylglutamine (PAG) and p-cresol sulfate (PCS) are high in elderly people, and it is associated with the intestinal microbiota (Ivanisevic et al., 2016; Swann et al., 2013). Levels of creatine and beta-hydroxy-beta-methylbutyrate (HMB) levels are decreased by age and it shows that muscle mass becomes less with age (Swann et al., 2013). Individuals with the same chronological age but different in biological age have different clinical risks, and morbidities. After detailed urine profiles, it is understood that lipid metabolism and lipoprotein particle size play an important role in a long-life span. In another research, they reported that low triglyceride (TG) levels were associated with long-lived families (Vaarhorst et al., 2011). In another study about lipidomes it is found that higher levels of phosphocholine and sphingomyelin, phosphoethano-lamine (PE) and long chain triglycerides lower levels are also related with long lived families (Gonzalez-Covarrubias et al., 2013). Increased monounsaturated/polyunsaturated fatty acids ratio associated with long life span and associated with less oxidative stress in women (Gonzalez-Covarrubias et al., 2013). When studying about sex and age-specific metabolites, significant differences were found in lipoproteins, cholesterol, and triglyceride levels in both genders and specifically in women after menopause atherogenic metabolites and certain amino acids increased (Auro et al., 2014). In a large study, it is found that in women specifically C18, serine, tyrosine and in men diacylphosphatidylcholine and phosphatidyl-choline altered with age; but in both sexes arginine decreased and ornithine levels increased with age (Chak et al., 2019).

One of the age-related diseases is sarcopenia. In sarcopenia, the patient has low physical performance, easily gets fatigued and has muscle weakness

(Cruz-Jentoft et al., 2010; Cruz-Jentoft et al., 2019; Gingrich et al., 2019). It affects the quality of life in elderly people and is associated with serious health problems such as falls, fractures, hospitalization, disability, and mortality (Beaudart et al., 2017). Thus, it is important to do research to turn back the effects of years or to decrease the effects of aging to increase a healthy life period. By age, the loss of muscle is associated with remodelling of the skeletal muscle structure again by genetic and environmental factors (Casati et al., 2019).

Mitochondrial dysfunction, oxidative stress, inflammation, and DNA methylation are some of the factors that can affect muscle cell metabolism. These processes can result with muscle cell damage and aging and can lead to skeletal muscle quality destruction. Mitochondria play an important role in oxidative phosphorylation, ATP synthesis, and energy production in skeletal muscle cells (Marzetti et al., 2013). With aging, muscle cell quality and function disturb, and degeneration of mitochondria, decreased maximal oxygen consumption, decreased activities of tricarboxylic acid cycle enzymes, and oxidative phosphorylation (OXPHOS) activity occur (Crane et al., 2010; Petersen et al., 2003; Short et al., 2004). With the aging of muscle, it is found that many metabolites are associated as BCAA, tryptophan, serine, methionine, sarcosine, aspartate, glutamate, taurine, and vitamin D (Gu et al., 2022). BCAA, which cannot be synthesized by the human being and must be taken from diets, decreased by age (Lustgarten et al., 2014; Meng et al., 2022). They are involved in protein synthesis and proteolysis inhibition (le Couteur et al., 2020). BCAA is degraded in muscle tissues by mitochondrial dehydrogenase and branch-chain ketoacid dehydrogenase enzymes (Holeček, 2018). After they degraded, especially glutamine and alanine increase in the blood. BCAA also play a role in signal transduction, especially leucine, in regulating the mammalian target of the rapamycin (mTOR) pathway. The mTOr pathway increases mitochondiral biogenesis by increasing the nitric oxide system (Biswas et al., 2019; D'Antona et al., 2010; Neinast et al., 2019; Zhang et al., 2020). BCAA also associated with other pathophysiological processes in skeletal muscle aging (Li et al., 2022). Therefore, the impairment of BCAA metabolism is one of the basic composing factors of sarcopenia.

Several molecular changes, including defects in mitochondrial biogenesis, and mechanisms contribute to the deterioration of muscle structure and function during aging (Cartee et al., 2016; Chabi et al., 2008; Conley et al., 2000). To start the protein synthesis and mammalian target of rapamycin complex-1 (mTORC1) against insulin and growth factors is reduced in skeletal muscle of elderly people (Cuthbertson et al., 2005). Insulin resistance in elderly people's skeletal muscle contributes to impaired glucose homeostasis and metabolic dysfunction (Uchitomi et al., 2019). Skeletal muscle lipid accumulation has also been associated with age, and we see that skeletal muscle glucose and lipid metabolism change by age (Goodpaster et al., 2001; Uchitomi et al., 2019).

Routine physical exercise can prevent many chronic diseases associated with aging (Booth et al., 2012). Doing exercise properly affects all systems against the metabolic dysfunction and also skeletal muscle becomes stronger (Navas-Enamorado et al., 2017). Investigations about the way exercises affect muscles reveal that muscle protein synthesis stimulated by exercises, controlled insulin resistance and increased induction of mTORC1 signalling (Fujita et al., 2007; Harber et al., 2009).

Regular physical exercise induces skeletal muscle ATP production, NAD+ homeostasis, and pyrimidine nucleotide biosynthesis (Hawley et al., 2014). Exercise can improve skeletal muscle quality and strength. Carbohydrate-derived substrates provide most of the energy during high-intensity exercises, whereas plasma fatty acids supply the energy during low-intensity exercises (Hargreaves & Spriet, 2020). By the beginning of exercise, oxidation of intramuscular glycogen and triglyceride starts but if it prolongs uptake and oxidation of plasma glucose and fatty acids from the liver and adipose tissue have to start (Hargreaves & Spriet, 2020). Metabolic waste products from skeletal muscle after exercise, those named as lactate and glycerol, can be used in gluconeogenesis in the liver (Hargreaves & Spriet, 2020). Generally, with aging people started to do less exercise, less physical activity and by the way come over the metabolic dysfunction. With a continuous and not so high intensity exercise program, muscle function and metabolic health will be better in the elderly people.

By age according to lipid metabolism disturbance, cell membrane composition changes. These changes mostly occur in functional organs such as brain and heart (Almeida et al., 2021). Like age, genetic factors, diet, and gender affect the lipid compositions (Nam et al., 2017; Wong et al., 2020). The investigations about lipidomes revealed that there are systematic changes in the metabolism of organisms and membrane lipid profile changes during aging (Almeida et al., 2021). For example, in women triglyceride and phospholipid levels increase by age and after menopause brain lipidome compositions change and Alzheimer's disease is seen more often in these elderly women (Díaz et al., 2018; Jové et al., 2016b).

Polyunsaturated fatty acids (PUFAs), short-chained sphingolipids, cholesterol and phospholipid levels decrease in human brains by aging, whereas long-chained sphingolipids and monounsaturated fatty acid (MUFAs) levels increase (Hwangbo et al., 2020; Pamplona et al., 2019; Tu et al., 2018). These cerebral lipidome alterations contribute to age-related neuronal disorientation by the way of mitochondrial dysfunction, increased oxidative stress, and membrane changes. Decrease in PUFA, and other phospholipid levels, decrease in the fluidity of neuronal membranes causes a reduction in the diffusion of membrane proteins, alterations in protein-protein interaction, and neuronal transmission alterations that cause cognitive dysfunction in elderly people (Céspedes et al., 2021; Das, 2021). PUFAs come from either the diet or synthesized in liver, pass the brain-blood barrier (BBB) and composize cerebral cell membranes. In elderly people, PUFA levels increase in serum, but cerebral membranes contain less PUFAs. This is because of alterations of BBB transport capacity with ages (Chappus-McCendie et al., 2019). The BBB undergoes many morphological and functional changes during aging that result with decreased transportation of lipids (Pifferi et al., 2021).

Lower levels of phospholipid cardiolipin in mitochondiral membranes are associated with electron transport chain activity reduction in elderly people diagnosed Alzheimer's disease (Kao et al., 2020). Age-related lipidome alterations, especially reduction in cholesterol, and impaired neuronal functions are associated with Alzheimer's disease and Parkinson disease (Jové et al., 2021; Mesa-Herrera et al., 2019). Down-regulation of the transport system and up-regulation of cholesterol removing enzyme CYP46 in elderly people, contributes to low cholesterol levels in the brain (Jové et al., 2021).

The age-dependent mechanism is related with age dependent neuromelanin production in Parkinson disease (Carballo-Carbajal et al., 2019). Glycine, serine, and threonin metabolism have an age dependency in Parkinson disease that suggests it is associated with neurodegenerative processes (Hashizume et al., 2015). But this age-dependent effect occurs in the advanced stages of the disease (Hunsberger et al., 2020).

Choline is the product of these metabolites and increases directly with age in Parkinsonian patients. Choline has a critical role in the synthesis of phospholipids and in the synthesis of acetylcholine. And its deficiency disturbs cell proliferation, differentiation, and apoptosis (Michel et al., 2006). If we check young and old fibroblasts, the down-regulation of glycine C-acetyltransferase (GCAT) and serine hydroxymethyltransferase-2 (SHMT2) genes involved in mitochondrial glycine synthesis correspond to the aging-related decrease in cellular respiration (Hashizume et al., 2015).

By aging, many systematic mechanisms are disturbed and degenerated. Reactions to vaccines also change with age. In a prospective cohort research in 2022, they performed untargeted metabolomics on blood samples from patients between 21-30 ages and older than 65 years old who received the seasonal trivalent inactivated influenza vaccine in the last season (Chou et al., 2022). In blood samples that are taken before vaccination in the younger group, fatty acid, linoleic acids, glycerophospholipids were higher, whereas amino acids and triacylglycerols were lower. The purine metabolism pathway increased after vaccination, especially in older people. Metabolites from glycine and serine pathway also increased but it does not have any meaningful difference between young and old people. Sarcosine was persistently increased in older people but in young people, it increased only on the 28th day. These are about increased metabolism in young people and dendritic cell migration, and, by this property, they can respond to dendritic-based vaccines (Dastmalchi et al., 2019; Obata et al., 2014). Sarcosine was higher in older people after the vaccine, but this is not an indicator of the response to a vaccine. As we know that serine requires T-cell proliferation to regulate immunity, it seems serine level is higher in older people (Ma et al., 2017). In elderly people, fatty acyl carnitines and cholesterol esters increased predominantly, triacylglycerol and products of amino acid metabolism increases. As finally, in the younger group adenosine, guanine and phosphatidylinositol metabolism increased, fatty acyl carnitines decreased. This suggests that fatty acid oxidation is increased in young people. In older people serine and glycine are also a component of glutathione metabolism which is essential for regulatory T-cell function. Elderly people have an effective response to the influenza vaccine by this T-cell memory and regulatory T cells.

Conclusion

As we know the omics enable us to analyse many biological process and diseases and the field of metabolomics is the most powerful section of omics. But the details of the mechanisms, and how metabolites regulate aging, are yet unknown. Targeted and untargeted metabolomics have a highly predicted value for research in aging and also can be studied from body fluids with a small sample, so it is so easy to reach the sample. In the future metabolomics will be used clinical practice, in the diagnosis and screening of diseases, and in preventive medicine to improve human health care, decrease chronic diseases, and reach a long-life span.

References

Almeida, I., Magalhães, S., & Nunes, A. (2021). Lipids: biomarkers of healthy aging. *Biogerontology*, *22*(3), 273–295. https://doi.org/10.1007/s10522-021-09921-2

Auro, K., Joensuu, A., Fischer, K., Kettunen, J., Salo, P., Mattsson, H., Niironen, M., Kaprio, J., Eriksson, J. G., Lehtimäki, T., Raitakari, O., Jula, A., Tiitinen, A., Jauhiainen, M., Soininen, P., Kangas, A. J., Kähönen, M., Havulinna, A. S., Ala-Korpela, M., Salomaa, V., Metspalu, A., & Perola, M. (2014). A metabolic view on menopause and ageing. *Nature Communications*, *5*(1), 4708. https://doi.org/10.1038/ncomms5708

Avanesov, A. S., Ma, S., Pierce, K. A., Yim, S. H., Lee, B. C., Clish, C. B., & Gladyshev, V. N. (2014). Age- and diet-associated metabolome remodeling characterizes the aging process driven by damage accumulation. *ELife*, *3*. https://doi.org/10.7554/eLife.02077

Beaudart, C., Zaaria, M., Pasleau, F., Reginster, J.-Y., & Bruyère, O. (2017). Health Outcomes of Sarcopenia: A Systematic Review and Meta-Analysis. *PLOS ONE*, *12*(1), e0169548. https://doi.org/10.1371/journal.pone.0169548

Biagi, E., Rampelli, S., Turroni, S., Quercia, S., Candela, M., & Brigidi, P. (2017). The gut microbiota of centenarians: Signatures of longevity in the gut microbiota profile. *Mechanisms of Ageing and Development*, *165*, 180–184. https://doi.org/10.1016/j.mad.2016.12.013

Biswas, D., Duffley, L., & Pulinilkunnil, T. (2019). Role of branched-chain amino acid–catabolizing enzymes in intertissue signaling, metabolic remodeling, and energy homeostasis. *The FASEB Journal*, *33*(8), 8711–8731. https://doi.org/10.1096/fj.201802842RR

Booth, F. W., Roberts, C. K., & Laye, M. J. (2012). Lack of Exercise Is a Major Cause of Chronic Diseases. In *Comprehensive Physiology* (pp. 1143–1211). Wiley. https://doi.org/10.1002/cphy.c110025

Carballo-Carbajal, I., Laguna, A., Romero-Giménez, J., Cuadros, T., Bové, J., Martinez-Vicente, M., Parent, A., Gonzalez-Sepulveda, M., Peñuelas, N., Torra, A., Rodríguez-Galván, B., Ballabio, A., Hasegawa, T., Bortolozzi, A., Gelpi, E., & Vila, M. (2019). Brain tyrosinase overexpression implicates age-dependent neuromelanin production in Parkinson's disease pathogenesis. *Nature Communications*, *10*(1), 973. https://doi.org/10.1038/s41467-019-08858-y

Cartee, G. D., Hepple, R. T., Bamman, M. M., & Zierath, J. R. (2016). Exercise Promotes Healthy Aging of Skeletal Muscle. *Cell Metabolism*, *23*(6), 1034–1047. https://doi.org/10.1016/j.cmet.2016.05.007

Casati, M., Costa, A. S., Capitanio, D., Ponzoni, L., Ferri, E., Agostini, S., & Lori, E. (2019). The Biological Foundations of Sarcopenia: Established and Promising Markers. *Frontiers in Medicine*, *6*, 184. https://doi.org/10.3389/fmed.2019.00184

Céspedes, P. F., Beckers, D., Dustin, M. L., & Sezgin, E. (2021). Model membrane systems to reconstitute immune cell signaling. *The FEBS Journal*, *288*(4), 1070–1090. https://doi.org/10.1111/febs.15488

Chabi, B., Ljubicic, V., Menzies, K. J., Huang, J. H., Saleem, A., & Hood, D. A. (2008). Mitochondrial function and apoptotic susceptibility in aging skeletal muscle. *Aging Cell*, *7*(1), 2–12. https://doi.org/10.1111/j.1474-9726.2007.00347.x

Chak, C., Lacruz, M., Adam, J., Brandmaier, S., Covic, M., Huang, J., Meisinger, C., Tiller, D., Prehn, C., Adamski, J., Berger, U., Gieger, C., Peters, A., Kluttig, A., & Wang-Sattler, R. (2019). Ageing Investigation Using Two-Time-Point Metabolomics Data from KORA and CARLA Studies. *Metabolites*, *9*(3), 44. https://doi.org/10.3390/metabo9030044

Chaleckis, R., Murakami, I., Takada, J., Kondoh, H., & Yanagida, M. (2016). Individual variability in human blood metabolites identifies age-related differences. *Proceedings of the National Academy of Sciences of the United States of America*, *113*(16), 4252–4259. https://doi.org/10.1073/pnas.1603023113

Chappus-McCendie, H., Chevalier, L., Roberge, C., & Plourde, M. (2019). Omega-3 PUFA metabolism and brain modifications during aging. *Progress in Neuro-Psychopharmacology and Biological Psychiatry*, *94*, 109662. https://doi.org/10.1016/j.pnpbp.2019.109662

Chen, B. H., Marioni, R. E., Colicino, E., Peters, M. J., Ward-Caviness, C. K., Tsai, P.-C., Roetker, N. S., Just, A. C., Demerath, E. W., Guan, W., Bressler, J., Fornage, M., Studenski, S., Vandiver, A. R., Moore, A. Z., Tanaka, T., Kiel, D. P., Liang, L., Vokonas, P., Schwartz, J., Lunetta, K. L., Murabito, J. M., Bandinelli, S., Hernandez, D. G., Melzer, D., Nalls, M., Pilling, L. C., Price, T. R., Singleton, A. B., Gieger, C., Holle, R., Kretschmer, A., Kronenberg, F., Kunze, S., Linseisen, J., Meisinger, C., Rathmann, W., Waldenberger, M., Visscher, P. M., Shah, S., Wray, N. R., McRae, A. F., Franco, O. H., Hofman, A., Uitterlinden, A. G., Absher, D., Assimes, T., Levine, M. E., Lu, A. T., Tsao, P. S., Hou, L., Manson, J. E., Carty, C. L., LaCroix, A. Z., Reiner, A. P., Spector, T. D., Feinberg, A. P., Levy, D., Baccarelli, A., van Meurs, J., Bell, J. T., Peters, A., Deary, I. J., Pankow, J. S., Ferrucci, L., & Horvath, S. (2016). DNA methylation-based measures of biological age: meta-analysis predicting time to death. *Aging*, *8*(9), 1844–1865. https://doi.org/10.18632/aging.101020

Chou, C., Mohanty, S., Kang, H. A., Kong, L., Avila-Pacheco, J., Joshi, S. R., Ueda, I., Devine, L., Raddassi, K., Pierce, K., Jeanfavre, S., Bullock, K., Meng, H., Clish, C., Santori, F. R., Shaw, A. C., & Xavier, R. J. (2022). Metabolomic and transcriptomic signatures of influenza vaccine response in healthy young and older adults. *Aging Cell*, *21*(9). https://doi.org/10.1111/acel.13682

Conley, K. E., Jubrias, S. A., & Esselman, P. C. (2000). Oxidative capacity and ageing in human muscle. *The Journal of Physiology*, *526 Pt 1*, 203–210. https://doi.org/10.1111/j.1469-7793.2000.t01-1-00203.x

Crane, J. D., Devries, M. C., Safdar, A., Hamadeh, M. J., & Tarnopolsky, M. A. (2010). The Effect of Aging on Human Skeletal Muscle Mitochondrial and Intramyocellular Lipid Ultrastructure. *The Journals of Gerontology Series A: Biological Sciences and Medical Sciences*, *65A*(2), 119–128. https://doi.org/10.1093/gerona/glp179

Cruz-Jentoft, A. J., Baeyens, J. P., Bauer, J. M., Boirie, Y., Cederholm, T., Landi, F., Martin, F. C., Michel, J.-P., Rolland, Y., Schneider, S. M., Topinkova, E., Vandewoude, M., & Zamboni, M. (2010). Sarcopenia: European consensus on definition and diagnosis: Report of the European Working Group on Sarcopenia in Older People. *Age and Ageing*, *39*(4), 412–423. https://doi.org/10.1093/ageing/afq034

Cruz-Jentoft, A. J., Bahat, G., Bauer, J., Boirie, Y., Bruyère, O., Cederholm, T., Cooper, C., Landi, F., Rolland, Y., Sayer, A. A., Schneider, S. M., Sieber, C. C., Topinkova, E., Vandewoude, M., Visser, M., Zamboni, M., & Writing Group for the European Working Group on Sarcopenia in Older People 2 (EWGSOP2), and the E. G. for E. (2019). Sarcopenia: revised European consensus on definition and diagnosis. *Age and Ageing*, *48*(4), 601. https://doi.org/10.1093/ageing/afz046

Cuthbertson, D., Smith, K., Babraj, J., Leese, G., Waddell, T., Atherton, P., Wackerhage, H., Taylor, P. M., & Rennie, M. J. (2005). Anabolic signaling deficits underlie amino acid resistance of wasting, aging muscle. *FASEB Journal: Official Publication of the Federation of American Societies for Experimental Biology*, *19*(3), 422–424. https://doi.org/10.1096/fj.04-2640fje

D'Antona, G., Ragni, M., Cardile, A., Tedesco, L., Dossena, M., Bruttini, F., Caliaro, F., Corsetti, G., Bottinelli, R., Carruba, M. O., Valerio, A., & Nisoli, E. (2010). Branched-Chain Amino Acid Supplementation Promotes Survival and Supports Cardiac and Skeletal Muscle Mitochondrial Biogenesis in Middle-Aged Mice. *Cell Metabolism*, *12*(4), 362–372. https://doi.org/10.1016/j.cmet.2010.08.016

Das, U. N. (2021). "Cell Membrane Theory of Senescence" and the Role of Bioactive Lipids in Aging, and Aging Associated Diseases and Their Therapeutic Implications. *Biomolecules*, *11*(2), 241. https://doi.org/10.3390/biom11020241

Dastmalchi, F., Karachi, A., Yang, C., Azari, H., Sayour, E. J., Dechkovskaia, A., Vlasak, A. L., Saia, M. E., Lovaton, R. E., Mitchell, D. A., & Rahman, M. (2019). Sarcosine promotes trafficking of dendritic cells and improves efficacy of anti-tumor dendritic cell vaccines via CXC chemokine family signaling. *Journal for ImmunoTherapy of Cancer*, *7*(1), 321. https://doi.org/10.1186/s40425-019-0809-4

de Guzman, J. M., Ku, G., Fahey, R., Youm, Y.-H., Kass, I., Ingram, D. K., Dixit, V. D., & Kheterpal, I. (2013). Chronic caloric restriction partially protects against age-related alteration in serum metabolome. *Age (Dordrecht, Netherlands)*, *35*(4), 1091–1104. https://doi.org/10.1007/s11357-012-9430-x

Díaz, M., Fabelo, N., Ferrer, I., & Marín, R. (2018). "Lipid raft aging" in the human frontal cortex during nonpathological aging: gender influences and potential implications in Alzheimer's disease. *Neurobiology of Aging*, *67*, 42–52. https://doi.org/10.1016/j.neurobiolaging.2018.02.022

Fuchs, S., Bundy, J. G., Davies, S. K., Viney, J. M., Swire, J. S., & Leroi, A. M. (2010). A metabolic signature of long life in Caenorhabditis elegans. *BMC Biology*, *8*, 14. https://doi.org/10.1186/1741-7007-8-14

Fujita, S., Rasmussen, B. B., Cadenas, J. G., Drummond, M. J., Glynn, E. L., Sattler, F. R., & Volpi, E. (2007). Aerobic exercise overcomes the age-related insulin resistance of muscle protein metabolism by improving endothelial function and Akt/mammalian target of rapamycin signaling. *Diabetes*, *56*(6), 1615–1622. https://doi.org/10.2337/db06-1566

Gingrich, A., Volkert, D., Kiesswetter, E., Thomanek, M., Bach, S., Sieber, C. C., & Zopf, Y. (2019). Prevalence and overlap of sarcopenia, frailty, cachexia and malnutrition in older medical inpatients. *BMC Geriatrics*, *19*(1), 120. https://doi.org/10.1186/s12877-019-1115-1

Golubev, A., Hanson, A. D., & Gladyshev, V. N. (2017). Non-enzymatic molecular damage as a prototypic driver of aging. *Journal of Biological Chemistry*, *292*(15), 6029–6038. https://doi.org/10.1074/jbc.R116.751164

Gonzalez-Covarrubias, V., Beekman, M., Uh, H.-W., Dane, A., Troost, J., Paliukhovich, I., van der Kloet, F. M., Houwing-Duistermaat, J., Vreeken, R. J., Hankemeier, T., & Slagboom, E. P. (2013). Lipidomics of familial longevity. *Aging Cell*, *12*(3), 426–434. https://doi.org/10.1111/acel.12064

Goodpaster, B. H., Carlson, C. L., Visser, M., Kelley, D. E., Scherzinger, A., Harris, T. B., Stamm, E., & Newman, A. B. (2001). Attenuation of skeletal muscle and strength in the elderly: The Health ABC Study. *Journal of Applied Physiology*, *90*(6), 2157–2165. https://doi.org/10.1152/jappl.2001.90.6.2157

Gu, X., Wang, W., Yang, Y., Lei, Y., Liu, D., Wang, X., & Wu, T. (2022). The Effect of Metabolites on Mitochondrial Functions in the Pathogenesis of Skeletal Muscle Aging. *Clinical Interventions in Aging*, *17*, 1275–1295. https://doi.org/10.2147/CIA.S376668

Harber, M. P., Crane, J. D., Dickinson, J. M., Jemiolo, B., Raue, U., Trappe, T. A., & Trappe, S. W. (2009). Protein synthesis and the expression of growth-related genes are altered by running in human vastus lateralis and soleus muscles. *American Journal of Physiology. Regulatory, Integrative and Comparative Physiology*, *296*(3), R708-14. https://doi.org/10.1152/ajpregu.90906.2008

Hargreaves, M., & Spriet, L. L. (2020). Skeletal muscle energy metabolism during exercise. *Nature Metabolism*, *2*(9), 817–828. https://doi.org/10.1038/s42255-020-0251-4

Hashizume, O., Ohnishi, S., Mito, T., Shimizu, A., Ishikawa, K., Nakada, K., Soda, M., Mano, H., Togayachi, S., Miyoshi, H., Okita, K., & Hayashi, J.-I. (2015). Epigenetic regulation of the nuclear-coded GCAT and SHMT2 genes confers human age-associated mitochondrial respiration defects. *Scientific Reports*, *5*(1), 10434. https://doi.org/10.1038/srep10434

Hawley, J. A., Hargreaves, M., Joyner, M. J., & Zierath, J. R. (2014). Integrative biology of exercise. *Cell*, *159*(4), 738–749. https://doi.org/10.1016/j.cell.2014.10.029

Holeček, M. (2018). Branched-chain amino acids in health and disease: metabolism, alterations in blood plasma, and as supplements. *Nutrition & Metabolism*, *15*(1), 33. https://doi.org/10.1186/s12986-018-0271-1

Hunsberger, H. C., Greenwood, B. P., Tolstikov, V., Narain, N. R., Kiebish, M. A., & Denny, C. A. (2020). Divergence in the metabolome between natural aging and Alzheimer's disease. *Scientific Reports*, *10*(1), 12171. https://doi.org/10.1038/s41598-020-68739-z

Hwangbo, D.-S., Lee, H.-Y., Abozaid, L. S., & Min, K.-J. (2020). Mechanisms of Lifespan Regulation by Calorie Restriction and Intermittent Fasting in Model Organisms. *Nutrients*, *12*(4), 1194. https://doi.org/10.3390/nu12041194

Ivanisevic, J., Stauch, K. L., Petrascheck, M., Benton, H. P., Epstein, A. A., Fang, M., Gorantla, S., Tran, M., Hoang, L., Kurczy, M. E., Boska, M. D., Gendelman, H. E., Fox, H. S., & Siuzdak, G. (2016). Metabolic drift in the aging brain. *Aging*, *8*(5), 1000–1020. https://doi.org/10.18632/aging.100961

Jin, K. (2010). Modern Biological Theories of Aging. *Aging and Disease*, *1*(2), 72–74.

Jové, M., Maté, I., Naudí, A., Mota-Martorell, N., Portero-Otín, M., de la Fuente, M., & Pamplona, R. (2016a). Human Aging Is a Metabolome-related Matter of Gender. *The Journals of Gerontology. Series A, Biological Sciences and Medical Sciences*, *71*(5), 578–585. https://doi.org/10.1093/gerona/glv074

Jové, M., Maté, I., Naudí, A., Mota-Martorell, N., Portero-Otín, M., de la Fuente, M., & Pamplona, R. (2016b). Human Aging Is a Metabolome-related Matter of Gender. *The Journals of Gerontology Series A: Biological Sciences and Medical Sciences*, *71*(5), 578–585. https://doi.org/10.1093/gerona/glv074

Jové, M., Mota-Martorell, N., Torres, P., Portero-Otin, M., Ferrer, I., & Pamplona, R. (2021). New insights into human prefrontal cortex aging with a lipidomics approach. *Expert Review of Proteomics*, *18*(5), 333–344. https://doi.org/10.1080/14789450.2021.1940142

Kao, Y.-C., Ho, P.-C., Tu, Y.-K., Jou, I.-M., & Tsai, K.-J. (2020). Lipids and Alzheimer's Disease. *International Journal of Molecular Sciences*, *21*(4), 1505. https://doi.org/10.3390/ijms21041505

Ke, Z., Mallik, P., Johnson, A. B., Luna, F., Nevo, E., Zhang, Z. D., Gladyshev, V. N., Seluanov, A., & Gorbunova, V. (2017). Translation fidelity coevolves with longevity. *Aging Cell*, *16*(5), 988–993. https://doi.org/10.1111/acel.12628

Lawton, K. A., Berger, A., Mitchell, M., Milgram, K. E., Evans, A. M., Guo, L., Hanson, R. W., Kalhan, S. C., Ryals, J. A., & Milburn, M. v. (2008). Analysis of the adult human plasma metabolome. *Pharmacogenomics*, *9*(4), 383–397. https://doi.org/10.2217/14622416.9.4.383

Laye, M. J., Tran, V., Jones, D. P., Kapahi, P., & Promislow, D. E. L. (2015). The effects of age and dietary restriction on the tissue-specific metabolome of *<scp>D</scp> rosophila*. *Aging Cell*, *14*(5), 797–808. https://doi.org/10.1111/acel.12358

le Couteur, D. G., Solon-Biet, S. M., Cogger, V. C., Ribeiro, R., de Cabo, R., Raubenheimer, D., Cooney, G. J., & Simpson, S. J. (2020). Branched chain amino acids, aging and age-related health. *Ageing Research Reviews*, *64*, 101198. https://doi.org/10.1016/j.arr.2020.101198

Li, C., Yu, K., Shyh-Chang, N., Jiang, Z., Liu, T., Ma, S., Luo, L., Guang, L., Liang, K., Ma, W., Miao, H., Cao, W., Liu, R., Jiang, L., Yu, S., Li, C., Liu, H., Xu, L., Liu, R., Zhang, X., & Liu, G. (2022). Pathogenesis of sarcopenia and the relationship with fat mass: descriptive review. *Journal of Cachexia, Sarcopenia and Muscle*, *13*(2), 781–794. https://doi.org/10.1002/jcsm.12901

López-Otín, C., Blasco, M. A., Partridge, L., Serrano, M., & Kroemer, G. (2013). The hallmarks of aging. *Cell*, *153*(6), 1194–1217. https://doi.org/10.1016/j.cell.2013.05.039

Lustgarten, M. S., Price, L. L., Chale, A., Phillips, E. M., & Fielding, R. A. (2014). Branched Chain Amino Acids Are Associated With Muscle Mass in Functionally

Limited Older Adults. *The Journals of Gerontology Series A: Biological Sciences and Medical Sciences*, *69*(6), 717–724. https://doi.org/10.1093/gerona/glt152

Ma, E. H., Bantug, G., Griss, T., Condotta, S., Johnson, R. M., Samborska, B., Mainolfi, N., Suri, V., Guak, H., Balmer, M. L., Verway, M. J., Raissi, T. C., Tsui, H., Boukhaled, G., Henriques da Costa, S., Frezza, C., Krawczyk, C. M., Friedman, A., Manfredi, M., Richer, M. J., Hess, C., & Jones, R. G. (2017). Serine Is an Essential Metabolite for Effector T Cell Expansion. *Cell Metabolism*, *25*(2), 345–357. https://doi.org/10.1016/j.cmet.2016.12.011

Marzetti, E., Calvani, R., Cesari, M., Buford, T. W., Lorenzi, M., Behnke, B. J., & Leeuwenburgh, C. (2013). Mitochondrial dysfunction and sarcopenia of aging: From signaling pathways to clinical trials. *The International Journal of Biochemistry & Cell Biology*, *45*(10), 2288–2301. https://doi.org/10.1016/j.biocel.2013.06.024

Meng, L., Yang, R., Wang, D., Wu, W., Shi, J., Shen, J., Dang, Y., Fan, G., Shi, H., Dong, J., Xi, H., & Yu, P. (2022). Specific lysophosphatidylcholine and acylcar-nitine related to sarcopenia and its components in older men. *BMC Geriatrics*, *22*(1), 249. https://doi.org/10.1186/s12877-022-02953-4

Menni, C., Kastenmüller, G., Petersen, A. K., Bell, J. T., Psatha, M., Tsai, P.-C., Gieger, C., Schulz, H., Erte, I., John, S., Brosnan, M. J., Wilson, S. G., Tsaprouni, L., Lim, E. M., Stuckey, B., Deloukas, P., Mohney, R., Suhre, K., Spector, T. D., & Valdes, A. M. (2013). Metabolomic markers reveal novel pathways of ageing and early development in human populations. *International Journal of Epidemiology*, *42*(4), 1111–1119. https://doi.org/10.1093/ije/dyt094

Mesa-Herrera, Taoro-González, Valdés-Baizabal, Diaz, & Marín. (2019). Lipid and Lipid Raft Alteration in Aging and Neurodegenerative Diseases: A Window for the Development of New Biomarkers. *International Journal of Molecular Sciences*, *20*(15), 3810. https://doi.org/10.3390/ijms20153810

Michel, V., Yuan, Z., Ramsubir, S., & Bakovic, M. (2006). Choline Transport for Phospholipid Synthesis. *Experimental Biology and Medicine*, *231*(5), 490–504. https://doi.org/10.1177/153537020623100503

Nam, K. N., Mounier, A., Wolfe, C. M., Fitz, N. F., Carter, A. Y., Castranio, E. L., Kamboh, H. I., Reeves, V. L., Wang, J., Han, X., Schug, J., Lefterov, I., & Koldamova, R. (2017). Effect of high fat diet on phenotype, brain transcriptome and lipidome in Alzheimer's model mice. *Scientific Reports*, *7*(1), 4307. https://doi.org/10.1038/s41598-017-04412-2

Navas-Enamorado, I., Bernier, M., Brea-Calvo, G., & de Cabo, R. (2017). Influence of anaerobic and aerobic exercise on age-related pathways in skeletal muscle. *Ageing Research Reviews*, *37*, 39–52. https://doi.org/10.1016/j.arr.2017.04.005

Neinast, M., Murashige, D., & Arany, Z. (2019). Branched Chain Amino Acids. *Annual Review of Physiology*, *81*(1), 139–164. https://doi.org/10.1146/annurev-physiol-020518-114455

Obata, F., Kuranaga, E., Tomioka, K., Ming, M., Takeishi, A., Chen, C.-H., Soga, T., & Miura, M. (2014). Necrosis-Driven Systemic Immune Response Alters SAM Metabolism through the FOXO-GNMT Axis. *Cell Reports*, *7*(3), 821–833. https://doi.org/10.1016/j.celrep.2014.03.046

Pamplona, R., Borras, C., Jové, M., Pradas, I., Ferrer, I., & Viña, J. (2019). Redox lipidomics to better understand brain aging and function. *Free Radical Biology and Medicine*, *144*, 310–321. https://doi.org/10.1016/j.freeradbiomed.2019.03.016

Parkhitko, A. A., Jouandin, P., Mohr, S. E., & Perrimon, N. (2019). Methionine metabolism and methyltransferases in the regulation of aging and lifespan extension across species. *Aging Cell*, *18*(6). https://doi.org/10.1111/acel.13034

Petersen, K. F., Befroy, D., Dufour, S., Dziura, J., Ariyan, C., Rothman, D. L., DiPietro, L., Cline, G. W., & Shulman, G. I. (2003). Mitochondrial Dysfunction in the Elderly: Possible Role in Insulin Resistance. *Science*, *300*(5622), 1140–1142. https://doi.org/10.1126/science.1082889

Pifferi, F., Laurent, B., & Plourde, M. (2021). Lipid Transport and Metabolism at the Blood-Brain Interface: Implications in Health and Disease. *Frontiers in Physiology*, *12*. https://doi.org/10.3389/fphys.2021.645646

Short, K. R., Vittone, J. L., Bigelow, M. L., Proctor, D. N., & Nair, K. S. (2004). Age and aerobic exercise training effects on whole body and muscle protein metabolism. *American Journal of Physiology-Endocrinology and Metabolism*, *286*(1), E92–E101. https://doi.org/10.1152/ajpendo.00366.2003

Srivastava, S. (2017). The Mitochondrial Basis of Aging and Age-Related Disorders. *Genes*, *8*(12). https://doi.org/10.3390/genes8120398

Swann, J. R., Spagou, K., Lewis, M., Nicholson, J. K., Glei, D. A., Seeman, T. E., Coe, C. L., Goldman, N., Ryff, C. D., Weinstein, M., & Holmes, E. (2013). Microbial-mammalian cometabolites dominate the age-associated urinary metabolic phenotype in Taiwanese and American populations. *Journal of Proteome Research*, *12*(7), 3166–3180. https://doi.org/10.1021/pr4000152

Tomás-Loba, A., Bernardes de Jesus, B., Mato, J. M., & Blasco, M. A. (2013). A metabolic signature predicts biological age in mice. *Aging Cell*, *12*(1), 93–101. https://doi.org/10.1111/acel.12025

Tu, J., Yin, Y., Xu, M., Wang, R., & Zhu, Z.-J. (2018). Absolute quantitative lipidomics reveals lipidome-wide alterations in aging brain. *Metabolomics*, *14*(1), 5. https://doi.org/10.1007/s11306-017-1304-x

Uchitomi, R., Hatazawa, Y., Senoo, N., Yoshioka, K., Fujita, M., Shimizu, T., Miura, S., Ono, Y., & Kamei, Y. (2019). Metabolomic Analysis of Skeletal Muscle in Aged Mice. *Scientific Reports*, *9*(1), 10425. https://doi.org/10.1038/s41598-019-46929-8

Vaarhorst, A. A. M., Beekman, M., Suchiman, E. H. D., van Heemst, D., Houwing-Duistermaat, J. J., Westendorp, R. G. J., Slagboom, P. E., Heijmans, B. T., & Leiden Longevity Study (LLS) Group. (2011). Lipid metabolism in long-lived families: the Leiden Longevity Study. *Age (Dordrecht, Netherlands)*, *33*(2), 219–227. https://doi.org/10.1007/s11357-010-9172-6

Valdes, A. M., Glass, D., & Spector, T. D. (2013). Omics technologies and the study of human ageing. *Nature Reviews Genetics*, *14*(9), 601–607. https://doi.org/10.1038/nrg3553

Wei, M., Brandhorst, S., Shelehchi, M., Mirzaei, H., Cheng, C. W., Budniak, J., Groshen, S., Mack, W. J., Guen, E., di Biase, S., Cohen, P., Morgan, T. E., Dorff, T., Hong, K., Michalsen, A., Laviano, A., & Longo, V. D. (2017). Fasting-mimicking diet and markers/risk factors for aging, diabetes, cancer, and cardiovascular disease. *Science Translational Medicine*, *9*(377). https://doi.org/10.1126/scitranslmed.aai8700

Wong, M. W., Thalamuthu, A., Braidy, N., Mather, K. A., Liu, Y., Ciobanu, L., Baune, B. T., Armstrong, N. J., Kwok, J., Schofield, P., Wright, M. J., Ames, D., Pickford, R., Lee, T., Poljak, A., & Sachdev, P. S. (2020). Genetic and environmental determinants of variation in the plasma lipidome of older Australian twins. *ELife*, *9*. https://doi.org/10.7554/eLife.58954

Yu, Z., Zhai, G., Singmann, P., He, Y., Xu, T., Prehn, C., Römisch-Margl, W., Lattka, E., Gieger, C., Soranzo, N., Heinrich, J., Standl, M., Thiering, E., Mittelstraß, K., Wichmann, H., Peters, A., Suhre, K., Li, Y., Adamski, J., Spector, T. D., Illig, T., & Wang-Sattler, R. (2012). Human serum metabolic profiles are age dependent. *Aging Cell*, *11*(6), 960–967. https://doi.org/10.1111/j.1474-9726.2012.00865.x

Zhang, L., Li, F., Guo, Q., Duan, Y., Wang, W., Zhong, Y., Yang, Y., & Yin, Y. (2020). Leucine Supplementation: A Novel Strategy for Modulating Lipid Metabolism and Energy Homeostasis. *Nutrients*, *12*(5), 1299. https://doi.org/10.3390/nu12051299

Chapter 4

Geno-Metabolomics: Genotype Effects on Metabolites

Şeyda Kaya*, PhD

Department of Medical Services and Techniques, Health Services Vocational School, Gaziantep Islam Science and Technology University, Gaziantep, Turkey

Abstract

The integrative science of metabolites, metabolomics, today encompasses life sciences in every aspect, ranging from the discovery of metabolic pathways in species to the identification of significant biomarkers for various physiological and pathological conditions. Metabolism is the foundation of living systems that contains small and low molecular weight substances called metabolites in its entirety, which is an intricate network of numerous molecular pathways working seamlessly. As a discipline, metabolomics studies the metabolome, which is the integrative whole of all the steps of metabolism and its interactions in a living system. The entire DNA existence of a living system is called the genome, which contains all the genes responsible for functional units of transcripts and proteins. The genome also has its own set of modifications primarily on genes called the epigenome, which adds to its complexity. Metabolites as substances differ from gene-encoded products of transcripts and proteins by their intermediary and transitive natures, which are not well-defined as the gene-encoded products. In this chapter, the genetic basis of metabolomics and its possible applications in the research are reviewed.

Keywords: gene, genome, genetics, metabolomics, metabolite

* Corresponding Author's Email: sydkaya58@gmail.com.

In: Metabolomics and Clinical Approach
Editors: Sevgi Durna Daştan and Taner Daştan
ISBN: 979-8-89113-095-1

Introduction

All known metabolites are formed in the line of their metabolic pathways, which represent the metabolic network. Differing from pathways, metabolic networks contain all reactions simultaneously as a whole, and in all its layers, enzymes function to direct metabolic cascades in their routes associated with pathways. Since enzymes are macro-molecular products of genes, there is an evident interconnection between the genes and the metabolic network in their functioning, which is termed as the Gene-to-Protein Reaction (GPR). Therefore, the metabolome is an open framework for the application of multiple omics methodologies for gaining integrative results representing the final status of a living system. Metabolomics, in this aspect, mainly aims at mapping metabolites to the metabolome. By using computational tools, researchers can establish genome-wide metabolic networks that use annotated reference genomes from databases to reveal associated enzymes functioning in a given metabolic pathway mainly through investigating responsible genes by using sequence homology-based methods (Frainay and Jourdan, 2020; Thiele and Palsson, 2010; Wehrens and Sale, 2020).

Either spontaneously or enzyme-catalyzed, all metabolic reactions transform metabolites into other metabolites. Enzyme-catalyzed reactions in a particular metabolic reaction can be further assessed by establishing connections between genes and enzymes as dictated by the GPR, which leads to interconnection between genomic and proteomic data. Based on the genetic directive, all metabolic pathways form around sets of input and output variables for the particular metabolic function (Frainay and Jourdan, 2020; Wehrens and Sale, 2020). In particular, genome-wide molecular networks are only indicative of the global profile and are not specialized for tissue levels. All tissues that make up a living system contribute to the global metabolic profile in part by utilizing metabolic pathways differentially to achieve their tissue-specific functions. Therefore, meaningful data from branches of omics are used in different methods to specifically reveal which part(s) of the global network is active for the investigated reaction (Frainay and Jourdan, 2020; Jerby et al., 2010; Shlomi et al., 2008; Wehrens and Sale, 2020). On a more basic level, it can be stated that metabolic networks are metabolic superstructures that are formed by various numbers of metabolic pathways that function as a module for sets of reactions and their associated metabolites. Such a perspective enables the sub-structuring complex natures of networks into particular pathways to focus on and monitor, which leads to the pathway-specific discovery of metabolites and their associated genes.

The application of different omics methodologies for integrative research of species is a multidisciplinary framework of research, which requires the harmonious working of different specializations. Up to this point, present studies that used the genome-wide association study (GWAS) approach for metabolomics and their genomic connections have provided convincing results for their potential to unlock the hidden aspects of the molecular mechanisms of diseases and gene-to-environment interactions. Such results would certainly add up to the development of personalized medicine by combining the genotype with the metabolite profiles. Initially identified SNPs (Single Nucleotide Polymorphisms) are now being employed for clinical monitoring procedures and developing treatment strategies in various pathological conditions. It is very likely that GWAS in the near future would integrate more than one omics approach into a single unified study to reveal and identify significant markers and associated genes that are clinically and physiologically important and represent themselves in the metabolome. By integrating regulatory transcripts such as microRNAs and epigenetic modifications of DNA into the research framework, it would become possible in the future to make clear associations in all aspects of complex and chronic diseases (Suhre, 2012).

From Genomics to Metabolomics

The genome of a cell is its blueprint represented by the sequential combination of nitrogenous organic bases of nucleotides that are adenine (A), thymine (T), guanine (G), and cytosine (C), which are continuously transcribed and translated to make the living system function as it should from the very conception to the moment of death. The enormous four-letter cryptography that is the genome represents the information that is necessary for life to exist in its sequential structure, and some parts of this sequential structure contain information that are more directly active than others, called genes. Genes, while critical, do not answer by themselves how the entirety of the system would function; instead, genes are differentially used by different tissues to achieve particular outcomes that complement each other into a seamless whole that is the living system (Fanos, 2016).

Genomics is the systematic and integrative study of the genome with all its constituents, from nucleotide sequences to gene structures to gene interactions. Ultimately, genomics aims to completely cover the entire form and function of all genes that are present in a genome to link the blueprint to the final product. With advancements in high-throughput DNA sequencing platforms and available bioinformatics approaches for analysis, systems biology has gained a significant focus in research and newer aspects of living systems were discovered (Arjmand, 2019; Larijani et al., 2019).

In summary, the reconstruction of a metabolic network is the meaningful compilation of individual metabolic pathways into a functional module by using all associated metabolites in a given system. Individually testing each reaction is a laborious way of determination their existence, but there are now metabolic models formed by using high-quality data from respective omics that represent a model living system with interconnections between genes, biochemical reactions, and associated phenotype (Gille et al., 2010; Orth et al., 2011). Outside of the model species, verified and recognized metabolic reactions are still limited, but this has its own prospective nature of rapid development as increasing numbers of genome projects are present for less typical species, which would lead to gene annotations and their associations with biochemical reactions. To simplify the framework of gene-to-metabolic reaction association discoveries, different protocols have been developed in recent years (Krumsiek et al., 2012; Suhre, 2012). While not as reliable as the reconstructed networks from model species, such draft networks from non-model species have the prospect of revealing novel metabolic pathways together with their metabolites and associated phenotypes, which would then be integrated into more detailed integrative research for metabolomics (Durot et al., 2009; Gehlenborg et al., 2010; Krumsiek et al., 2012; Suhre, 2012).

To have a genome-wide metabolic network, the very first need is the assembly of the genome sequence, which then should be annotated for genes both for their localization and function. Dedicated tools and pipelines are used for gene prediction in the sequence that reveal coding domain sequences by determining open reading frames (ORFs) using different algorithms. These determined raw ORF sequences are subjected to filtering algorithms that evaluate the coding potential based on the inherent properties of the sequence. Filtered sequences are then subjected to functional annotations by associating the coding domains with biological functions, which would reveal the function of the product encoded by that sequence. Consequently, annotations based on this principle require the discovery of similar sequences in drafts that correspond to already annotated sequences and functions of proteins as references. Therefore, the main focus is on the identification of orthologies from reference protein annotations by using typical sequence alignment algorithms of BLAST (Altschul et al., 1990) or FASTA (Pearson, 1990) in well-established databases for proteomic data such as UniProtKB/Swiss-Prot

(Krumsiek et al., 2012; Médigue and Moszer, 2007). Determined orthologies based on sequence similarities are further complemented with the analysis of structure by revealing conserved and functional domains within the sequence (Apweiler et al., 2000; Claudel-Renard et al., 2003). While the principle of annotation transfer is currently the routine, it is also a limiting factor in protein characterization in draft genome assemblies due to the fact of reliance on presently documented annotations, which often means no functional similarity between the orthologous sequence and the transferred annotation (Palmer et al., 1999; Seffernick et al., 2001). This is seen as either sequential gaps or errors in auto-annotations that use already known annotations from databases. However, automatic annotations for functions are provided for draft sequences in databases with already established annotations. Consequently, a draft sequence can be annotated for functions either by using annotation transfer from already present annotations or using proprietary processing methods for functional annotations (Krumsiek et al., 2012).

Conclusion

The entirety of metabolites in a living system in a given time is the metabolome of that system, which includes all the gene-encoded and non-genic substances simultaneously present. Ultimately, the metabolome has the potential to represent all the different phenotypes that can arise by crosslinking the metabolite profiles that are subjects of environmental variables to gene functions and genome properties. Therefore, metabolomics has become a significant part of systems biology that aims to understand cellular behavior by analyzing all the cellular components as a whole rather than focusing on separate components, which would identify how metabolic trafficking directs or affects the cellular behavior. Ultimately, this requires the unification of mathematical models, computational algorithms, and experimental protocols into an integrative framework to process and analyze the system as a whole. The advances contributing to systems biology have the potential of transforming conventional medical and biotechnology practices. Currently, such potential is mostly evident in increasing research in stem-cells that contribute greatly to the advancement of regenerative medicine because different omics are used in conjunction with each other to better understand stem-cell biology. Naturally and hopefully, different branches of omics will transform into transomics in the future that unifies different branches into a global whole that can globally analyze and evaluate living systems to reveal mechanisms behind the most intricate molecular interactions.

References

Altschul, S. F., Gish, W., Miller, W., Myers, E. W., & Lipman, D. J. (1990). Basic local alignment search tool. *Journal of molecular biology*, *215*(3), 403-410. https://doi.org/10.1016/S0022-2836(05)80360-2.

Apweiler, R., Attwood, T. K., Bairoch, A., Bateman, A., Birney, E., Biswas, M., Bucher, P., Cerutti, L., Corpet, F., Croning, M. D., Durbin, R., Falquet, L., Fleischmann, W., Gouzy, J., Hermjakob, H., Hulo, N., Jonassen, I., Kahn, D., Kanapin, A., Karavidopoulou, Y., Lopez, R., Marx, B., Mulder, N. J., Oinn, T. M., Pagni, M., Servant, F., Sigrist, C. J., & Zdobnov, E. M. (2000). InterPro—an integrated documentation resource for protein families, domains and functional sites. *Bioinformatics*, *16*(12), 1145-1150. https://doi.org/10.1093/bioinformatics/16.12.1145.

Arjmand, B. (2019). *Genomics, proteomics, and metabolomics*. Springer, Cham.

Claudel-Renard, C., Chevalet, C., Faraut, T., & Kahn, D. (2003). Enzyme-specific profiles for genome annotation: PRIAM. *Nucleic acids research*, *31*(22), 6633-6639. https://doi.org/10.1093/nar/gkg847.

Durot, M., Bourguignon, P. Y., & Schachter, V. (2008). Genome-scale models of bacterial metabolism: reconstruction and applications. *FEMS microbiology reviews*, *33*(1), 164-190. https://doi.org/10.1111/j.1574-6976.2008.00146.x.

Fanos, V. (2016). *Metabolomics and microbiomics: personalized medicine from the fetus to the adult*. London: Academic Press.

Frainay, C., & Jourdan, F. (2020). Genome-Scale Metabolic Networks. In Wehrens, R., Sale, R. (Eds.), *Metabolomics: Practical Guide to Design and Analysis* (pp: 177-189). CRC Press, Taylor & Francis Group.

Gehlenborg, N., O'donoghue, S. I., Baliga, N. S., Goesmann, A., Hibbs, M. A., Kitano, H., Kohlbacher, O., Neuweger, H., Schneider, R., Tenenbaum, D., & Gavin, A. C. (2010). Visualization of omics data for systems biology. *Nature methods*, *7*(Suppl 3), S56-S68. https://doi.org/10.1038/nmeth.1436.

Gille, C., Bölling, C., Hoppe, A., Bulik, S., Hoffmann, S., Hübner, K., Karlstädt, A., Ganeshan, R., König, M., Rother, K., Weidlich, M., Behre, J., & Holzhütter, H. G. (2010). HepatoNet1: a comprehensive metabolic reconstruction of the human hepatocyte for the analysis of liver physiology. *Molecular systems biology*, *6*(1), 411. https://doi.org/10.1038/msb.2010.62.

Jerby, L., Shlomi, T., & Ruppin, E. (2010). Computational reconstruction of tissue-specific metabolic models: application to human liver metabolism. *Molecular systems biology*, *6*(1), 401. https://doi.org/10.1038/msb.2010.56.

Krumsiek, J., Stückler, F., Kastenmüller, G., & Theis, F.J. (2012). Systems Biology Meets Metabolism. In Suhre, K. (Ed.), *Genetics Meets Metabolomics from Experiment to Systems Biology* (pp. 281-312). Springer.

Larijani, B., Goodarzi, P., Hosseini, M. S., Nejad, S. M., Alavi-Moghadam, S., Sarvari, M., Abedi, M., Arabi, M., Rahim, F., Heravani, N. F., Hadavandkhani, M., & Payab, M. (2019). OMICs Profiling of Cancer Cells. In Arjmand, B. (Ed.), *Genomics, Proteomics, and Metabolomics Stem Cells Monitoring in Regenerative Medicine.* Switzerland: Humana Press, Springer Nature.

Médigue, C., & Moszer, I. (2007). Annotation, comparison and databases for hundreds of bacterial genomes. *Research in microbiology*, *158*(10), 724-736. https://doi.org/10.1016/j.resmic.2007.09.009.

Orth, J. D., Conrad, T. M., Na, J., Lerman, J. A., Nam, H., Feist, A. M., & Palsson, B. Ø. (2011). A comprehensive genome-scale reconstruction of Escherichia coli metabolism—2011. *Molecular systems biology*, *7*(1), 535. https://doi.org/10.1038/msb.2011.65.

Palmer, D. R., Garrett, J. B., Sharma, V., Meganathan, R., Babbitt, P. C., & Gerlt, J. A. (1999). Unexpected divergence of enzyme function and sequence: "N-acylamino acid racemase" is o-succinylbenzoate synthase. *Biochemistry*, *38*(14), 4252-4258. https://doi.org/10.1021/bi990140p.

Pearson, W. R. (1990) Rapid and sensitive sequence comparison with FASTP and FASTA. *Methods Enzymol*, *183*, 63–98 https://doi.org/10.1016/0076-6879(90)83007-v.

Seffernick, J. L., de Souza, M. L., Sadowsky, M. J., & Wackett, L. P. (2001). Melamine deaminase and atrazine chlorohydrolase: 98 percent identical but functionally different. *Journal of bacteriology*, *183*(8), 2405-2410. https://doi.org/10.1128/JB.183.8.2405-2410.2001.

Shlomi, T., Cabili, M. N., Herrgård, M. J., Palsson, B. Ø., & Ruppin, E. (2008). Network-based prediction of human tissue-specific metabolism. *Nature biotechnology*, *26*(9), 1003-1010. https://doi.org/10.1038/nbt.1487.

Suhre, K. (2012). Genome-Wide Association Studies with Metabolomics. In Suhre, K. (Ed.). *Genetics Meets Metabolomics from Experiment to Systems Biology* (pp: 265-280). Springer.

Thiele, I., & Palsson, B. Ø. (2010). A protocol for generating a high-quality genome-scale metabolic reconstruction. *Nature protocols*, *5*(1), 93-121. https://doi.org/10.1038/nprot.2009.203.

Wehrens, R., Sale, R. (2020). *Metabolomics: Practical Guide to Design and Analysis*. CRC Press, Taylor & Francis Group.

Chapter 5

Pharmaco-Metabolomics: Drug Effects on Metabolites

Eda Sonmez Gurer*, PhD
Department of Pharmacognosy, Faculty of Pharmacy,
Sivas Cumhuriyet University, Sivas, Turkey

Abstract

The development and advancements in technology, artificial intelligence, and fields of bioinformatics, enabled the use of enormous data coming from genes, transcripts, and proteins processed by the omics in medicine as biomarkers. Scientists are improving different methods, such as stem-cell therapies, applications of regenerative medicine, and enhanced drug interactions in personalized medicine, using omics technologies in a broad scope of biology. Thus, the omics can discern functions of individual genes, proteins, and metabolites; to evaluate drug effects of drugs made or derived from such substances; and analyze differences in cellular pathways that occur from these drugs. The combined use of omics with system biology in regenerative medicine research, and pharmacology fields increases the information regarding concealed molecular mechanisms of diseases, their potential therapies, and personalized applications of stem-cell applications. Improved characterization of living systems along with a detailed evaluation of clinical and pharmacological data are required aspects for the further development of studies containing multiple omics methodologies. The application of data mining on the present data from the literature would enable to obtain experimental evidence in a cost-effective manner by reducing the prior experimental research. Metabolomics in

* Corresponding Author's Email: edagurer@cumhuriyet.edu.tr.

In: Metabolomics and Clinical Approach
Editors: Sevgi Durna Daştan and Taner Daştan
ISBN: 979-8-89113-095-1

pharmacology serves to attain personalization in medicinal treatments to preserve health and prevent diseases. Different branches of omics, such as metabolomics, transcriptomics, proteomics, and toxicogenomics, would lead to improved and easier use of pharmacometabolites in treatment protocols.

Keywords: biomarkers, diagnosis, individual therapy, pharmacology, metabolomics, pharmaco-metabolomics

Introduction

Changes in the amount of messenger RNA do not always respond to variations in protein levels and/or protein activities in the cell. Therefore, metabolites better represent actual outcomes of gene expression than proteomics information. Therefore, changes in the concentrations of metabolites may be more relevant for describing the physiological regulatory processes of organisms, diagnosing diseases, and treating the individual. Likewise, the biological effects that occur with the use of a drug cannot be decreased to the effect of just one compound. Metabolomics studies involve the sequential and combined use of many analytical techniques to create metabolite profiling and create relevant bioinformatics equipment. Currently, NMR technology is the generally used tool for metabolomics. Another important instrumental tool for pharmaco-metabolomics is MS-based proteomics technology. With MS instruments, all organic soluble components can be profiled quantitatively and with high precision (Zhang et al., 2010; Fiehn et al., 2000; Watkins and German, 2002). In addition, HPLC and UPLC technologies are also included in the field of metabolomics. Compared to conventional HPLC-TOF-MS systems, UPLC-TOF-MS systems appear to have a significant reduction in time with peak capacity and sensitivity. For metabolomic studies, it is a noteworthy problem that the experimental profile is affected by gender, genotype, age, nutritional status, drugs, lifestyle, and stress (Zhang et al., 2010). Individual metabolic fingerprinting creates new perspectives for metabolomics studies in determining personalised therapies and drug interaction profiles. Existing statistical studies of morbidity and mortality from the use of drugs reveal the urgent need for individual pharmaco-genomic and pharmaco-metabolomic profiling studies (Chadwick, 2010). Metabonomics/metabolomics and pharmaco-metabolomics technologies also provide a possibility for quality control (Wang and Tang, 2010).

Metabonomics involves metabolic responses from the multivariate analysis of organisms to physiological or pathological stimuli (Nicholson et al., 1999; 2002; 2004; Nicholson and Wilson, 2003). Metabonomics analyses NMR or mass data. In the target organism, all chemical components within a process under investigation are revealed as a "metabolic fingerprint" visualised by applying statistical data to identify the pattern of change of environmental or genetically induced variations in metabolite composition (Wang and Tang, 2010). The science of metabolomics has begun to create striking effects on biological, biomedical, and pharmacological studies. Researchers also use metabolomic approaches to elucidate xenobiotic toxicity mechanisms, pathophysiological processes, diagnosis and improvement of disease states, and the discovery of herbal or synthetic drugs (Whitfield and Kirwan, 2010; Lindon et al., 2005; Kaddurah-Daouk et al., 2008; Griffin ve Shockor 2004; Denkert et al., 2006; Whitfield et al., 2005; Marchesi et al., 2007; Kenny et al., 2008). Metabolomics studies on the determination of metabolic pathways related to normal physiology and pathophysiological conditions, including cancer (Trujillo et al., 2006; Barnes, 2008; Kim et al., 2008). The metabolome is the most comprehensive evaluation process for internally or produced low molecular weight metabolites externally such as vitamins, small peptides, amino acids, lipids, and carbohydrates, which are the most common metabolites in biological systems. At the same time, these metabolites can be sensitive indicators of various states of the disease and drug use (Jenab et al., 2009; Barnes, 2008; Kim et al., 2008; Emenaker and Milner, 2010). With the developments from many fields such as transcriptomics, genomics, metabolomics, and proteomics, it has been possible to benefit from all kinds of data from different sources in every field of biological sciences, and advances have been seen with bioinformatic analyses on the discovery of drug targets and understanding of pathways (Chen et al., 2005). More than 80% of current pharmaceutical drugs target enzymes such as G-protein coupled receptors (GPCR), kinases, and pathways belonging to several gene classes, such as proteases, nuclear hormone receptors, and ion channels. Studies on the development of new therapeutic drugs for these target genes for therapeutic use have gained weight. Regarding drug metabolism and drug transport, it can be said that the in-vivo response to a chemical component or drug treatment taken by the organism is very complex. As a matter of fact, the changes that occur within the cell and within the organism after the drugs are taken by the organism are an extremely dynamic process and consist of many sub-steps. For example, a large number of molecules consisting of at least 50 proteins participate in the pharmacodynamic process for metabolized drugs. Also, various genes contain different polymorphisms to encode such proteins, control activity, or alter expression level (Pirmohamed and Park, 2001). Thus, the individual response to a drug reflects the interaction of multiple genetic variations involving multiple pathways, such as drug metabolism, toxicity, and drug delivery. Additionally, metabolic changes occur rapidly. When necessary or due to a physiological or pathological stimulus, there is the formation of target metabolites in the cell within seconds or minutes, with the expression of the messenger RNA changing, directing the focus on metabolomics research (Fanos, 2016). Liver metabolism is an essential center for drug elimination of (Rushmore and Kong, 2001). These metabolisms are generally dependent on the cytochrome P450 isoenzyme, which is presented in the biotransformation of drugs. More than 100 isoforms for P450 have been identified in humans (Nelson, 1998; Chen et al., 2005; Sensen, 2005).

Pharmaceutical Metabolomics

The field of pharmaco-metabolomics and pharmaco-metabonomics is an approach that aims to provide predictions of drug effects such as efficacy, toxicity, and drug metabolism using mathematical models created from pre-dose metabolic profiles. As a matter of fact, urine profiles determined before the administration of the toxin are used to estimate the toxicity profiles resulting from the administration of toxins in rats (Clayton et al., 2006). There is an important relationship between the metabolic profile before the application of an active substance and the metabolic profile that may occur after the application. Similarly, a strong correlation was determined between post-dose outcomes and pre-dose urinary metabolite profiles, both in terms of toxicity and metabolic aspects. Such pharmacometabolomic profiling to screen patients in drug trials is an extremely important area, but significant efforts are required to obtain knowledge of the metabolic profiling and outcomes of drug metabolism. The potential of metabonomics and pharmaco-metabolomics to illuminate systems-level responses is currently under investigation in a variety of complex multicellular and multiorgan animals such as rodents and humans. Combined with data at other levels, integrating biomolecular organization with metabolomic changes at the proteome and genome level appears promising for producing new pharmacometabolomic insights. Identification of better biomarkers in areas such as toxicity and disease detection will certainly bring about a fundamental understanding of monitoring disease processes and a better understanding of molecular organization (Wilson and Nicholson, 2008). Together with pharmaco-metabolomics, it will be possible to diagnose diseases and monitor drug therapy for humans on pharmaceutical metabolomics. However, research is intense and clinical applications will change rapidly in the future with pharmacometabolomic profiling and monitoring studies compared to many preclinical samples. One of the factors that will positively affect this is the emergence of huge biological bank capacity to comparison (Dumas et al., 2006; Everett, 2007; Lindon et al., 2007).

Pharmaco-Metabolomics and Cancer Drugs

The genetic and metabolic pathways used as drug targets. The interconversion of metabolites is expressed as extreme pathways of the metabolic network, and these pathways are used for drug screening. In the current century of genomic studies, scientists are keen to apply genomic knowledge from molecular engineering research in medicinal trials. In the field of pharmacogenomics, a genetic signal is thought to act as an on-off switch in metabolic control. However, the genotype-phenotype correlation must be established in drug screening to successfully implement genetic switches. Gene expression and peptides are signaling switches for metabolism. So, the effect of drugs on metabolic regulation is related to genetic translation. Cancer cells generally have different metabolic properties from normal cells and synthesize macromolecules for cell growth and proliferation. The deficiency of the tumor suppressor gene or the overexpression of an oncogene is sufficient to generate the genetic signals to modulate metabolic pathways in the formation of the cancer phenotype (Lee et al., 2012; Roessner, 2012).

Overall, pharmacometabolomic approaches have been observed to be quite successful in cancer studies. It is expected that 'personalized medicine' studies will benefit greatly from pharmaco-metabolomics, along with data from all omics sciences. The goal of chemotherapy is to both cure the disease and reduce symptoms. Chemotherapeutic-induced cytotoxicities may occur in the patient shortly after administration or chronically. The aim of pharmaco-metabolomic approaches is to conduct profiling studies on the metabolite differentiations that occur at the onset of the disease, in the diagnosis, treatment stages and depending on drug use, by providing small amounts of samples that can be taken from all body fluids, or by the samples that can be obtained quickly without harming the patient, and, accordingly, directing the treatment (Chiang et al., 2018).

The Dynamic Nature of Metabolism

There is increasing interest in drug transport, spatial distribution, and analysis of drug metabolites in a target cell or in various cell cultures. The imaging, monitoring, and analysis of drug metabolisms are generally based on the LC-MS method. The LC-MS method makes it possible to detect trace amounts of molecules and to determine the localization of drugs within a cell. Primary cultures of human hepatocyte cells are used as a basis for estimating drug-related metabolism pathways. Therefore, hepatocytes are preferred as suitable cell line systems for metabolomics. In addition, LC-MS techniques are quite successful even in determining the heterogeneity of drugs even in a single cell. This approach has the potential to identify correlations between drug metabolism in cells cultured from a single cell and at subcellular levels, and between pharmacological studies, pharmacometabolomic analyses, and even toxicological effects (Fukano et al., 2012; Emara et al., 2017). However, more detailed studies are required with very large sample groups. In the preclinical phase of biomarker discovery, several technical challenges need to be overcome, and mass spectrometry data needs to be analyzed very carefully. In fact, there may be a high degree of correlation between metabolites in LC-MS data, making it difficult to distinguish between metabolites with similar chemical properties or significant correlations based on shared metabolic pathways. On the other hand, the identification of informative and specific biomarkers is an important limitation of pharmaco-metabolomics as a health technology. Identifying which metabolites could be potentially useful biomarkers is a much more difficult process than previously thought. The dynamic nature of metabolism, which can be significantly affected by genetic differences and environmental exposure, is quite complex. Furthermore, prior to inclusion in clinical practice, clinical validation is required to determine whether a particular metabolic test is sensitive enough to identify those at risk or affected by a disease and whether it is specific enough to a particular disease process.

Conclusion

Metabolomics research plays an increasingly important role in the sciences, in the diagnosis and treatment of nutritional-related chronic and systemic diseases, and in the profiling of physiological processes. Additionally, studies that search for metabolite clues that can express the symptoms or treatment processes of the disease in all body tissues or fluids of individuals in the diagnosis or treatment processes of common or rare diseases occupy a large place in the field of pharmaco-metabolomics. Pharmaco-metabolic strategies that have the ability to describe pharmaco-metabolomics create a great opportunity to obtain knowledge of the molecular basis of metabolic processes. It is likely that with future technological developments studies on the effects of drugs on physiological processes and the profiling of formed metabolites in various diseases will be sought in the field of pharmaco-metabolomics. On the other hand, with the effect of the drugs or herbal or synthetic active substances used, metabolite changes that occur in individuals before or after their use seem to be the focus of research for all diseases or pathological processes. However, with the increased capacity to determine metabolite profiles and technologies to develop them, it will support a more detailed understanding of direct control mechanisms and improve our understanding of the effects of different environmental or internal stimuli on individuals. Similarly, pharmaco-metabolomics makes it possible to help develop functional nutrients and follow and classify the effects of drugs or active substances to be used before and after treatment. This may ultimately improve personalized medicine and individualized therapeutic approaches where pharmaco-metabolomics exists.

References

Barnes, S. (2008). Nutritional genomics, polyphenols, diets, and their impact on dietetics. *Journal of the American Dietetic Association*, *108*(11), 1888-1895. https://doi.org/10.1016/j.jada.2008.08.014.

Chadwick, R. (2010). Nutrigenomics and statistical power: The ethics of genetically informed nutritional advice. In Debasis, B., Francis, L., & Manashi, B. (Eds.) *Genomics, proteomics and Metabolomics in nutraceuticals and Functional foods* (pp. 23-35). USA: Wiley- Blackwell Publishing.

Chen, J., Wu, S., & Daviso, D. B. (2005). Applied Bioinformatics for Drug Discovery and Development p:353-383. In Sensen, C. W. (Ed.) *Handbook of Genome Research. Genomics, Proteomics, Metabolomics, Bioinformatics, Ethical and Legal Issues.* Weinheim: Wiley-VCH.

Chiang, T. E., Ho, C. L., Lin, C. S., & Chen, Y. W. (2018). Complete remission in very advanced oral cancer by docetaxel, cisplatin, 5-fluorouracil based induction chemotherapy followed by concurrent chemoradiation. *Journal of Dental Sciences*, *13*(1), 82. https://doi.org/10.1016/j.jds.2017.05.004.

Clayton, T.A., Lindon, J. C., Cloarec, O., Antti, H., Charuel, C., Hanton, G., Provost, J-P., Le Net, J-L., Baker, D., Walley, R. J., Everett, J. R., & Nicholson, J. K. (2006). Pharmaco-metabonomic phenotyping and personalized drug treatment. *Nature*, *440*(7087), 1073-1077. https://doi.org/10.1038/nature04648.

Denkert, C., Budczies, J., Kind, T., Weichert, W., Tablack, P., Sehouli, J., Niesporek, S., Konsgen, D., Dietel, M., & Fiehn, O. (2006). Mass spectrometry–based metabolic profiling reveals different metabolite patterns in invasive ovarian carcinomas and ovarian borderline tumors. *Cancer research*, *66*(22), 10795-10804. https://doi.org/10.1158/0008-5472.CAN-06-0755.

Dumas, M. E., Maibaum, E. C., Teague, C., Ueshima, H., Zhou, B., Lindon, J. C., Nicholson, J. K., Stamler, J., Elliott, P., Chan, Q., & Holmes, E. (2006). Assessment of analytical reproducibility of 1H NMR spectroscopy based metabonomics for large-scale epidemiological research: the INTERMAP Study. *Analytical chemistry*, *78*(7), 2199-2208. https://doi.org/10.1021/ac0517085.

Emara, S., Amer, S., Ali, A., Abouleila, Y., Oga, A., & Masujima, T. (2017). Single-Cell Metabolomics. In Sussulini, A., Martins-de-Souza, D. (Eds.), *Advances in Experimental Medicine and Biology Proteomics, Metabolomics, Interactomics and Systems Biology*. Springer International Publishing.

Emenaker, N. J., & Milne, J. A. (2010). Contribution of omics revolution to cancer prevention research. In Debasis, B., Francis, L. Manashi, B. (Eds.), *Genomics, proteomics and Metabolomics in nutraceuticals and Functional foods* (pp. 315-329). USA: Wiley- Blackwell Publishing

Everett, J. R. (2007). Applications of Metabonomics in Clinical Pharmaceutical R&D. In Lindon, J. C., Nicholson, J. K., Holmes, E. (Eds.), *The Handbook of Metabonomics and Metabolomics*. Elsevier B.V.

Fanos, V. (2016). *Metabolomics and Microbiomics Personalized Medicine from the Fetus to the Adult*. London, UK: Academic Press, Elsevier.

Fiehn, O., Kopka, J., Dörmann, P., Altmann, T., Trethewey, R. N., & Willmitzer, L. (2000). Metabolite profiling for plant functional genomics. *Nature biotechnology*, *18*(11), 1157-1161. https://doi.org/10.1038/81137.

Fukano, Y., Tsuyama, N., Mizuno, H., Date, S., Takano, M., & Masujima, T. (2012). Drug metabolite heterogeneity in cultured single cells profiled by pico-trapping direct mass spectrometry. *Nanomedicine*, *7*(9), 1365-1374. https://doi.org/10.2217/nnm.12.34.

Griffin, J. L., & Shockcor, J. P. (2004). Metabolic profiles of cancer cells. *Nature reviews cancer*, *4*(7), 551-561. https://doi.org/10.1038/nrc1390.

Jenab, M., Slimani, N., Bictash, M., Ferrari, P., & Bingham, S. A. (2009). Biomarkers in nutritional epidemiology: applications, needs and new horizons. *Human genetics*, *125*, 507-525. https://doi.org/10.1007/s00439-009-0662-5.

Kaddurah-Daouk, R., Kristal, B. S., & Weinshilboum, R. M. (2008). Metabolomics: a global biochemical approach to drug response and disease. *Annu. Rev. Pharmacol. Toxicol.*, *48*, 653-683. https://doi.org/10.1146/annurev.pharmtox.48.113006.094715.

Kenny, L. C., Broadhurst, D., Brown, M., Dunn, W. B., Redman, C. W., Kell, D. B., & Baker, P. N. (2008). Detection and identification of novel metabolomic biomarkers in preeclampsia. *Reproductive Sciences*, *15*(6), 591-597. https://doi.org/10.1177/1933719108316908.

Kim, Y. S., Maruvada, P., & Milner, J. A. (2008). Metabolomics in biomarker discovery: future uses for cancer prevention. *Future Oncol., 4*(1), 93–102. https://doi.org/10.2217/14796694.4.1.93.

Lee, W. N. P., Boros, L. G., Go, V. L. W. (2012). Metabolic Pathways as Targets for Drug Screening. In Roessner, U. (Ed.), *Metabolomics.* Crotia: InTech.

Lindon, J. C., Nicholson, J. K., & Holmes, E. (2007). *The Handbook of Metabonomics and Metabolomics*. Netherlands: Elsevier.

Lindon, J. C., Keun, H. C., Ebbels, T. M., Pearce, J. M., Holmes, E., & Nicholson, J. K. (2005). The Consortium for Metabonomic Toxicology (COMET): aims, activities and achievements. *Pharmacogenomics*, *6*(7), 691-699. https://doi.org/10.2217/14622416.6.7.691.

Marchesi, J. R., Holmes, E., Khan, F., Kochhar, S., Scanlan, P., Shanahan, F., Wilson, I. D., Wang, Y. (2007). Rapid and noninvasive metabonomic characterization of inflammatory bowel disease. *Journal of proteome research*, *6*(2), 546-551. https://doi.org/10.1021/pr060470d.

Nelson, D. R. (2006). Cytochrome P450 Nomenclature, 2004. *Cytochrome P450 protocols*, 1-10. https://doi.org/10.1385/1-59259-998-2:1.

Nicholson, J. K., Lindon, J. C., & Holmes, E. (1999). 'Metabonomics': understanding the metabolic responses of living systems to pathophysiological stimuli via multivariate statistical analysis of biological NMR spectroscopic data. *Xenobiotica*, *29*(11), 1181-1189. https://doi.org/10.1080/004982599238047

Nicholson, J. K., Connelly, J., Lindon, J. C., & Holmes, E. (2002). Metabonomics: a platform for studying drug toxicity and gene function. *Nature reviews Drug discovery*, *1*(2), 153-161. https://doi.org/10.1038/nrd728.

Nicholson, J. K., & Wilson, I. D. (2003). Understanding'global'systems biology: metabonomics and the continuum of metabolism. *Nature Reviews Drug Discovery*, *2*(8), 668-676. https://doi.org/10.1038/nrd1157.

Nicholson, J. K., Holmes, E., Lindon, J. C., & Wilson, I. D. (2004). The challenges of modeling mammalian biocomplexity. *Nature biotechnology*, *22*(10), 1268-1274. https://doi.org/10.1038/nbt1015.

Pirmohamed, M., & Park, B. K. (2001). Genetic susceptibility to adverse drug reactions. *Trends in pharmacological sciences*, *22*(6), 298-305. https://doi.org/10.1016/S0165-6147(00)01717-X.

Roessner, U. (2012). *Metabolomics*. Croatia: InTech.

Rushmore, T. H., & Tony Kong, A. (2002). Pharmacogenomics, regulation and signaling pathways of phase I and II drug metabolizing enzymes. *Current drug metabolism*, *3*(5), 481-490. https://doi.org/10.2174/1389200023337171.

Sensen, C. W. (2005). *Handbook of Genome Research. Genomics, Proteomics, Metabolomics, Bioinformatics, Ethical and Legal Issues*. Weinheim: Wiley-VCH.

Trujillo, E., Davis, C., & Milner, J. (2006). Nutrigenomics, proteomics, metabolomics, and the practice of dietetics. *Journal of the American dietetic association*, *106*(3), 403-413. https://doi.org/10.1016/j.jada.2005.12.002.

Wang, Y., and Tang, H. (2010). NMR-based-metabolomics strategy for the classification and quality control of nutraceuticals and functional foods. In Debasis, B., Francis, L.,

Manashi, B. (Eds.), *Genomics, proteomics and Metabolomics in nutraceuticals and Functional foods* (pp. 265-271). USA: Wiley- Blackwell Publishing.

Watkins, S. M., & German, J. B. (2002). Toward the implementation of metabolomic assessments of human health and nutrition. *Current opinion in biotechnology*, *13*(5), 512-516. https://doi.org/10.1016/S0958-1669(02)00363-4.

Whitfield, P. D., and Kirwan, J. (2010). Metabolomics: An emerging post-genomic tool for nutrition In Genomics, proteomics and Metabolomics in nutraceuticals and Functional foods. In Debasis, B., Francis, L., Manashi, B. (Eds.), *Genomics, proteomics and Metabolomics in nutraceuticals and Functional foods* (pp. 271-287). USA: Wiley-Blackwell Publishing.

Whitfield, P. D., Noble, P. J. M., Major, H., Beynon, R. J., Burrow, R., Freeman, A. I., & German, A. J. (2005). Metabolomics as a diagnostic tool for hepatology: validation in a naturally occurring canine model. *Metabolomics*, *1*, 215-225. https://doi.org/10.1007/s11306-005-0001-3.

Wilson, I. D., & Nicholson, J. K. (2008). Metabonomics and Global Systems Biology. In Griffiths, W. J. (Ed). *Metabolomics, Metabonomics and Metabolite Profiling. RSC Biomolecular Sciences.* The Royal Society of Chemistry.

Zhang, X., Wang, W., & Xiao, K. (2010). Novel omics technologies in nutraceutical and functional food research. In Debasis, B., Francis, L., Manashi, B. (Eds.), *Genomics, proteomics and Metabolomics in nutraceuticals and Functional foods.* USA: Wiley-Blackwell Publishing.

Chapter 6

The Use of HPLC in Metabolomics Research

Tunay Karan[1,*]
and Sinan Vicil[2]
[1]Department of Genetics, Yozgat Bozok University, Yozgat, Turkey
[2]Department of Biochemistry, Namik Kemal University, Tekirdag, Turkey

Abstract

Metabolomics detects, identifies, and quantifies small molecule-containing metabolites in cells, tissues, and physiological fluids through high-performance yielding technologies. Metabolomics is an integral part of biotechnology, which includes drug activity investigations, enzyme-to-substrate interactions, biomarker identifications, and metabolomic pathway analyses. Metabolite profiling can be achieved cost-effectively in a short time with high precision and specificity through High-Performance Liquid Chromatography (HPLC), one of the analytical methods. Metabolomics research is seen in different fields, including nutrition, toxicology, environmental pollution, drug research and development, and a broad spectrum of biochemical and industrial analyses. Here in this chapter, fundamental basics about HPLC will be given, and the use and importance of HPLC in metabolomics will be highlighted.

Keywords: chromatography, metabolomics, HPLC, industry

* Corresponding Author's Email: tunay.karan@bozok.edu.tr.

In: Metabolomics and Clinical Approach
Editors: Sevgi Durna Daştan and Taner Daştan
ISBN: 979-8-89113-095-1

Introduction

Chromatography was first used by Russian botanist Mikhail Tsvet in 1906 to elucidate plant pigment chlorophyll and is still being conducted as a powerful tool to detect biochemical substances. Zeolites were first used in 1913 to soften water. Palmer managed to separate carotenoids from fats in 1922. Taylor and Urey managed to fraction lithium isotopes in ion-exchange chromatography in 1937. Martin and Synge discovered liquid-liquid dispersion chromatography in 1941 and won the Nobel prize in Chemistry in 1952 for their research.

Csaba Horvath developed high-pressure liquid chromatography in 1965 at Yale University. Chromatography is a word of Greek origin and means color writing ("Chroma" means color, and "graph" means writing in Greek). Today, chromatography is a method where substances of a mixture are dissolved inside an appropriate solvent and separated according to their physical and chemical properties. This method utilizes the movement of various substances on a solid phase by an appropriate solvent. The mobile phase i.e., the carrier phase, can range from liquid to gas, and the solid phase can range from cellulose paper to capillary glass tubes (Dokoumetzidis & Macheras, 2006; Eser & Dincel, 2018).

High-Performance Liquid Chromatography

HPLC is the process of fractioning the dissolved substances (e.g., amino acids, vitamins, carbohydrates, pesticides, antibiotics, food flavorers, pigments, and derivatives of such substances) inside a liquid solvent under high pressure by passing through a column. The movement of the mobile phase is through the effect of high pressure and, thus, is called high-pressure liquid chromatography. In this method, substances inside the solvent separate from each other by leaving the column at different times per their molecular sizes, polarities, and ion charges, which alter the movement of substances through the column. HPLC is used in different fields, such as nutrition, environment, cosmetics, pharmaceuticals, and industry, to safely assess the substances of organic, inorganic, and biological specimens (Engelhardt, 2004).

Components of HPLC Apparatus

The HPLC apparatus contains various components with specialized functions of mobile phase chamber, pumps, columns, column heater, injectors, degasser, autosampler, and detector.

Mobile Phase Chamber

One or more chambers for the mobile phase are available in HPLC apparatus made of either glass or stainless steel, which are suitable for different pure solvents with different polarities ranging from watery buffers to hydrocarbons. Precautions should be taken to prevent contamination of the mobile phase from chambers.

Degasser

The degasser component preserves pumps and columns by eliminating air bubbles and dissociated air carried from the chambers. Otherwise, air bubbles in the column would result in peak widening and retention time (RT) deviations. There are suitable degassers for pumps and different numbers of mobile phases.

Pumps

The pumps direct the mobile phase solvents into the column by regulating the flow rate under high pressure. In other words, the pumps enable the circulation of liquids in the HPLC apparatus. Prolonged usage requires pump care and maintenance.

Autosampler and Injectors

Autosamplers enable the injection of samples inside solvents into columns in a determined volume through automatic injectors. The prolonged waiting times and increased error rates required using autosamplers. Today, automatic injectors have additional features, such as temperature control, dilution, and mixer properties.

The Column and Column Heater

The column is an integral part of the HPLC, where the substance separation occurs. Various analytical columns have a length between 30 to 300 mm and a caliber between 2 to 5 mm. An adequate column is necessary according to the method and the mobile phase used. Column infills, pore diameters, particle shapes and sizes, and silica purity are vital parameters. The column heater is critical to keep the column environment at a constant temperature.

Detector

Detectors enable the generation of chromatograms by recording as peaks the substances that left the column by measuring their existence and quantity. The use of different software packages readily evaluates the generated chromatograms. On an excellent chromatogram, it should have low noise, high specificity, and broad linear response. Chromatograms are expected to be preserved from deviations in temperature and flow rates. Various detectors are used, including ultraviolet (UV) visible field detectors, electrochemical detectors, fluorescence detectors, mass detectors, conductivity detectors, and photodiode array detectors, which are chosen depending on the sample analyzed (Boyer, 2003; Nikolin et al., 2004; Patwekar et al., 2015).

Advantages of the HPLC

Today, HPLC is indispensable in different fields of biology, biochemistry, pharmacology, medicine, agriculture, and any biotechnology field as an analytical method. It is a logical and trending choice for non-volatile and heat-intolerant substances. It can also fraction high-polarity samples without generating derivations. HPLC is advantageous compared to other liquid chromatography methods for the following reasons: shorter time in analysis; high resolution of peaks; picogram-grade specificity when used with fluorescence or electrochemical detectors; the possibility of multiple-analysis in a single column; adequateness for large particles and ion sizes; and sample recycling (Ren et al., 2006; Swartz, 2010).

The Usage Fields of the HPLC in Metabolomics Research

Prominent usage fields of the HPLC method in the analysis are described in detail under separate headings ranging from pharmaceutical research to industrial applications.

Pharmaceutical Applications

The HPLC method as an analytical tool has seen large-scale usage in pharmaceutical applications. Due to its inherent power in analysis, it can reveal the composition and impurities of a novel drug. Due to quality control regulations, it is crucial to reveal and determine the impurities of a drug before releasing it to consumers. The associated authorities validate drugs before release by evaluating different parameters of bioavailability, stability, and adverse effects. The simultaneous analysis of active substances of paracetamol, chlorpheniramine, and phenylephrine in commercial drugs was conducted by Marin et al. (2002) using the HPLC method. The HPLC has seen increased use in the assessment of blood levels for screening against adverse drug effects. Drug dosages should be carefully formulated to eliminate the overdose effects of chemicals that might occur in patients. In a study by Ge et al. (2004), the HPLC method was used to detect human blood plasma levels of pseudoephedrine and chlorpheniramine.

The HPLC method enables the investigations of the pharmacokinetics of a diverse array of drugs with its high specificity and selectivity. A dihydropyridine class calcium-channel blocker, Amlodipine, is prescribed for hypertension treatment and is used as a vascular muscle relaxant. The HPLC method was used for the fractionation and identification of enantiomers of amlodipine (Haria & Wagstaff, 1995). Additionally, the HPLC is effective in monitoring dosage and emergency diagnostics in hospitals. HPLC is prevalent in analyzing steroids, analgesics, and similar components (Sokolova & Chernyaev, 2002). An approved drug for influenza patients, favipiravir, is also prescribed for COVID-19 infections, primarily diagnosed with respiratory symptoms. An HPLC method was devised to detect favipiravir impurities (Marzouk et al., 2022).

Plant species contain large quantities of biologically active metabolites in their tissues, in addition to essential nutrient substances. Polyphenols are a class of abundant secondary metabolites with various plant biological functions, including growth and development, metabolism regulation, and protection against pathogens. The HPLC is an adequate method to characterize plant polyphenolic compounds with high selectivity when coupled with different detectors. Based on their chemical properties, plant polyphenols include phenolic acids, flavonoids, lignans, stilbenes, and others. Flavonoids, in particular, have seen the highest density in polyphenols investigations, including classes of flavones, flavanones, flavonols, flavanols, isoflavones, and anthocyanidins. Flavonoids are pharmacologically prominent because of their antioxidant properties (Luo et al., 2011; Niedzwiecki et al., 2016). It was reported that quercetin, known to have Anti-HIV properties, maintains blood LDL levels to protect against cardiovascular disease developments. Organoselenium in onions was reported to have anticancer and cholesterol regulatory properties (Amagase, 2006). Anthocyanidins were stated to have improving effects on sight-related activities and reducing properties on chronic cardiac disease developments. It was determined that taxifolin, one of the flavanones, has anti-inflammatory properties and might be effective on ovarian cancer. Daidzein and Genistein, both isoflavones, can be analyzed by HPLC and are effective in alleviating climacteric symptoms at 40 and 80 mg doses, respectively (Uesugi et al., 2004; Tarahovsky et al., 2007).

Phenolic acids include two groups of hydroxycinnamic and hydroxybenzoic acids, and derivatives of phenolic acids are formed by binding the -OH and -OCH_3 groups to these acids. Phenolic acid derivatives were extensively investigated for their alleged properties for anticancer, antioxidant, antiallergy, antithrombotic, antidiabetic, and anti-inflammatory effects (Pokorný, 1991). It was determined that caffeic acid, which is found prominently in coffee beans, sage flowers, mint and thyme leaves, and apricots, has antioxidant, anti-inflammatory, immunomodulatory, and tissue-protecting properties. Another study revealed sinapic acid's anticancer and antimicrobial effects (Cherng et al., 2013). Like aspirin, salicylic acid, isolated from willow bark, was reported to have analgesic, anti-inflammatory, and anticoagulant properties (Norn et al., 2009). Tannins are known as tannic acids, and they are known to have antiseptic properties. The HPLC method revealed their higher quantities in tea leaves and acorns used in pharyngitis, tonsillitis, and hemorrhoid prescriptions (Chowdhury et al., 2004).

Food Industry Applications

Nutriceutical foods, superfoods, therapeutical foods, and designed foods are trending concepts of late in the food industry. They are collectively named functional foods that are beneficial in maintaining and preserving the health status of humans. Polyphenol compounds in such foods are externally taken into the human body as they are not synthesized endogenously (Osés et al., 2016). Fruits are essential to human nutrition due to the overly rich nutrients. The flavor and taste of fruits and juices are directly related to organic acids. Certain juices are adjusted to mild souring by adding citric, ascorbic, or malic acids. Since the organic acid compositions of fruits and vegetables are related to associated chemical properties and freshness, it is imperative to determine the organic acid compositions. The HPLC identified the organic acid compositions of various fruits in nutritional research. The HPLC method revealed the existence of malic acid, fumaric acid, citric acid, isocitric acid, and gallic acid in persimmon fruit. Similarly, the existence of malic acid, citric acid, succinic acid, and oxalic acid in raspberry fruit; tartaric acid, oxalic acid, methylmalonic acid, malic acid, and succinic acid in blackberry fruit; L-malic acid, oxalic acid, quinic acid, and succinic acid in pineapple juice; tartaric acid, fumaric acid, quinic acid, oxalic acid, malic acid, pyruvic acid, and citric acid in apple juice was determined by HPLC method (Chinnici et al., 2005).

Flavanols are present in low concentrations in fruits and vegetables, and there are common types according to their glycosylation patterns. Rutin, fisetin, quercetin, myricetin, kaempferol, galangin, and isorhamnetin are important flavanols in onions, leek, broccoli, and blueberry (Kopustinskiene et al., 2020). Celery root, chamomile flowers, parsley, mint leaves, and tomato peels have high quantities of noteworthy flavanols of apigenin, luteolin, and chrysin (Ozcan et al., 2020). Naringenin is found in high concentrations in citrus fruits and is the flavanone responsible for the bittersweet taste of grapefruit (Khan & Dangles, 2014). Catechins in black and green tea leaves, apples, and pears are antioxidant-acting flavanols. The HPLC determined the presence of isoflavonoids in legumes such as soybeans, and they are named phytoestrogens due to their structural similarities to estrogen (Panche et al., 2016). Anthocyanins are water-soluble plant pigments that are rich in plants with red and purple plants, such as strawberries, cranberries, raspberries, and blueberries. They can be quantified using the HPLC method (Teng & Chen, 2019).

Phenolic acids are naturally present in plant-based products, vegetables, and fruits. They are used for altering the taste and flavor of foods by changing their colorization, odor, aroma, bitterness, and texture. The Reverse Phase (RP) HPLC is a popular method for profiling phenolic acids. Since the reported hepatic impairments and the alleged cancerous properties of synthetic antioxidant substances such as BHA (Butylated Hydroxyanisole), BHT (Butylated Hydroxytoluene), TBHQ (Tert-Butylhydroquinone), and PG (Propyl Gallate), natural phenolic antioxidant substances are favored in the food industry as of late. The conducted studies revealed a higher antioxidant capacity of rosmarinic acid compared to synthetic BHT and vitamin E. Rosmarinic acid is used for food preservation due to its antimicrobial properties in addition to its alleged therapeutic effects against ulcer, asthma, and cancer (Robbins & Bean, 2004; Saad et al., 2008). Gallic acid has an antioxidant potential close to tocopherols, and its antioxidant capacity is higher than ascorbic acid. Gallic acid is used for food packaging against rancidities caused by lipid peroxidation (Yen et al., 2002). Chemical structures, solubilities, and natural sources of antioxidants are essential in healthy nutrition (Kaur & Kapoor, 2001). A resin-like nutrient substance, propolis, is produced by honeybees (Apis mellifera) and has very high amounts of phenolic compounds, contributing to its potent antioxidant properties. The HPLC method was conducted on propolis samples gathered from different regions for characterization. Substances of phenolic acids, esters, flavonoids, and other chemicals were isolated from different propolis samples (Graikou et al., 2016). Mycotoxins are metabolites generated by different molds, including the Aspergillus, Fusarium, Alternaria, and Penicillium genera. The mycotoxin presence in foods is a serious concern for human health and economic viability; thus, its determination is of prime importance. Among the mycotoxins, the following are considered to be the most profound concern for health and economy due to their excessive contamination capabilities: aflatoxin, patulin, ochratoxin-A, fumonisin, and (deoxy) nivalenol. The HPLC method is the most widely applied approach to determine various toxins. The HPLC method was conducted to reveal the presence of ochratoxin-A in packaged pones, and grain-based infant feeds (Juan et al., 2007; Coronel et al., 2012). The most toxic of the mycotoxins, aflatoxin, was revealed to be present in unpasteurized milk by the HPLC method (Rodriguez et al., 2003).

Food additives have seen increased use in recent years for different reasons e.g., prolonged shelf life, preservation of nutrient values, increasing variety, and increasing appeal. Using HPLC, synthetic water- and fat-soluble food additives that give out colors were investigated in a study in non-alcoholic beverages. The presence of food dyes in fruit juices was revealed using the HPLC method containing the UV-DAD detector. The existence of tartrazine, known to damage the DNA structure and give yellow colorization, was confirmed in various drinks (Ma et al., 2006; Alves et al., 2008). The HPLC method is also the most widely used method to analyze the presence of monosodium glutamate (MSG), which is used in bouillons and soups as aroma enhancers (Populin et al., 2007).

Environmental Safety Applications

The HPLC method is utilized to determine organic pollutants in cases of environmental pollution. Due to its inherent selectivity and specificity, the HPLC method is preferred for detecting non-volatile, heavy molecular-weight substances and pesticides. Pesticides are severe concerns for environmental safety and ecosystem integrity due to their long-lasting presence and easy transmission to air, water, and soil. Pesticides are accepted as economic poisons and classed according to their intended targets e.g., insecticides, herbicides, rodenticides, fungicides, molluscicides, nematicides, and others. According to their chemical structures, the following convention is used: organophosphates, N-methyl carbamates, chlorine hydrocarbons, dithiocarbamates, organotins, arsenic, pyrethroids, phenoxy aliphatic acids, and phenol derivatives. These toxic pesticide substances should be tested in water sources, foods, and the environment to maintain the integrity of life quality. A study on pesticide determination in subterranean water sources using the HPLC method revealed the existence of nine distinct substances in water. The isolates of atrazine and simazine herbicides were obtained from various water samples and assessed by HPLC (Mezcua et al., 2006; Zhao et al., 2008). Carbendazim (Methyl-2-benzimidazol carbamate) is a benzimidazol derivative fungicide used in the cultivation of greenhouse and ornamental plant species. Chlorpyrifos is an organophosphate derivative pesticide used in agriculture and domestic pest control. Imizamox is an imidazolinone derivative herbicide used to cultivate peas, soybeans, clovers, peanuts, and corn. Due to their perceived hazardous nature to health and the environment as pesticides, various HPLC methods were devised to analyze them (Boudina et al., 2003; Panggabean, 2016; Torra et al., 2021).

The unresponsible use of pesticides against various pests inevitably leads to their inclusion in the food chain and, by their reach to humans, would cause carcinogenic effects, chromosome aberrations, and mutations. The HPLC method was used to investigate organophosphate pesticide fenthion on Carassius auratus (Kitamura et al., 2000). Pesticides applied by spraying evaporate and dissipate, but specific amounts would remain on the soil and plant surfaces. Two-dimensional mass spectrometry coupled with HPLC was used to determine pesticide residues and metabolites on several fruits, such as apples, cucumbers, and oranges. Pesticides in the air can recycle into the soil by weather phenomena such as winds, fog, or rainfall. The air concentration of a pesticide, fenhexamid, in a greenhouse for tomato cultivation was evaluated by HPLC with specialized sorbents and pumps (Tsiropoulos et al., 2006).

Research on toxic and carcinogen heavy metals is of prime importance for environmental safety concerns and assessing environmental pollution. Spectroscopic methods can evaluate total concentrations and oxidation determinations of heavy metals. The selectivity and specificity of HPLC can be utilized in heavy metal investigations by using various adsorbents and ion-exchange columns. Vanadium is present in various minerals at different oxidation levels and is associated with environmental pollution in regions of fuel consumption. Arsenic is greyish to yellow crystal in aquatic environments and is both toxic and carcinogenic. The increased concentrations of arsenic in the environment, water sources, and soil is an elevated concern for public health. The HPLC is an effective tool for fractionating vanadium, arsenic, and arsenic analogs (Tatár et al., 1999; Miyashita et al., 2009). Research for the preservation of water sources is accelerating in light of increased global warming and environmental pollution. Heavy metals such as Zn, Cu, Cd, Pb, Cr, and Ni pose the most significant risk to aquatic environments as they aggregate in sedimentation layers and pose health risks to humans and aquatic life. Lately, samples from sedimentation layers of water sources, reservoirs, and lakes have been subjected to routine analyses to eliminate chemical risks and preserve water sources (Žemberyová et al., 2006).

Industrial Applications

Natural dyes are increasingly popular in various industrial fields e.g., textile, cosmetics, foods, and pharmaceuticals. Coloring agents of alizarin and purpurin are obtained from the roots of the Rubia tinctorum plant. Different metabolites with coloring effects, such as luteolin and apigenin, are present in walnut shells, Cyprus oak, and buckthorns. HPLC analyses revealed the presence of gallic acid, ellagic acid derivatives, and alizarin in clothes treated with madders. According to the results, the dyes were from the Quercus and Rubia species of madders (Mouri & Laursen, 2012).

Surface-active agents of anionic (Dioctyl sulfosuccinate), cationic (Quaternary ammonium ethoxylate), and non-ionic (Nonylphenol ethoxylate) nature, which are widely used in various industrial fields, particularly in the textile and chemistry, are analyzed by HPLC using reverse phase C-18 columns (Liwarska-Bizukojc & Bizukojc, 2005).

Biochemical Analyses

As a preparative and analytical method, the HPLC method quickly and effectively identifies diverse molecules of amino acids, proteins, carbohydrates, lipids, hormones, and vitamins. The preparative aspect indicates the purification of a sample from a complex mixture, and the analytical aspect indicates the determination of the physical and structural properties of the chemical compounds.

Amino acids are the foundations of proteins that constitute the organism's framework and are active in metabolic pathways. Electrophoretic methods can identify amino acids by utilizing their neutral and ionic structures. The HPLC can also be used to efficiently determine amino acids. The amino acid compositions of Chlorella vulgaris incubated in different media were identified using HPLC. It was revealed that higher amounts of amino acid content, particularly arginine and glutamic acid, in nitrogen-rich media. Arginine is a crucial amino acid as it is the precursor for nitric oxide, and because of its anti-atherogenic properties make, it is a vasodilator agent. Glutamic acid is considered a specialized flavorer (Xie et al., 2017). Hemoglobin disorders are hereditary conditions caused by point mutations in genes that alter a single amino acid in one of the globulin chains. HPLC can precisely determine various hemoglobin fractions to identify abnormal hemoglobin variants (Fucharoen & Winichagoon, 2002).

Proteins are the fundamental molecules in organisms that drive growth and development. While plant organisms can synthesize their protein requirements, animals are primarily dependent on consuming rations, plants, and other animals to receive their essential needs. Fine-tuning animal feed protein content for farm animals is vital to maintain their health and improve their productivity. Unnecessary supplication of proteins in feeds would increase the expenses. Therefore, HPLC assessment of the protein content of feeds is becoming evident (Henderson et al., 2000).

Hormones are chemical substances with diverse regulatory roles in physiology that are produced in different parts of the body and transported through the blood and lymph circulation to target tissues. Numerous research is present in the literature that use the HPLC method to quantify growth hormone and insulin in commercial prescriptions. The HPLC method, coupled with a UV detector, was used to analyze recombinant human growth hormone. Investigations of bioavailability and quality control of recombinant growth hormone were investigated in monkeys using HPLC analysis. Insulin quantification in pharmaceutical preparations was obtained by using RP-

HPLC. Another study evaluated the relationship between different pressure and temperature adsorption and retention times of cattle, swine, and recombinant human insulin hormones using the HPLC method (Szabelski et al., 2002; Kim et al., 2005). Progesterone, a steroid hormone, prepares women for pregnancy and is released from the ovaries each month in cycles. Also, progesterone enhances mammary tissue development during adolescence. HPLC analysis can determine plasma levels and concentration differences of progesterone, which are critical for pregnancy. The progesterone and specific metabolites having the A-ring were purified by using the HPLC method. In a different study, progesterone and its metabolite, 5B-hydroxyprogesterone, were determined using the HPLC method (Sheehan et al., 2005).

Vitamins are essential organic compounds that are involved in various biochemical reactions and metabolic pathways, and they can be quantified by HPLC analysis. Pyridoxine, one of the B-complex vitamins, is vital in sodium-potassium equilibrium, cardiovascular care, and the production of various hormones and erythrocytes. Its deficiency is marked by metabolic disorders associated with anorexia, fatigue, anemia, and anxiety. Thiamine (vitamin B1) is essential in carbohydrate metabolism and the maintenance of the skeletomuscular system. Its deficiency manifests itself with weakness, gastrointestinal disorders, and depression. Nutritional research uses HPLC analysis for the determination of pyridoxine and thiamine quantities. Multivitamin supplements are subjected to HPLC analysis for pyridoxine, thiamine, and cyanocobalamine quantification; to RP-HPLC analysis for nicotinamide, pyridoxine, folic acid, riboflavin, and thiamine quantification (Markopoulou et al., 2002; Höller et al., 2003). In another study, the HPLC method was used to assess the status of vitamin C, thiamine, riboflavin, and pyridoxine in premature babies subjected to parenteral and enteral feeding. The HPLC-UV method determines and controls the total amount of vitamin C in infant feeds and purees. Due to its cost-effectiveness, HPLC is preferred for ascorbic acid and vitamin C determination in fruits and peas (Friel et al., 2001; Fontannaz et al., 2006).

Conclusion

Metabolomics is the high-performance quantification of metabolites e.g., oligonucleotides, nucleosides, peptides, amines, organic acids, aldehydes, ketones, steroids, alkaloids, and amino acids. Metabolomics is a multidisciplinary field that combines biology, chemistry, engineering, and mathematics.

The HPLC enables the purification, quantification, and quality analysis of metabolites. It is widely used in the scientific community due to its preparative and analytical aspects, specificity, precision, and speed. Aromatic plants have been used in alternative medicine for treatment purposes throughout history. The determination and quantification of biologically active substances existing in plant species are of vital importance. Again, large-scale analysis of pharmaceuticals, biomolecules, and polymers is necessary. Investigations of drugs and drug metabolites enable further studies in bioavailability and dosage regimes.

HPLC in the food industry has been outstanding in determining metabolites of carbohydrates, vitamins, additives, preservers, and toxins. Notably, in industrial agriculture and food processing, the chemicals used to improve the quality and prolong the shelf life pose risks to human health. Thus, HPLC is rigorously used in the food industry to determine various compounds.

Heavy metal contamination of the environment, which is a result of exceeding population increases and technological developments, is affecting the biological functions of organisms. Their analysis is necessary as they would act as toxins in the body when aggregating. Unresponsible and unregulated use of pesticides in agriculture to attain desired final products inevitably affects human health and environmental integrity. The HPLC makes the extraction and determination of such metabolites with high speed and high performance possible, and the application fields of HPLC are ever-increasing with the development of different detectors.

References

Alves, S. P., Brum, D. M., de Andrade, É. C. B., and Netto, A. D. P. (2008). Determination of synthetic dyes in selected foodstuffs by high performance liquid chromatography with UV-DAD detection. *Food chemistry*, 107(1), 489-496. https://doi.org/10.1016/j.foodchem.2007.07.054.

Amagase, H. (2006). Clarifying the real bioactive constituents of garlic. *The Journal of nutrition*, 136(3), 716S-725S. https://doi.org/10.1093/jn/136.3.716s.

Boudina, A., Emmelin, C., Baaliouamer, A., Grenier-Loustalot, M. F., and Chovelon, J. M. (2003). Photochemical behaviour of carbendazim in aqueous solution. *Chemosphere*, 50(5), 649-655. https://doi.org/10.1016/S0045-6535(02)00620-3.

Boyer, R. (2003). Concepts and skills in the biochemistry/molecular biology lab. *Biochemistry and Molecular Biology Education*, 31(2), 102-105. https://doi.org/10.1016/S0045-6535(02)00620-3.

Cherng, Y. G., Tsai, C. C., Chung, H. H., Lai, Y. W., Kuo, S. C., and Cheng, J. T. (2013). Antihyperglycemic action of sinapic acid in diabetic rats. *Journal of Agricultural and Food Chemistry*, 61(49), 12053-12059. https://doi.org/10.1021/jf403092b.

Chinnici, F., Spinabelli, U., Riponi, C., and Amati, A. (2005). Optimization of the determination of organic acids and sugars in fruit juices by ion-exclusion liquid chromatography. *Journal of food composition and analysis*, 18(2-3), 121-130. https://doi.org/10.1016/j.jfca.2004.01.005.

Chowdhury, S. P., Khanna, S., Verma, S. C., and Tripathi, A. K. (2004). Molecular diversity of tannic acid degrading bacteria isolated from tannery soil. *Journal of applied microbiology*, 97(6), 1210-1219. https://doi.org/10.1016/j.jfca.2004.01.005.

Coronel, M. B., Marín, S., Cano-Sancho, G., Ramos, A. J., and Sanchis, V. (2012). Exposure assessment to ochratoxin A in Catalonia (Spain) based on the consumption of cereals, nuts, coffee, wine, and beer. *Food Additives & Contaminants: Part A*, 29(6), 979-993. https://doi.org/10.1080/19440049.2012.660708.

Dokoumetzidis, A., and Macheras, P. (2006). A century of dissolution research: from Noyes and Whitney to the biopharmaceutics classification system. *International journal of pharmaceutics*, 321(1-2), 1-11. https://doi.org/10.1016/ j.ijpharm.2006.07.011.

Engelhardt, H. (2004). One century of liquid chromatography from Tswett's columns to modern high speed and high performance separations. *Journal of chromatography. B, Analytical technologies in the biomedical and life sciences*, 800(1), 3-6. https://doi.org/10.1016/j.jchromb.2003.09.064.

Eser, B., and Dincel, A. S. (2018). Introduction to Chromatography, Basic Working Tips for High Performance Liquid Chromatography (Kromatografiye giriş, yüksek performanslı sıvı kromatografi kullanımında basit ipuçları). *Journal of Health Services and Education*, 2(2), 51-57. https://doi.org/10.26567/JOHSE.2018250150.

Fontannaz, P., Kilinç, T., and Heudi, O. (2006). HPLC-UV determination of total vitamin C in a wide range of fortified food products. *Food chemistry*, 94(4), 626-631. https://doi.org/10.1016/j.foodchem.2005.02.012.

Friel, J. K., Bessie, J. C., Belkhode, S. L., Edgecombe, C., Steele-Rodway, M., Downton, G., and Aziz, K. (2001). Thiamine, riboflavin, pyridoxine, and vitamin C status in premature infants receiving parenteral and enteral nutrition. *Journal of pediatric gastroenterology and nutrition*, 33(1), 64-69. https://doi.org/10.1097/00005176-200107000-00011.

Fucharoen, S., and Winichagoon, P. (2002). Thalassemia and abnormal hemoglobin. *International journal of hematology*, 76(2), 83-89. https://doi.org/10.1007/ bf03165094.

Ge, Q. H., Zhou, Z., Zhi, X. J., and Wang, H. (2004). Simultaneous determination of Pseudoephedrine and chlorpheniramine in human plasma by HPLC-UV detection method. *Yao xue xue bao= Acta Pharmaceutica Sinica*, 39(4), 281-284. https://doi.org/10.1002/bmc.311.

Graikou, K., Popova, M., Gortzi, O., Bankova, V., and Chinou, I. (2016). Characterization and biological evaluation of selected Mediterranean propolis samples. Is it a new type? *LWT-Food Science and Technology*, 65, 261-267. https://doi.org/10.1016/j.lwt.2015.08.025.

Haria, M., and Wagstaff, A. J. (1995). Amlodipine. *Drugs*, 50(3), 560-586. https://doi.org/10.2165/00003495-199550030-00009.

Henderson, J. W., Ricker, R. D., Bidlingmeyer, B. A., and Woodward, C. (2000). Rapid, accurate, sensitive, and reproducible HPLC analysis of amino acids. *Amino acid analysis using Zorbax Eclipse-AAA columns and the Agilent*, 1100(1100), 1-10.

Höller, U., Brodhag, C., Knöbel, A., Hofmann, P., and Spitzer, V. (2003). Automated determination of selected water-soluble vitamins in tablets using a bench-top robotic system coupled to reversed-phase (RP-18) HPLC with UV detection. *Journal of pharmaceutical and biomedical analysis*, 31(1), 151-158. https://doi.org/10.1016/S0731-7085(02)00574-5.

Juan, C., Lino, C. M., Pena, A., Moltó, J. C., Mañes, J., and Silveira, I. (2007). Determination of ochratoxin A in maize bread samples by LC with fluorescence detection. *Talanta*, 73(2), 246-250. https://doi.org/10.1016/j.talanta.2007.03.029.

Kaur, C., and Kapoor, H. C. (2001). Antioxidants in fruits and vegetables–the millennium's health. *International journal of food science & technology*, 36(7), 703-725. http://dx.doi.org/10.1046/j.1365-2621.2001.00513.x.

Khan, M. K., and Dangles, O. (2014). A comprehensive review on flavanones, the major citrus polyphenols. *Journal of Food Composition and Analysis*, 33(1), 85-104. https://doi.org/10.1016/j.jfca.2013.11.004.

Kim, S. J., Hahn, S. K., Kim, M. J., Kim, D. H., and Lee, Y. P. (2005). Development of a novel sustained release formulation of recombinant human growth hormone using sodium hyaluronate microparticles. *Journal of controlled release*, 104(2), 323-335. https://doi.org/10.1016/j.jconrel.2005.02.012.

Kitamura, S., Kadota, T., Yoshida, M., Jinno, N., and Ohta, S. (2000). Whole-body metabolism of the organophosphorus pesticide, fenthion, in goldfish, Carassius auratus. *Comparative Biochemistry and Physiology Part C: Pharmacology, Toxicology and Endocrinology*, 126(3), 259-266. https://doi.org/10.1016/S0742-8413(00)00124-9.

Kopustinskiene, D. M., Jakstas, V., Savickas, A., and Bernatoniene, J. (2020). Flavonoids as anticancer agents. *Nutrients*, 12(2), 457. https://doi.org/10.3390/nu12020457.

Liwarska-Bizukojc, E., and Bizukojc, M. (2005). Digital image analysis to estimate the influence of sodium dodecyl sulphate on activated sludge flocs. *Process Biochemistry*, 40(6), 2067-2072. https://doi.org/10.1016/j.procbio.2004.07.020.

Luo, C., Zou, X., Li, Y., Sun, C., Jiang, Y., and Wu, Z. (2011). Determination of flavonoids in propolis-rich functional foods by reversed phase high performance liquid chromatography with diode array detection. *Food Chemistry*, 127(1), 314-320. https://doi.org/10.1016/j.foodchem.2011.01.006.

Ma, M., Luo, X., Chen, B., Su, S., and Yao, S. (2006). Simultaneous determination of water-soluble and fat-soluble synthetic colorants in foodstuff by high-performance liquid chromatography–diode array detection–electrospray mass spectrometry.

Journal of Chromatography A, 1103(1), 170-176. https://doi.org/10.1016/j.chroma.2005.11.061.

Marin, A., Garcıa, E., Garcıa, A., and Barbas, C. (2002). Validation of a HPLC quantification of acetaminophen, phenylephrine and chlorpheniramine in pharmaceutical formulations: capsules and sachets. *Journal of Pharmaceutical and Biomedical Analysis*, 29(4), 701-714. https://doi.org/10.1016/s0731-7085(02)00124-3.

Markopoulou, C. K., Kagkadis, K. A., and Koundourellis, J. E. (2002). An optimized method for the simultaneous determination of vitamins B1, B6, B12, in multivitamin tablets by high performance liquid chromatography. *Journal of Pharmaceutical and Biomedical Analysis*, 30(4), 1403-1410. https://doi.org/10.1016/S0731-7085(02)00456-9.

Marzouk, H. M., Rezk, M. R., Gouda, A. S., and Abdel-Megied, A. M. (2022). A novel stability-indicating HPLC-DAD method for determination of favipiravir, a potential antiviral drug for COVID-19 treatment; application to degradation kinetic studies and in-vitro dissolution profiling. *Microchemical Journal*, 172, 106917. https://doi.org/10.1016/j.microc.2021.106917.

Mezcua, M., Agüera, A., Lliberia, J. L., Cortés, M. A., Bagó, B., and Fernández-Alba, A. R. (2006). Application of ultra performance liquid chromatography–tandem mass spectrometry to the analysis of priority pesticides in groundwater. *Journal of Chromatography A*, 1109(2), 222-227. https://doi.org/10.1016/j.chroma.2006.01.024.

Miyashita, S., Shimoya, M., Kamidate, Y., Kuroiwa, T., Shikino, O., Fujiwara, S., and Kaise, T. (2009). Rapid determination of arsenic species in freshwater organisms from the arsenic-rich Hayakawa River in Japan using HPLC-ICP-MS. *Chemosphere*, 75(8), 1065-1073. https://doi.org/10.1016/j.chemosphere.2009.01.029.

Mouri, C., and Laursen, R. (2012). Identification of anthraquinone markers for distinguishing Rubia species in madder-dyed textiles by HPLC. *Microchimica Acta*, 179(1), 105-113. https://doi.org/10.1007/s00604-012-0868-4.

Niedzwiecki, A., Roomi, M. W., Kalinovsky, T., and Rath, M. (2016). Anticancer efficacy of polyphenols and their combinations. *Nutrients*, 8(9), 552. https://doi.org/10.1007/s00604-012-0868-4.

Nikolin, B., Imamović, B., Medanhodžić-Vuk, S., and Sober, M. (2004). High perfomance liquid chromatography in pharmaceutical analyses. *Bosnian journal of basic medical sciences*, 4(2), 5. https://doi.org/10.17305/bjbms.2004.3405.

Norn, S., Permin, H., Kruse, P. R., and Kruse, E. (2009). From willow bark to acetylsalicylic acid. *Dansk medicinhistorisk arbog* [*Danish medical history workbook*], 37, 79-98.

Osés, S. M., Pascual-Maté, A., Fernández-Muiño, M. A., López-Díaz, T. M., and Sancho, M. T. (2016). Bioactive properties of honey with propolis. *Food chemistry*, 196, 1215-1223. https://doi.org/10.1016/j.foodchem.2015.10.050.

Ozcan, Ö., Aldemir, O., and Karabulut, B. (2020). Flavones (apigenin, luteolin, chrysin) and their importance for health. *Mellifera*, 20(1), 16-27.

Panche, A. N., Diwan, A. D., and Chandra, S. R. (2016). Flavonoids: an overview. *Journal of nutritional science*, 5. https://doi.org/10.1017/jns.2016.41.

Panggabean, A. S. (2016). Analisis residu klorpirifos dalam sayur-sayuran dengan teknik high performance liquid chromatography (HPLC). *Jurnal Kimia Mulawarman* [*Journal of Mulawarman Chemistry*], 13(2).

Patwekar, S. L., Sakhare, R. S., and Nilesh, N. N. (2015). HPLC method development and validation-A general Concept. *International Journal of Chemical and Pharmaceutical Sciences*, 6(1), 8-14. http://dx.doi.org/10.7897/2230-8407.04407.

Pokorný, J. (1991). Natural antioxidants for food use. *Trends in Food Science & Technology*, 2, 223-227. https://doi.org/10.1016/0924-2244(91)90695-F.

Populin, T., Moret, S., Truant, S., and Conte, L. S. (2007). A survey on the presence of free glutamic acid in foodstuffs, with and without added monosodium glutamate. *Food chemistry*, 104(4), 1712-1717. https://doi.org/10.1016/j.foodchem.2007.03.034.

Ren, S., Chen, X. Y., Duan, X. T., and Zhong, D. F. (2006). Simultaneous determination of ephedrine and chlorpheniramine in human plasma by a highly sensitive liquid chromatography-tandem mass spectrometric method. *Yao xue xue bao= Acta Pharmaceutica Sinica* [*Y Aoxue Journal = act A pharmaceutical A sin ICA*], 41(2), 188-192. https://doi.org/10.1002/bmc.311.

Robbins, R. J., and Bean, S. R. (2004). Development of a quantitative high-performance liquid chromatography–photodiode array detection measurement system for phenolic acids. *Journal of chromatography A*, 1038(1-2), 97-105. https://doi.org/10.1016/j.chroma.2004.03.009.

Rodriguez, V. M. L., Calonge Delso, M. M., and Ordonez Escudero, D. (2003). ELISA and HPLC determination of the occurrence of aflatoxin M 1 in raw cow's milk. *Food Additives & Contaminants*, 20(3), 276-280. https://doi.org/10.1080/0265203021000045208.

Saad, B., Sing, Y. Y., Nawi, M. A., Hashim, N., Ali, A. S. M., Saleh, M. I., and Ahmad, K. (2007). Determination of synthetic phenolic antioxidants in food items using reversed-phase HPLC. *Food chemistry*, 105(1), 389-394. https://doi.org/10.1016/j.foodchem.2006.12.025.

Sheehan, P. M., Rice, G. E., Moses, E. K., and Brennecke, S. P. (2005). 5β-Dihydroprogesterone and steroid 5β–reductase decrease in association with human parturition at term. *Molecular human reproduction*, 11(7), 495-501. https://doi.org/10.1016/j.foodchem.2006.12.025.

Sokolova, L. I., and Chernyaev, A. P. (2002). Reversed-phase HPLC determination of antibiotics of the cephalosporin series in biological objects. *Pharmaceutical Chemistry Journal*, 36(5), 263-269. http://dx.doi.org/10.1023/A:1020525614433.

Swartz, M. (2010). HPLC detectors: a brief review. *Journal of Liquid Chromatography & Related Technologies*, 33(9-12), 1130-1150. https://doi.org/10.1080/10826076.2010.484356.

Szabelski, P., Cavazzini, A., Kaczmarski, K., Liu, X., Van Horn, J., and Guiochon, G. (2002). Experimental studies of pressure/temperature dependence of protein adsorption equilibrium in reversed-phase high-performance liquid chromatography. *Journal of Chromatography A*, 950(1-2), 41-53. https://doi.org/10.1016/S0021-9673(01)01614-4.

Tarahovsky, Y. S., Selezneva, I. I., Vasilieva, N. A., Egorochkin, M. A., and Kim, Y. A. (2007). Acceleration of fibril formation and thermal stabilization of collagen fibrils in the presence of taxifolin (dihydroquercetin). *Bulletin of Experimental Biology and Medicine*, 144(6), 791-794. https://doi.org/10.1007/s10517-007-0433-z.

Tatár, E., Mihucz, V. G., Varga, A., Záray, G., and Cseh, E. (1999). Effect of lead, nickel and vanadium contamination on organic acid transport in xylem sap of cucumber. *Journal of inorganic biochemistry*, 75(3), 219-223.

Teng, H., and Chen, L. (2019). Polyphenols and bioavailability: An update. *Critical reviews in food science and nutrition*, 59(13), 2040-2051. https://doi.org/10.1080/10408398.2018.1437023.

Torra, J., Rojano-Delgado, A. M., Menéndez, J., Salas, M., and de Prado, R. (2021). Cytochrome P450 metabolism-based herbicide resistance to imazamox and 2, 4-D in Papaver rhoeas. *Plant Physiology and Biochemistry*, 160, 51-61. https://doi.org/10.1016/j.plaphy.2021.01.007.

Tsiropoulos, N. G., Bakeas, E. B., Raptis, V., and Batistatou, S. S. (2006). Evaluation of solid sorbents for the determination of fenhexamid, metalaxyl-M, pyrimethanil, malathion and myclobutanil residues in air samples: application to monitoring malathion and fenhexamid dissipation in greenhouse air using C-18 or Supelpak-2 for sampling. *Analytica chimica acta*, 573, 209-215. https://doi.org/10.1016/j.aca.2006.03.091.

Uesugi, S., Watanabe, S., Ishiwata, N., Uehara, M., and Ouchi, K. (2004). Effects of isoflavone supplements on bone metabolic markers and climacteric symptoms in Japanese women. *Biofactors*, 22(1-4), 221-228. https://doi.org/10.1002/biof.5520220145.

Xie, T., Xia, Y., Zeng, Y., Li, X., and Zhang, Y. (2017). Nitrate concentration-shift cultivation to enhance protein content of heterotrophic microalga Chlorella vulgaris: Over-compensation strategy. *Bioresource technology*, 233, 247-255. https://doi.org/10.1016/j.biortech.2017.02.099.

Yen, G. C., Duh, P. D., and Tsai, H. L. (2002). Antioxidant and pro-oxidant properties of ascorbic acid and gallic acid. *Food chemistry*, 79(3), 307-313. https://doi.org/10.1016/S0308-8146(02)00145-0.

Zhao, R. S., Yuan, J. P., Jiang, T., Shi, J. B., and Cheng, C. G. (2008). Application of bamboo charcoal as solid-phase extraction adsorbent for the determination of atrazine and simazine in environmental water samples by high-performance liquid chromatography-ultraviolet detector. *Talanta*, 76(4), 956-959. https://doi.org/10.1016/j.talanta.2008.04.029.

Žemberyová, M., Bartekova, J., and Hagarova, I. (2006). The utilization of modified BCR three-step sequential extraction procedure for the fractionation of Cd, Cr, Cu, Ni, Pb and Zn in soil reference materials of different origins. *Talanta*, 70(5), 973-978. https://doi.org/10.1016/j.talanta.2006.05.057.

Chapter 7

The Scope of LC-MS-Based Metabolomics

Pelin Koparir[1,*], PhD
and İnanç Baral[2], PhD
[1]Department of Medical Services and Techniques, Health Services Vocational School, Fırat University, Elazıg, Turkey
[2]Department of Zootechnics and Animal Nutrition, Faculty of Veterinary Medicine, Sivas Cumhuriyet University, Sivas, Turkey

Abstract

The field of metabolomics is becoming an indispensable part of clinical research with its potential for the discovery of biomarkers and diagnostic molecules along with its potential for revealing concealed aspaects of pathophysiological conditions. Basically, metabolomics aims to objectively identify and quantify all metabolites present in a living system at a particular state or point of time. In summary, all metabolomics research contains steps of sample collection and processing, detection, and analysis of raw data, and evaluation of the results. A frame of the metabolic state of a eukaryotic living system can be understood by using various biological samples ranging from cerebospinal fluid to tissues to blood plasma. Each biological sample contains a large set of endogenous compounds that are classified under various compounds, e.g., organic acids, amino acids, peptides, carbohydrates, etc. Both internal (gender, age, health, physiological state, etc.) and external (diet, lifestyle, pollution, environment, etc.) stimuli affect the metabolite composition, sometimes quite strikingly. A large number of variables are effective in the composition of metabolites, which requires a careful design of the research and the use of standardized experimental procedures encompassing all the steps. There

* Corresponding Author's Email: mpelin23@hotmail.com.

In: Metabolomics and Clinical Approach
Editors: Sevgi Durna Daştan and Taner Daştan
ISBN: 979-8-89113-095-1

are conventional standardized methods for the individual identification of particular metabolites based on their compound classes. Metabolomics methods, however, aim to detect and profile the global metabolite context by applying pattern recognition and profiling on complex sets of metabolite data. Currently, there is no single approach to achieve such a daunting task. Therefore, different analytical approaches are used according to the intended metabolomics study. An analytical method should be both sensitive and comprehensive to cover large data series of metabolites in a robust and specific manner. Of the available methods, nuclear magnetic resonance (NMR) and mass spectrometry are the best instrumental and analytical methods frequently used for metabolomics research. The high sensitivity and wide dynamic range provided by mass spectrometry (MS) can be coupled with chromatography methods to achieve large-scale analysis of metabolites from biological samples. Mass spectrometry can be coupled with liquid chromatography (LC) for the metabolite profiling of thermolabile or involatile compounds. The LC-MS-based metabolomics research that used the liquid chromatography-mass spectrometry (LC-MS) approach was reviewed in this chapter.

Keywords: liquid chromatography, lc, mass spectrometry, ms, metabolomics, metabolite, spectrometry

Introduction

For the discovery of biomarkers and investigations of metabolic pathways in various biological samples, mass spectrometry is the commonly used method in metabolomics (Dunn et al., 2011a; Kell and Oliver, 2016). Furthermore, mass spectrometry is a prominent tool in the field of precision medicine (Beger et al., 2016). However, difficulties in associating metabolomic data with biochemical reactions and their functional annotations are still solid challenges (Dias et al., 2016; Viant et al., 2017). Liquid chromatography-mass spectrometry (LC-MS) is an effective and constantly advancing analytical tool for non-targeted metabolomics that has the capacity to analyse thousands of compounds in a given sample (Chaleckis et al., 2018; Giera, 2018) with its extensive coverage of metabolites and high sensitivity (Dunn et al., 2011b). Despite these qualities, LC-MS requires to be supported with tandem mass spectrometry (MS/MS) spectra to increase the validity of identifications due to the presence of metabolites with similar molecular characteristics in a given pool of metabolites and the possibility of co-elution of metabolites during the separation (Chaleckis et al., 2018; Giera, 2018). Therefore, the metabolite confirmation requires the use of spectral databases to compare. While databases containing and dedicated to molecular spectra are increasing in number and improving in quality, precise identification and validation of metabolites still need comprehensive tools that can be used by researchers to confidently validate their findings. To better introduce this concept, it would be beneficial to discuss the AIF (all-ion fragmentation) technique that is part of the LC-MS procedure, which uses low-energy CID (collision-induced dissociation) to detect mass spectra for precursor ions, while high-energy CID is used for MS/MS to detect the actual product by ion contrasting (Plumb et al., 2006). Following the ion contrasting, the analysis then commences with extracted ion chromatograms (EIC) that would reveal the target ions from low and high-energy spectra. Once the target ion was revealed from the EIC, it would be used for relative quantification of the target metabolite. Subsequently, other ions extracted from the same compound can be utilized as qualifiers. This particular technique has its own dedicated database based on established analytical standards and enables the spectral fragmentation of the data extensively, which can be clarified and validated by using MS/MS spectra from databases (Chaleckis et al., 2018; Giera, 2018; Naz et al., 2017).

LC-Based Metabolomics Studies

Non-targeted metabolomics studies for profiling that use LC-MS methodology frequently employ MS systems of triple quadrupole (QqQ), Time-of-Flight (TOF), quadrupole time-of-flight (Q-TOF), and Orbitrap. TOF-MS is generally used in cases where capillary electrophoresis (CE) was used due to its fast-scanning properties. QqQ-MS is considered an appropriate MS system for targeted metabolite profiling in tandem mode of operation due to its extensive dynamic range, which makes it powerful for quantitative analysis (Hyotylainen and Wiedmer, 2013; Poho and Hyotylainen, 2013). Metabolite identification by LC-MS and CE-MS requires precise measurements for the determination of elemental and molecular properties that are necessary for validation. Nevertheless, just a single metabolite can provide multiple detection peaks in both LC-MS and CE-MS due to the existence of isotopes or fragment deviations. This requires the ion annotation of detected metabolites to associate related ions with their parent metabolites, and for this purpose, spectral libraries are present in metabolomics databases

(Horai et al., 2010; Hyotylainen and Wiedmer, 2013; Poho and Hyotylainen, 2013; Wishart et al., 2009).

Liquid chromatography is also used by itself as conventional high-performance (HPLC) and ultra-high-pressure (UHPLC) and as newer supercritical fluid chromatography (SFC) methods with variable selectivity for separation (3 to 5 µm for HPLC, less than 2 µm for UHPLC). Again, both miniaturized and capillary LC systems are existing. Mass spectrometry can be used by itself, resulting in significantly reduced analytical prowess and complexity, yet such an approach is quite disadvantageous for complex matrices, where ion suppression and ion enhancement would distort the profiles. Consequently, with such distorted profiles, it would be almost impossible to distinguish isobaric and isomeric metabolites. LC integration to MS effectively eliminates ion-based distortions and enables the individual identification of isobaric and isomeric structures. While it is apparent in the scientific community that the major desire is the analysis of the maximum number of compounds as quickly as possible and obtain comprehensive results, the practical experience suggests otherwise to obtain detailed, validated, and comprehensive profiles, which can be acquired by longer run times (10 to 20 minutes on average) and higher resolutions in chromatography. To achieve the most comprehensive and detailed profile that is possible, emphasis should be placed on resolution and run times, which significantly limit the possible number of outcomes. Overall, a generalized approach for global metabolite profiling can be utilized with a balance of resolution and run times (Naz et al., 2017; Theodoridis et al., 2013), while highly detailed profiling requires the maximum possible chromatographic resolution, such as capillary LC and longer run times (Theodoridis et al., 2013).

For the determination, identification, and characterization of very small organic molecules present in biological samples, mass spectrometry was integrated into the UPLC method, and this approach provided striking efficiency with very high levels of resolution, speed, and sensitivity (Li et al., 2013; Qi et al., 2014; Raftery, 2014). UPLC is already a well-known method for the efficient separation of less than 2 µm small particles under very high pressure (12k to 15k PSI) (MacNair et al., 1997). By combining UPLC with Q-TOF-MS, researchers achieved a much larger dynamic range of detection for non-targeted profiling coupled with enhanced selectivity and potential for identification. Integration of ESI (electrospray ionization) into UPLC-MS, thus forming UPLC-ESI-Q-TOF-MS, is today regarded the most advanced analytical tool of metabolomics research for global metabolite profiling in high-complexity biological systems (Qi et al., 2014; Raftery, 2014).

MS-Based Metabolomics Studies

Today, LC-MS is the most frequently used analytical model method for metabolomics studies. However, LC-MS has its downfalls, despite its frequent use, which requires alternative approaches to overcome the inherent limitations of MS systems. The first of these limitations are the distorted ionization efficiency that is the result of variations in compound structures. It is known that the ionization efficiency is quite variable between even structurally similar compounds. To cover the entire metabolome and for global metabolite profiling, the dual operation of the ESI with positive and negative modes in LC-MS has seen increased usage. For the specified detection of apolar substances in a metabolite pool, the APCI (Atmospheric Pressure Chemical Ionization) method was proposed as advantageous but was not received little use in metabolite profiling. High-resolution LC like UHPLC is quite suitable for coupled with TOF-MS due to its analytical qualities of higher sensitivity and accuracy that are complementary to narrow chromatic peaks obtained from UHPLC. Overall, UHPLC-TOF-MS provided fast, sensitive, and accurate analysis of metabolites for profiling. TOF-MS systems can be combined with ion traps for metabolomics research such as IT-TOF-MS (Loftus et al., 2008; Theodoridis et al., 2013) and QTRAP (Gika et al., 2007; Gika et al., 2010; Theodoridis et al., 2013). Advanced systems of Fourier Transform-Ion Cyclotron (FT-ICR) MS and Orbitrap MS can be utilized for much higher resolution and mass accuracy, which can lead to highly detailed and comprehensive metabolite profiling (Forcisi et al., 2013; Zhang et al., 2012). Of particular note are the difficulties in data comparisons and data contrasting when different MS systems were used, even for the same sample. Indeed, metabolite profiles obtained from the same samples using LC-Q-TOF-MS and LC-QTRAP-MS provided significantly different results that proved to be quite difficult to compare. Therefore, MS system-specific multivariate statistical analysis algorithms (such as Principal Component Analysis) are necessary to enable comparisons and contrasting of data obtained by using different MS systems (Theodoridis et al., 2013; Zhang et al., 2012).

Metabolomics research that used MS systems was most apparent in investigations of drug and toxin effects on metabolism, identification of metabolic pathways, metabolic fluctuation measurements, and the metabolic layering of different diseases. The impact of MS-based metabolomics and the successes of MS systems were highlighted in various cancer types (breast cancer, colorectal cancer, prostate cancer, and gastric cancer), in congenital metabolic disorders, in chronic and complex diseases, and in evaluations of nutrients and toxins in a living system (Gowda and Djukovich, 2014; Raftery, 2014; Wishart et al., 2009).

Conclusion

Without a doubt, metabolomics has the potential to be an indispensable tool in medicine and biotechnology. By deciphering metabolite profiles from diverse populations of humans and thus revealing metabolic phenotypes, which are termed as metabotypes, metabolomics would contribute greatly to the development of personalized medicine and personalized pharmaceutical agents. Nevertheless, at this stage, this remains a possibility and requires further advancements in analytical systems and data processing tools. While rigorous and time-consuming, the LC-MS methodology for metabolite profiling and its use in metabolomics are widely and frequently applied in different research frameworks. Different analysis systems are developed to overcome the inherent difficulties in MS systems, but the identification and validation of biomarkers are still challenges to overcome, which necessitate novel protocols and algorithms for the identification and validation of important biomarkers that might be used in clinical practice.

References

Beger, R. D., Dunn, W., Schmidt, M. A., Gross, S. S., Kirwan, J. A., Cascante, M., Brennan, L., Wishart, D. S., Oresic, M., Hankemeier, T., Broadhurst, D. I., Lane, A. N., Suhre, K., Kastenmüller, G., Sumner, S. J., Thiele, I., Fiehn, O., & Kaddurah-Daouk, R.; for "Precision Medicine and Pharmacometabolomics Task Group"-Metabolomics Society Initiative. (2016). Metabolomics enables precision medicine:"a white paper, community perspective." *Metabolomics*, *12*, 1-15. https://doi.org/10.1007/s11306-016-1094-6.

Chaleckis, R., Naz, S., Meister, I., Wheelock, C.E. (2018). LC-MS-Based Metabolomics of Biofluids Using All-Ion Fragmentation (AIF) Acquisition. In Giera, M. (Ed). *Clinical Metabolomics Methods and Protocols* (pp: 45-59). USA: Humana Press, Springer Nature.

Dias, D. A., Jones, O. A., Beale, D. J., Boughton, B. A., Benheim, D., Kouremenos, K. A., Wolfender, J.L., & Wishart, D. S. (2016). Current and future perspectives on the structural identification of small molecules in biological systems. *Metabolites*, *6*(4), 46. https://doi.org/10.3390/metabo6040046.

Dunn, W.B., Broadhurst, D., Begley, P., Zelena, E., Francis-McIntyre, S., Anderson, N., Brown, M., Knowles, J. D., Halsall, A., Haselden, J. N., Nicholls, A. W., Wilson, I.

D., Kell, D. B., Goodacre, R. & Human Serum Metabolome (HUSERMET) Consortium (2011a). Procedures for large-scale metabolic profiling of serum and plasma using gas chromatography and liquid chromatography coupled to mass spectrometry. *Nature protocols*, *6*(7), 1060-1083. https://doi.org/10.1038/nprot.2011.335.

Dunn, W. B., Broadhurst, D. I., Atherton, H. J., Goodacre, R., & Griffin, J. L. (2011b). Systems level studies of mammalian metabolomes: the roles of mass spectrometry and nuclear magnetic resonance spectroscopy. *Chemical society reviews*, *40*(1), 387-426. https://doi.org/10.1039/b906712b.

Forcisi, S., Moritz, F., Kanawati, B., Tziotis, D., Lehmann, R., & Schmitt-Kopplin, P. (2013). Liquid chromatography–mass spectrometry in metabolomics research: Mass analyzers in ultra high pressure liquid chromatography coupling. *Journal of Chromatography A*, *1292*, 51-65. https://doi.org/10.1016/j.chroma.2013.04.017.

Giera, M. (2018). *Clinical Metabolomics Methods and Protocols*. USA: Humana Press, Springer Nature,

Gika, H. G., Theodoridis, G. A., Wingate, J. E., & Wilson, I. D. (2007). Within-day reproducibility of an HPLC− MS-based method for metabonomic analysis: application to human urine. *Journal of proteome research*, *6*(8), 3291-3303. https://doi.org/10.1021/pr070183p.

Gika, H. G., Theodoridis, G. A., Earll, M., Snyder, R. W., Sumner, S. J., & Wilson, I. D. (2010). Does the mass spectrometer define the marker? A comparison of global metabolite profiling data generated simultaneously via UPLC-MS on two different mass spectrometers. *Analytical chemistry*, *82*(19), 8226-8234. https://doi.org/10.1021/ac1016612.

Gowda, G.A.N., Djukovic, D. (2014). Overview of Mass Spectrometry-Based Metabolomics: Opportunities and Challenges. In Raftery, D. (Ed), *Mass Spectrometry in Metabolomics Methods and Protocols* (pp. 1-15). Humana Press. Springer.

Horai, H., Arita, M., Kanaya, S., Nihei, Y., Ikeda, T., Suwa, K., Ojima, Y., Tanaka, K., Tanaka, S., Aoshima, K., Oda, Y., Kakazu, Y., Kusano, M., Tohge, T., Matsuda, F., Sawada, Y., Hirai, M. Y., Nakanishi, H., Ikeda, K., Akimoto, N., Maoka, T., Takahashi, H., Ara, T., Sakurai, N., Suzuki, H., Shibata, D., Neumann, S., Iida, T., Tanaka, K., Funatsu, K., Matsuura, F., Soga, T., Taguchi, R., Saito, K., & Nishioka, T. (2010). MassBank: a public repository for sharing mass spectral data for life sciences. *Journal of mass spectrometry, 45*(7), 703-714.

Hyotylainen, T., & Wiedmer, S. (2013). *Chromatographic Methods in Metabolomics*. UK: The Royal Society of Chemistry Press.

Kell, D. B., & Oliver, S. G. (2016). The metabolome 18 years on: a concept comes of age. *Metabolomics*, *12*, 1-8. https://doi.org/10.1007/ s11306-016-1108-4

Li, F., Patterson, A. D., Krausz, K. W., Jiang, C., Bi, H., Sowers, A. L., Cook, J. A., Mitchell, J. B., & Gonzalez, F. J. (2013). Metabolomics reveals that tumor xenografts induce liver dysfunction. *Molecular & Cellular Proteomics*, *12*(8), 2126-2135. https://doi.org/10.1074/mcp.M113.028324.

Loftus, N., Miseki, K., Iida, J., Gika, H. G., Theodoridis, G., & Wilson, I. D. (2008). Profiling and biomarker identification in plasma from different Zucker rat strains via high mass accuracy multistage mass spectrometric analysis using liquid chromatography/mass spectrometry with a quadrupole ion trap-time of flight mass spectrometer. *Rapid Communications in Mass Spectrometry: An International Journal Devoted to the Rapid Dissemination of Up-to-the-Minute Research in Mass Spectrometry*, *22*(16), 2547-2554. https://doi.org/10.1002/rcm.3640.

MacNair, J. E., Lewis, K. C., & Jorgenson, J. W. (1997). Ultrahigh-pressure reversed-phase liquid chromatography in packed capillary columns. *Analytical chemistry*, *69*(6), 983-989. https://doi.org/10.1021/ac961094r.

Naz, S., Gallart-Ayala, H., Reinke, S., Mathon, C., Blankley, R., Chaleckis, R., & Wheelock, C. E. (2017). Development of an LC-HRMS metabolomics method with high specificity for metabolite identification using all ion fragmentation (AIF) acquisition. *Analytical Chemistry*.. https://doi.org/10.1021/acs.analchem.7b00925.

Plumb, R. S., Johnson, K. A., Rainville, P., Smith, B. W., Wilson, I. D., Castro-Perez, J. M., & Nicholson, J. K. (2006). UPLC/MSE; a new approach for generating molecular fragment information for biomarker structure elucidation. *Rapid Communications in Mass Spectrometry: An International Journal Devoted to the Rapid Dissemination of Up-to-the-Minute Research in Mass Spectrometry*, *20*(13), 1989-1994. https://doi.org/10.1002/rcm.2550.

Poho, P., & Hyotylainen, T. (2013). Mass Spectrometric Detection for Chromatography. In Hyotylainen, T., Wiedmer, S. (Eds). *Chromatographic Methods in Metabolomics* (pp. 43-63). UK: The Royal Society of Chemistry Press.

Qi, Y., Song,Y., Gu, H., Fan, G., & Chai, Y. (2014). Global Metabolic Profiling Using Ultra-Performance Liquid Chromatography/Quadrupole Time-of-Flight Mass Spectrometry. In Raftery, D. (Ed). *Mass Spectrometry in Metabolomics Methods and Protocols* (pp. 15-28). Humana Press, Springer

Raftery, D. (2014). *Mass Spectrometry in Metabolomics Methods and Protocols*. Humana Press, Springer.

Theodoridis, G.A., Michopoulos, F., Gika, H.G., Plumb, R.S., Wilson, I.D. (2013). Liquid Chromatographic Techniques in Metabolomics. In Hyotylainen, T., Wiedmer, S. (Eds). *Chromatographic Methods in Metabolomics* (pp:64-86). UK: The Royal Society of Chemistry Press.

Viant, M. R., Kurland, I. J., Jones, M. R., & Dunn, W. B. (2017). How close are we to complete annotation of metabolomes? *Current opinion in chemical biology*, *36*, 64-69. https://doi.org/10.1016/j.cbpa.2017.01.001.

Wishart, D. S., Knox, C., Guo, A.C., Eisner, R., Young, N., Gautam, B., Hau, D.D., Psychogios, N., Dong, E., Bouatra, S., Mandal, R., Sinelnikov, I., Xia, J., Jia, L., Cruz, J.A., Lim, E., Sobsey, C.A., Shrivastava, S., Huang, P., Liu, P., Fang, L., Peng, J. Fradette, R., Cheng, D., Tzur, D., Clements, M., Lewis, A., De Souza, A., Zuniga, A., Dawe, M., Xiong, Y., Clive, D., Greiner, R., Nazyrova, A., Shaykhutdinov, R., Li, L., Vogel, H. J., & Forsythe, I. (2009). HMDB: a knowledgebase for the human metabolome. *Nucleic acids research, 37*(suppl_1), D603-D610. https://doi.org/10.1093/nar/gkn810.

Zhang, T., Creek, D. J., Barrett, M. P., Blackburn, G., & Watson, D. G. (2012). Evaluation of coupling reversed phase, aqueous normal phase, and hydrophilic interaction liquid chromatography with Orbitrap mass spectrometry for metabolomic studies of human urine. *Analytical chemistry*, *84*(4), 1994-2001. https://doi.org/10.1021/ac2030738.

Chapter 8

Databases for Metabolomics Research

Dilek Arslan Ateşşahin[1,*], PhD
and Yusuf Muhammed Durna[2], MD
[1]Department of Plant and Animal Production, Baskil Vocational School, Firat University, Elazığ, Turkey
[2]Department of Otolaryngology and Head and Neck Surgery, Private Practice, Istanbul, Turkey

Abstract

All biochemical elements that are part of the metabolism are represented in their entirety as the metabolome. It enables researchers to link the phenotype to the function provided as a whole from the genome and environmental variables. Cellular investigations of different components, e.g., DNA, mRNA, proteins, and their interactions, are now largely complemented with metabolomic research for revealing the function and interactions of individual metabolites. Different repositories for various molecules and molecular pathways are present for researchers. The metabolism itself is a vast network of intricate biochemical interactions, and mathematical models are required for a detailed analysis of particular pathways. Such a complex network of interactions can be better assessed using computational algorithms employing precise mathematical models. Metabolomics is already a noteworthy field in discovering novel therapeutic agents. In response to the increased demand for metabolomics research in various fields, different in silico tools were developed for the integrative analysis of metabolic systems, which have their own algorithms and pipelines for data simulation and evaluation. Some of the noteworthy metabolomic databases and associated software are introduced in this chapter.

* Corresponding Author's Email: datessahin@firat.edu.tr.

In: Metabolomics and Clinical Approach
Editors: Sevgi Durna Daştan and Taner Daştan
ISBN: 979-8-89113-095-1

Keywords: database, data mining, metabolite, metabolome, metabolomic, network

Introduction

Multi-cellular organisms are part of an intricate network of numerous mechanisms that made their phenotype differences the results of integrative outcomes from all levels of the biochemical structure instead of relegating it to a change of expression in a single or group of genes. Metabolism itself has a strict regulatory mechanism in its functioning, which eliminates the possibility of a linear correlation between gene expression and metabolic changes. Therefore, there are intertwining pathways with their cascades to form the complexity of the mechanism, which requires the precise understanding of the form and function of individual pathways (Knapp and Cabrera, 2011; Wiwanikit, 2011).

Identification and quantification of the entire metabolite inventory are the primary aims of metabolome analysis, which used one of two analytical approaches for this purpose (Villas-Bôas et al., 2005). Different platforms for detection seek to profile metabolites for qualitative classification (Villas-Bôas et al., 2005) by directly employing mass spectrophotometry or nuclear magnetic resonance methods or coupling them with a suitable separation method that includes capillary electrophoresis (CE) and liquid or gas chromatographies (Nielsen and Jewett, 2007). Metabolite profiling is supportive in functional genomics by linking metabolites to gene expressions (Fiehn 2001; Trethewey 2001).

Metabolomic Data Mining

It is evident that there is a gradual transition to quantitative approaches in integrative research, as seen from the ever-increasing amounts of data sets accumulated from different branches of the omics. Metabolite profiling is a pronounced method in systems biology with constantly advancing approaches for the determination and quantification of countless amounts of metabolites, which recently started to be reposited in developing databases. Despite the major efforts, only a fraction of the possible metabolites is known, while they remain unknown at large. However, advancements in analytical tools for metabolite detection are ongoing. Strategies and applications employed to extract meaningful data from a huge pool of raw data define data mining. Data mining is evident in metabolite profiling, which is the main theme of both metabolomics and metabonomics. Metabolite profiling seeks to identify and quantify metabolites from biological specimens by interpreting untargeted measurement data into meaningful associations. Both unsupervised and supervised statistical methods can be used to reveal potentially significant biomarkers from large data sets, and initial sets of revealed metabolites can be used to establish frameworks for newer research (Nordstrom, 2008). However, the obtained results should be evaluated based on different variable values to determine the significance of the extracted results. Various variables that should be considered include the statistical distribution of results, concentrations, amount folds, and significance results of applied tests (e.g., p-value, score value, and loading value). These variables would lead to the formation of relationship networks and clustural heat maps, which are used for data mining approaches (Nordstrom, 2008).

Metabolomic Databases

In their raw form, the data obtained from the omics, which usually indicates changes in metabolite pools, require standardized formatting for computational analysis and for being represented in databases. More than one analytical method is used in metabolomics to cover all aspects of metabolites resulting from different layers of metabolism, which lead to the emergence of methodology-based databases for metabolomics data. A particular database designed for the GC-TOF-MS methodology to detail metabolic fingerprints and profiles can be considered a model for metabolic database designing and modeling (Hummel et al., 2007). Comprehensive analysis of all existing databases is not the aim here, but a generalized overview of the current state by using a database provided by the Metabolomics Society (http://www.metabolomicssociety.org/) was intended.

Databases are integral parts of the data mining procedure, and databases in the field of metabolomics belong to one of five different classes of databases. In summary, these classes are (1) databases for detailed raw and meta-data for metabolites; (2) databases for species-specific metabolite data; (3) databases for metabolite data representing different physiological conditions from different species; (4) repositories of all known metabolomes of different species; and (5) databases that contain fact sheets and current understandings about the metabolomics (Mendes, 2002).

The very first use of a database would be the identification of an unknown metabolite after the initial detection. Currently, there are more than 100 different databases for the coverage of metabolic pathways. Some databases are specialized in mass spectrometry data, such as molecular weight and exact mass values, which enable comparisons of obtained data. Notable examples of such databases are METLIN; KEGG; ChemDB; ZINC; PubChem; ChemBank; and KNApSAcK (Smith et al., 2005; Kanehisa et al., 2002; Chen et al., 2005; Irwin and Shoichet, 2005; Wheeler et al., 2006; Strausberg and Schreiber, 2003; Shinbo et al., 2006). Among the present databases, KEGG, BRENDA, and BioCyc (Kanehisa 1997, 2006; Kanehisa and Goto 2000; Schomburg et al., 2002; Karp et al., 2005; Krummenacker et al., 2005; Keseler et al., 2005; Zhang et al., 2005) are known to be the most frequently used databases for metabolite information (Bader et al., 2006). Once the identification of a metabolite is established, existing servers such as KEGG, BRENDA, or BioCyc can be used to establish connections between the metabolite and gene expression or protein structure. Particularly, the BRENDA database can be utilized to establish crosslinks between metabolites and enzymes, which is based on the internationally recognized standards put forward by the IUPAC and the IUBMB (the International Union of Biochemistry and Molecular Biology). Previously documented experimental results can be directly used for data evaluations by using databases of classes 1, 2, and 3 as they mainly focus on raw and meta-data aspects. Therefore, scientifically acceptable and internationally recognized standards for data reporting that can be used universally at different levels of research are a significant requirement. Similar standards are already facilitated by existing databases for microarray analysis seen in MIAME and ARRAY EXPRESS (Brazma et al., 2001; Brazma et al., 2003); for gene expression profiles seen in GEO (Wheeler et al., 2006).

A tool called MSFACTS can be used for the spectral formatting, alignment, and conversion of metabolites for metabolite profiling (Duran et al., 2003; Wiwanikit, 2011). HybGFS is a hybrid method for metabolite identification, which combines sequence-based genomic information with elution time values from liquid chromatography that ultimately enables peptide mapping without needing coding sequence information (Shinoda et al., 2006). As of writing, the most complete and integrative database for metabolism and metabolites is the Human Metabolome Database (HMDB), which includes the known metabolome of humans in its entirety (Lange and

Ghassemian, 2005; Wishart et al., 2007). Again, another database with an integrative structure is aMAZE which includes gene expression, chemical reactions, assembly information, interactions, and pathway relations, which can be used in studies by using the web-based aMAZE LightBench interface (http://www.amaze.ulb.ac.be/) (Lemer et al., 2004). For the search and analysis of metabolic pathways, BioSilico can be used as a web-based database (Hou et al., 2004). Some databases enable researchers to retrieve data in a more comprehensive way by establishing systematic approaches such as LIGAND, ENZYME, EcoCyc, and MetaCyc (Hou et al., 2004). Among these, EcoCyc is a species-specific database for *Escherichia coli* by including all species-specific metabolic and signal-transduction pathways (Karp et al., 1996; 1997; 1999). On the other hand, MetaCyc is intended to be an encyclopedia of metabolites as a complete reference for metabolism, which collects and dissects experimental data reported (Caspi et al., 2006; Zhang et al., 2005). For the purposes of retrieving metabolomic information already present in other databases and building a pathway from retrieved integrals of the metabolism, a tool called PathAligner can be used (Chen and Hofestaedt, 2004). A web-based platform known as the Patikaweb can be used for retrieving and analyzing metabolic pathways that are located in the Patika database, which derives its data from other databases (Dogrusoz et al., 2006). As a publicly accessible database for metabolomics data, the Golm Metabolome Database (GMD) aims to be a complete database for researchers by including custom libraries for mass spectrometry, metabolite profiling protocols, and relevant information about metabolites coupled with tools that can be used for metabolomics research (Zhang et al., 2005; Kopka et al., 2005). For the visualization of metabolomic pathways, several tools can be used. Among these, PathFinder enables the interactive visualization of metabolomic pathways, which creates dynamic pathways from annotation data (Goesmann et al., 2002). For a genome-wide representation of metabolic pathways with pathway branchings, MetaViz can be used (Bourqui et al., 2007). A MATLAB package called the FluxAnalyzer can be utilized for analyzing metabolic fluxes from metabolic pathways (Klamt et al., 2003). For the publication of pathways, 3D illustrations of pathways can be designed using the ePath3D tool (Wiwanikit, 2011).

The Metabolite Profiling

Databases dedicated to non-targeted metabolite profiling that can be used for identifying low molecular weight compounds from biological specimens based on GC-MS methodology are present and widely used, such as the metabolite profiles from the Fiehn laboratory based on the BinBase tool (Fiehn et al., 2005), and the GMD with its custom libraries (Kopka et al., 2005; Schauer et al., 2005). METLIN and KNApSAcK databases are similarly designed for other high-resolution methods of Fourier Transform Mass Spectrometry, Tandem Mass Spectrometry, and LC/MS (Smith et al., 2005; Shinbo et al., 2006). For NMR methodology, the COMET database from the Consortium for Metabonomic Toxicology can be used (Lindon et al., 2005). In recent years, the Taverna system was postulated as a bioinformatics intermediary of abridging workflows for information interchangeability between different platforms (Oinn et al., 2004). There are increasing numbers of available analysis tools and databases for scientists to use, which require them to carefully analyze their research framework and integrate them into a pipeline accordingly for a desired result. Web frameworks for integrating diverse computational tools and repositories of different databases into a seamless interface are in development, and one of them is the standard called Resource Description Framework (RDF) (Stein 2002; Booth et al., 2003). Other than such unifying frameworks, there are other frameworks that create layered structures known as abstraction layers, which actually hide the structure and formats being used under the layer as seen in BioMOBY and BioMart systems (Wilkinson and Links 2002; Durinck et al., 2005). Despite the prospective nature of such unifying frameworks, they are currently limited in functions such as ontological gene annotations.

Conclusion

The data mining protocol being applied depends on the context of the metabolomics or metabonomics research since the metabolites are the bottom lines for any research to be conducted. In their bare forms, databases, and data repositories are invaluable for their systematic representation of large data sets inherently heterogeneous in nature. With the advancements of machine learning algorithms and artificial intelligence-based systems, databases will certainly be critical components for applied bioinformatics that focus on biomarker identifications and metabolomic pathway modeling.

References

Bader, G. D., Cary, M. P., & Sander, C. (2006). Pathguide: a pathway resource list. *Nucleic acids research*, *34*(suppl_1), D504-D506. https://doi.org/10.1093/nar/gkj126.

Booth, D., Haas, H., McCabe, F., Newcomer, E., Champion, M., Ferris, C., Orchard, D. (2003) *Web Services Architecture.* Retrieved from http://www.w3.org/TR/ws-arch/.

Bourqui, R., Cottret, L., Lacroix, V., Auber, D., Mary, P., Sagot, M. F., & Jourdan, F. (2007). Metabolic network visualization eliminating node redundance and preserving metabolic pathways. *BMC systems biology*, *1*, 1-19. https://doi.org/10.1186/1752-0509-1-29.

Brazma, A., Hingamp, P., Quackenbush, J., Sherlock, G., Spellman, P., Stoeckert, C., Aach, J., Ansorge, W., Ball, C A., Causton, HC., Gaasterland, T., Glenisson, P., Holstege, FC., Kim, I., Markowitz, V., Matese, J C., Parkinson, H., Robinson, A., Sarkans, U., Schulze-Kremer, S., Stewart, J., Taylor, R., Vilo, J., Vingron, M. (2001). Minimum information about a microarray experiment (MIAME)—toward standards for microarray data. *Nature genetics, 29*(4), 365-371. https://doi.org/10.1038/ng1201-365.

Brazma, A., Parkinson, H., Sarkans, U., Shojatalab, M., Vilo, J., Abeygunawardena, N., Holloway, E., Kapushesky, M., Kemmeren, P., Lara, G. G., Oezcimen, A., Rocca-Serra, P., Sansone, S. A. (2003). ArrayExpress—a public repository for microarray gene expression data at the EBI. *Nucleic acids research*, *31*(1), 68-71. https://doi.org/10.1093/nar/gkg091.

Caspi, R., Foerster, H., Fulcher, C. A., Hopkinson, R., Ingraham, J., Kaipa, P., Krummenacker, M., Paley, S., Pick, J., Rhee, S. Y., Tissier, C., Zhang, P., Karp, P.D. (2006). MetaCyc: a multiorganism database of metabolic pathways and enzymes. *Nucleic acids research*, *34*(suppl_1), D511-D516. https://doi.org/10.1093/nar/gkj128.

Chen, M., & Hofestaedt, R. (2004). PathAligner: metabolic pathway retrieval and alignment. *Applied Bioinformatics*, *3*, 241-252. https://doi.org/10.2165/00822942-200403040-00006.

Chen, J., Swamidass, S. J., Dou, Y., Bruand, J., & Baldi, P. (2005). ChemDB: a public database of small molecules and related chemoinformatics resources. *Bioinformatics*, *21*(22), 4133-4139. https://doi.org/10.1093/bioinforma tics/bti683.

Dogrusoz, U., Erson, E. Z., Giral, E., Demir, E., Babur, O., Cetintas, A., & Colak, R. (2006). PATIKA web: a web interface for analyzing biological pathways through advanced querying and visualization. *Bioinformatics*, *22*(3), 374-375. https://doi.org/10.1093/bioinformatics/bti776.

Duran, A. L., Yang, J., Wang, L., Sumner, L. W. (2003). Metabolomics spectral formatting, alignment and conversion tools (MSFACTs). *Bioinformatics. 19*(17), 2283-2293. https://doi.org/10.1093/bioinformatics/btg315.

Durinck, S., Moreau, Y., Kasprzyk, A., Davis, S., De Moor, B., Brazma, A., & Huber, W. (2005). BioMart and Bioconductor: a powerful link between biological databases and microarray data analysis. *Bioinformatics*, *21*(16), 3439-3440. https://doi.org/10.1093/bioinformatics/bti525.

Fiehn, O. (2001). Combining genomics, metabolome analysis, and biochemical modelling to understand metabolic networks. *Comparative and functional genomics*, *2*(3), 155-168. https://doi.org/10.1002/cfg.82.

Fiehn, O., Wohlgemuth, G., & Scholz, M. (2005). Automatic annotation of metabolomic mass spectra by integrating experimental metadata. *Proc Lect Notes Bioinformatics*, *615*, 224-239.

Goesmann, A., Haubrock, M., Meyer, F., Kalinowski, J., & Giegerich, R. (2002). PathFinder: reconstruction and dynamic visualization of metabolic pathways. *Bioinformatics*, *18*(1), 124-129.

Hou, B. K., Kim, J. S., Jun, J. H., Lee, D. Y., Kim, Y. W., Chae, S., Roh, M., In, Y-H., & Lee, S. Y. (2004). BioSilico: an integrated metabolic database system. *Bioinformatics*, *20*(17), 3270-3272.

Hummel, J., Selbig, J., Walther, D., & Kopka, J. (2007). The Golm Metabolome Database: a database for GC-MS based metabolite profiling. In Nielsen, J., Jewett, MC. (Eds.) *Topics in Current Genetics. Metabolomics A Powerful Tool in Systems Biology,* (pp:75-90). Springer-Verlag Berlin Heidelberg.

Irwin, J. J., & Shoichet, B. K. (2005). ZINC− a free database of commercially available compounds for virtual screening. *Journal of chemical information and modeling*, *45*(1), 177-182. https://doi.org/10.1021/ci049714+.

Kanehisa, M. (1997). A database for post-genome analysis. *Trends Genet*. 13:375-376. https://doi.org/10.1016/s0168-9525(97)01223-7.

Kanehisa, M., & Goto, S. (2000). KEGG: kyoto encyclopedia of genes and genomes. *Nucleic acids research*, *28*(1), 27-30. https://doi.org/10.1093/nar/28.1.27.

Kanehisa, M., Goto, S., Kawashima, S., & Nakaya, A. (2002). The KEGG databases at GenomeNet. *Nucleic acids research*, *30*(1), 42-46. https://doi.org/10.1093/nar/30.1.42.

Kanehisa, M., Goto, S., Hattori, M., Aoki-Kinoshita, K. F., Itoh, M., Kawashima, S., Katayama, T., Araki, M., Hirakawa, M. (2006). From genomics to chemical genomics: new developments in KEGG. *Nucleic Acids Res., 34*, D354-D357. https://doi.org/10.1093/nar/gkj102.

Karp, P. D., Riley, M., Paley, S. M., Pellegrini-Toole, A., & Krummenacker, M. (1997). EcoCyc: enyclopedia of Escherichia coli genes and metabolism. *Nucleic acids research*, *25*(1), 43-50. https://doi.org/10.1093/nar/25.1.43.

Karp, P. D., Riley, M., Paley, S. M., & Pelligrini-Toole, A. (1996). EcoCyc: an encyclopedia of Escherichia coli genes and metabolism. *Nucleic acids research*, *24*(1), 32-39. https://doi.org/10.1093/nar/24.1.32.

Karp, P. D. Riley, M., Paley, S. M., Pellegrini-Toole, A., Krummenacker, M. (1999). Eco Cyc: encyclopedia of *E. coli* genes and metabolism. *Nucleic acids research, 27*(1), 55-58. https://doi.org/10.1093/nar/27.1.55.

Karp, P. D., Ouzounis, C. A., Moore-Kochlacs, C., Goldovsky, L., Kaipa, P., Ahren, D., Tsoka, S., Darzentas, N., Kunin, V., Lopez-Bigas, N. (2005). Expansion of the BioCyc collection of pathway/genome databases to 160 genomes. *Nucleic acids research*, *33*(19), 6083-6089. https://doi.org/10.1093/nar/gki892.

Keseler, I.M., Collado-Vides, J., Gama-Castro, S., Ingraham, J., Paley, S., Paulsen, I.T., Peralta-Gill, M., & Karp, P.D. (2005). EcoCyc: a comprehensive database resource for Escherichia coli. *Nucleic acids research*, *33*(suppl_1), D334-D337. https://doi.org/10.1093/nar/gki108.

Klamt, S., Stelling, J., Ginkel, M., & Gilles, E. D. (2003). FluxAnalyzer: exploring structure, pathways, and flux distributions in metabolic networks on interactive flux maps. *Bioinformatics*, *19*(2), 261-269. https://doi.org/10.1093/bioinformatics/19.2.261.

Knapp, J. S., & Cabrera, W. L. (2011). *Metabolomics: Metabolites, Metabonomics, and Analytical Technologies*. New York: Nova Science Publishers

Kopka, J., Schauer, N., Krueger, S., Birkemeyer, C., Usadel, B., Bergmüller, E., Dörmann, P., Gibon,Y., Stitt, M., Willmitzer, L., Fernie, A.R., & Steinhauser, D. (2005) GMD@CSB. DB: the Golm metabolome database. *Bioinformatics*, *21*(8), 1635-1638. https://doi.org/10.1093/bioinformatics/bti236.

Krummenacker, M., Paley, S., Mueller, L., Yan, T., & Karp, P. D. (2005). Querying and computing with BioCyc databases. *Bioinformatics*, *21*(16), 3454-3455. https://doi.org/10.1093/bioinformatics/bti546.

Lange, B. M., & Ghassemian, M. (2005). Comprehensive post-genomic data analysis approaches integrating biochemical pathway maps. *Phytochemistry*. 66(4), 413-451. https://doi.org/10.1016/j.phytochem.2004.12.020.

Lemer, C., Antezana, E., Couche, F., Fays, F., Santolaria, X., Janky, R., Deville, Y., Richelle, J., & Wodak, S.J. (2004). The aMAZE LightBench: a web interface to a relational database of cellular processes. *Nucleic Acids Research*, *32*(suppl_1), D443-D448. https://doi.org/10.1093/nar/gkh139.

Lindon, J.C., Keun, H.C., Ebbels, T.M.D., Pearce, J.M.T., Holmes, E., & Nicholson, J.K. (2005). The Consortium for Metabonomic Toxicology (COMET): aims, activities and achievements. *Pharmacogenomics*, *6*(7), 691-699. https://doi.org/10.2217/ 14622416.6.7.691.

Mendes, P. (2002). Emerging bioinformatics for the metabolome. *Brief Bioinform*. *3*(2), 134-145. https://doi.org/10.1093/bib/3.2.134.

Nielsen, J., & Jewett, MC. (2007). The role of metabolomics in systems biology. In Nielsen, J., Jewett, MC. (Eds.) *Topics in Current Genetics. Metabolomics A Powerful Tool in Systems Biology* (pp. 1-20). Springer-Verlag Berlin Heidelberg.

Nordstrom, A. (2008). Data Mining for metabolomics. In Griffiths, W.J. (Ed), *Metabolomics, Metabonomics and Metabolite Profiling. The Royal Society of Chemistry* (pp: 273-280). RSC Biomolecular Sciences. ISBN: 978-0-85404-299-9.

Oinn, T., Addis, M., Ferris, J., Marvin, D., Senger, M., Greenwood, M., Carver, T., Glover, K., Pocock, M.R., Wipat, A., & Li, P. (2004). Taverna: a tool for the composition and enactment of bioinformatics workflows. *Bioinformatics*, *20*(17), 3045-3054. https://doi.org/10.1093/bioinformatics/bth361.

Schauer, N., Steinhauser, D., Strelkov, S., Schomburg, D., Allison, G., Moritz, T., Lundgren, K., Roessner-Tunali, U., Forbes, M.G., Willmitzer, L., Fernie, A.R., & Kopka, J. (2005). GC–MS libraries for the rapid identification of metabolites in complex biological samples. *FEBS letters*, *579*(6), 1332-1337. https://doi.org/10.1016/j.febslet.2005.01.029.

Schomburg, I., Chang, A., & Schomburg, D. (2002). BRENDA, enzyme data and metabolic information. *Nucleic acids research,* 30(1), 47-49. https://doi.org/10.1093/ nar/30.1.47.

Shinbo, Y., Nakamura, Y., Altaf-Ul-Amin, M., Asahi, H., Kurokawa, K., Arita, M., Saito, K., Ohta, D., Shibata, D., & Kanaya, S. (2006). KNApSAcK: A Comprehensive Species-Metabolite Relationship Database. In Saito, K., Dixon, R.A., Willmitzer, L. (Eds.), *Biotechnology in Agriculture and Forestry* (pp. 165-181). Springer.

Shinoda, K., Yachie, N., Masuda, T., Sugiyama, N., Sugimoto, M., Soga, T., & Tomita, M. (2006). HybGFS: a hybrid method for genome-fingerprint scanning. *BMC bioinformatics*, *7*, 1-8. https://doi.org/10.1186/1471-2105-7-479 https://doi.org/10.1186/ 1471-2105-7-479.

Smith, C. A., O'Maille, G., Want, E.J., Qin, C., Trauger, S.A., Brandon, T.R., Custodio, D.E., Abagyan, R., & Siuzdak, G. (2005). METLIN: a metabolite mass spectral database. *Therapeutic drug monitoring*, *27*(6), 747-751. https://doi.org/10.1097/01.ftd.0000179845.53213.39.

Stein, L. (2002). Creating a bioinformatics nation. *Nature*, *417*(6885), 119-120. https://doi.org/10.1038/417119a.

Strausberg, R. L., & Schreiber, S. L. (2003). From knowing to controlling: a path from genomics to drugs using small molecule probes. *Science*, *300*(5617), 294-295. https://doi.org/10.1126/science.1083395 .

Trethewey, R. N. (2001). Gene discovery via metabolic profiling. *Current Opinion in Biotechnology*, *12*(2), 135-138. https://doi.org/10.1016/S0958-1669(00)00187-7.

Villas-Bôas, S. G., Mas, S., Åkesson, M., Smedsgaard, J., & Nielsen, J. (2005). Mass spectrometry in metabolome analysis. *Mass spectrometry reviews*, *24*(5), 613-646. https://doi.org/10.1002/mas.20032.

Wheeler, D. L., Barrett, T., Benson, D.A., Bryant, S.H., Canese, K., Chetvernin, V., Church, D. M., DiCuccio, M., Edgar, R., Federhen, S., Geer, L. Y., Helmberg, W., Kapustin, Y., Kenton, D. L., Khovayko, O., Lipman, D. J., Madden, T. L., Maglott, D. R., Ostell, J., Pruitt, K. D., Schuler, G. D., Schriml, L.M., Sequeira, E., Sherry, S.T., Sirotkin, K., Souvorov, A., Starchenko, G., Suzek, T. O., Tatusov, R., Tatusova, T.A., Wagner, L., & Yaschenko, E. (2006). Database resources of the national center for biotechnology information. *Nucleic acids research*, *34*(suppl_1), D173-D180. https://doi.org/10.1093/nar/gkj158.

Wilkinson, M. D., & Links, M. (2002). BioMOBY: an open source biological web services proposal. *Briefings in bioinformatics*, *3*(4), 331-341. https://doi.org/10.1093/bib/3.4.331.

Wishart, D.S., Tzur, D., Knox, C., Eisner, R., Guo, A.C., Young, N., Cheng, D., Jewell, K., Arndt, D., Sawhney, S., Fung, C., Nikolai, L., Lewis, M., Coutouly, M.A., Forsythe, I., Tang, P., Shrivastava, S., Jeroncic, K., Stothard, P., Amegbey, G., Block, D., Hau, D.D., Wagner, J., Miniaci, J., Clements, M., Gebremedhin, M., Guo, N., Zhang, Y., Duggan, G.E., Macinnis, G.D., Weljie, A.M., Dowlatabadi, R., Bamforth, F., Clive, D., Greiner, R., Li, L., Marrie, T., Sykes, B.D., Vogel, H.J., & Querengesser, L.

(2007). HMDB: the human metabolome database. *Nucleic acids research, 35* (suppl_1), D521-D526. https://doi.org/10.1093/nar/gkl923.

Wiwanikit, V. (2011). Metabolomics. In Knapp, J.S., Cabrera, W.L. (Eds.). *Metabolomics: Metabolites, Metabonomics, and Analytical Technologies* (pp:225-242). New York: Nova Science Publishers

Zhang, P., Foerster, H., Tissier, C. P., Mueller, L., Paley, S., Karp, P. D., & Rhee, S. Y. (2005). MetaCyc and AraCyc. Metabolic pathway databases for plant research. *Plant physiology, 138*(1), 27-37. https://doi.org/10.1104/pp.105.060376.

Chapter 9

Metabolomic Research: Past, Present, and Future

Gonca Gulbay*, PhD

Department of Medical Biology, Faculty of Medicine, Ordu University, Ordu, Turkey

Abstract

Metabolomics is a field of omics that developed after genomics, transcriptomics, and proteomics as an important study area of systems biology. Metabolomic studies have gained an important place in various research areas, especially in the early diagnosis and treatment of diseases. For this purpose, metabolites are identified through software databanks using various separation and detection methods. Thanks to the development of software and computer and analytical device technology, new ones are added to what we know about the metabolome and metabolites every day. This chapter aims to guide researchers in a sequential manner on the past, present, and future goals of metabolomics studies.

Keywords: metabolite, metabolomic, metabolome database

Introduction

The "Human Genome Project" revealed the entire map of the human genome, enabling the investigation of the links of diseases with genome sequences (Bentley 2000). With the end of this project, the "post-genomic era" has

* Corresponding Author's E-mail: goncagulbay@odu.edu.tr.

In: Metabolomics and Clinical Approach
Editors: Sevgi Durna Daştan and Taner Daştan
ISBN: 979-8-89113-095-1

begun, and a new era has begun that examines the transcription and translation of genes, genome-proteome, and genome-metabolome relationships (Trifonova et al., 2013).

Low molecular weight chemical compounds (small particles) are formed in the cell as a result of enzymatic reactions. The chemical compounds formed are called metabolites. Together with these small particles and their connections in an organic framework, it is called the metabolome. Metabolomics, on the other hand, is the broad study of small particles (metabolites) in cells, biological fluids, tissues, or living organisms (Koçak et al., 2020). Metabolomics deals with the global assessment of metabolites present in a biological system to evaluate the development of disease, select potential biomarkers, and provide information about its pathophysiology (Tolstikov et al., 2020; Zhang et al., 2015). Metabolomics is a powerful technique that involves establishing links between phenotype and metabolic signature and elucidating associated metabolic pathways to improve diagnosis and treatment (Zhang et al., 2015; Ziarek et al., 2018). Metabolomic studies include identifying the metabolites in the cell, determining their amounts and comparing them with each other over the variables determined within the scope of the study (Ziarek et al., 2018).

Metabolomics for Biomarker Discovery

Metabolites are synthesized in living forms (endogenous) or imported from outside (exogenous) (Trifonova et al., 2013). Metabolites are not like DNA or proteins. Metabolites are not similar to each other in terms of their chemical structures and physical properties (Kaplan et al., 2020). The only common feature of the metabolites is that their molecular mass is less than 1.5 kDa and they are organic compounds (Koçak et al., 2020). Oligonucleotides, sugars, nucleosides, organic acids, amino acids, lipids, and peptides are metabolites. Metabolites are indicators of functional information about the cell and its intercellular relationships. As a result of this information, it defines the phenotype of the cell or tissue. The phenotype emerges as a combination of environmental conditions and genetic characteristics. Although genetic features are dominant in the phenotype, environmental factors can affect the one-to-one compatibility between genotype and phenotype. Metabolite levels reflect this compliance. The transcriptome, proteome, and metabolome are indicative of the physiological, developmental, and pathological characteristics of the living form and show variability. However, although there is a direct relationship between mRNA and proteins, this relationship does not exist between metabolites and genes (Kaplan & Çelebier, 2020; Solmaz et al., 2022). The high diversity of metabolites makes the analysis of metabolites very difficult due to the difference in their chemical structures.

Metabolite analyzes have been performed for a long time for diagnostic and therapeutic purposes. The analysis of intracellular metabolites illuminates the mechanisms of action of various diseases at the molecular level. The number of studies that find biomarkers at the metabolome level related to disease processes is increasing rapidly (Becker, et al., 2012; Zhou, et al., 2012). In clinical metabolomics studies, the goal is to identify metabolites that can be used as biomarkers (Kaplan & Çelebier, 2020; Zhang, et al., 2015).

The determination of biomarkers of preclinical disease will be very important for the development of disease-modifying and preventive treatment methods. Early diagnosis is very important for successful treatment and effective treatment management (Zhang et al., 2015). With the development of advanced technologies, the discovery of biomarkers has become the subject of many studies (Yoshida et al., 2012; Zhang et al., 2012). Metabolite changes are indicative of variations in the pathophysiology of diseases (Zhang et al., 2015).

Metabolomic studies can be divided into two main topics:

1. Targeted studies 2. Untargeted studies (metabolite profile)

Targeted studies are utilized for the absolute detection of currently focused metabolites. Metabolite profiling is used to determine the relative amount of metabolites affected by environmental conditions (age, nutrition, diseases, etc.) (Kaplan et al., 2020).

Historical Process of Metabolomic Studies

Although omic sciences are new fields of study, their history essentially dates back to ancient times. The origin of metabolomic studies also goes back to Antiquity. Between 1500 and 2000 BC, traditional Chinese physicians used ants as an indicator of diabetes to determine whether urine contains high doses of glucose. A similar practice has been observed in Ayurvedic medicine. It was stated that the urine of some people attracts insects and flies, and the taste of the urine is sweet and may be associated with some diseases. In principle, this application is a bodily fluid scan. Diabetes was mentioned in the Egyptian papyrus in 1552 BC, and the diagnosis was made based on a clinical symptom such as polyuria. In the late 1940s, the issue of normality in alcoholics and schizophrenic patients was investigated, and individual changes in body fluids and pathological conditions were examined. In the 1960s, when technological progress began, inborn errors of metabolism were studied in the clinic. In 1978, various techniques were discussed for obtaining quantitative metabolic profiles of volatile components of organic acids in human biological fluids. For this purpose, the use of gas chromatography/mass spectrometry/computer systems was emphasized (Van der Greef, & Smilde, 2005). In 1984, Games et al., identified the main components of black pepper and red pepper oil resins using a combination of high-performance 'liquid chromatography and mass spectrometry' (LC-MS) (Games et al.,1984). By the 1900s, 'capillary electrophoresis' research began (Koçak et al., 2020; Plumb et al., 2004). In the early 2000s, a brand new HPLC system with leading technology was designed and involved in studies such as ultra high-performance liquid chromatography (UPLC) (Nenni et al., 2022). In 2005, the first studies began for the Human Metabolome Project. The main objectives of this project were specified in 4 titles. These are:

a) Diagnosis and treatment of diseases, establishing a relationship between the metabolome and the disease in response to treatment through metabolic pathways,
b) Evaluation of drug metabolism and toxicology,
c) Establishing a link between human metabolism and the genome,
d) Development of a software program (Wishart et al., 2018).

Metabolomics Applications Today

Metabolomics is a powerful tool in the comprehensive and large-scale investigation of biomarkers. The metabolome contains more than 15,000 endogenous metabolites associated with diseases. Although there is no technique capable of examining the metabolome by injection, metabolomics research techniques for sample preparation and analysis, interpretation of results, and databases are constantly evolving (Solmaz et al., 2022).

The Human Metabolome Database (HMDB, www.hmdb.ca) is a database containing human metabolites and their biological roles, physiological properties, relationships with diseases, and chemical reactions of metabolites. In addition, this database contains comprehensive information on metabolic pathways, single nucleotide polymorphisms, and the effects of drugs on metabolites and their interactions. In HMDM, the number of metabolites has been expanded from 6408 to 114.100 (HMDB, 2022). This database has now become an important resource for human metabolomics studies (Solmaz et al., 2022).

Metabolomics is a multidisciplinary science in which biology, chemistry, and mathematics are combined by combining various analytical techniques with multivariate data analysis methods (Gu et al., 2011; Madsen et al., 2010). The separation of metabolites is done by gas and liquid chromatography and capillary electrophoresis methods, and the analysis of metabolites is done using mass spectroscopy and nuclear magnetic resonance spectroscopy (Patti et al., 2012).

Metabolite Separation Techniques

Gas Chromatography

Gas chromatography (GC) is one of the frequently used techniques in metabolomics studies. It provides the separation of volatile metabolites. However, derivatization is needed for most non-volatile biomolecules. It is used in combination with mass spectrometry. The most important advantage of this method is that it can be repeated (Haggarty & Burgess, 2017).

Liquid Chromatography

High performance liquid chromatography (HPLC) is one of the most dominant methods. In the early 2000s, a new HPLC system was designed with advanced technology. This system was called ultra high-performance liquid chromatography (UPLC) (Nenni et al., 2022). The HPLC method allows the separation of more metabolites than GC (Lei et al., 2011; Ramautar et al., 2009).

Capillary Electrophoresis

Capillary electrophoresis (CE) is a method that requires the application of high voltage to produce the electrophoretic flux of different ionic species in a narrow diameter capillary (Kawai 2021; Kostal et al., 2008). With the capillary electrophoresis (CE) technique, especially charged molecules are separated. It allows the analysis of more metabolites than LC and GC. Low sensitivity and reliability are among their disadvantages (Lei et al., 2011).

Metabolite Detection Methods

Mass Spectrometry

Mass spectrometry-based metabolomic analyzes allow the properties of thousands of metabolites to be detected and quantified simultaneously. MS analysis facilitates the obtaining of original results thanks to its high discrimination power. Therefore, it has an indispensable area of use in metabolomics studies. The only disadvantage of its routine use in metabolomic studies is its high cost (Alseekh et al., 2021; Han et al., 2008).

Nuclear Magnetic Resonance Spectroscopy

Nuclear Magnetic Resonance (NMR) spectroscopy techniques typically allow the observation of relatively fast-rolling species in an isotropic environment (Ramautar et al., 2009). It has been widely applied to many different types of samples for cell-based studies. NMR is one of the methods in which metabolomic studies can be performed without the need to separate metabolites. It can analyze multiple metabolites simultaneously. Thanks to its large number of databases, it is on the way to a universal metabolite detector (Beltran et al., 2012). It has advantages, especially in clinical studies. Visualizing post-translational modifications of protein structures, conformations, and interaction sites at the atomic level forms the basis for the development of new therapeutics in diseases (Ramautar et al., 2009).

Software and Database Support in Metabolomics Studies

The data obtained from the techniques used for metabolite profiling studies need to be processed by a computer. This process prevents wasted time and possible errors. Various software is available for this purpose. Some of this software are: BioSpider, Colmar, FiD (Fragment iDentificator), HORA (Human blOod Range vAlidator), MeltDB, MetaboloAnalyst, MetaboMiner, OpenMS, SetupX, and XCMS. Examination of the mass values of metabolites and their degradation products, the need to access data on the physical and chemical properties, clinical information, and pathways associated with each identified metabolite has increased the need for databases (Tsoka & Ouzounis, 2003). HMDB (Human Metabolome Database), Metlin, MMCD (Madison Metabolomics Consortium Database), Fiehn GC-MS Database, BML-NMR (Birmingham Metabolite Library Nuclear Magnetic Resonance database), Golm Metabolome Database, PubChem ChEBI ChemSpider, DrugBank PharmGKB STITCH databases are used according to different needs (Hastings et al., 2013; Knox et al., 2011; Kopka et al., 2005; Kuhn et al., 2010; Smith et al., 2005; Wang et al., 2012; Wishart et al., 2013; Zhu et al., 2010;).

Future Perspective

As one of the important members of systems biology, metabolomics provides "functional" information among omic studies and represents the final omics level (Ren et al., 2018). Metabolomics is a growing and rapidly evolving field for understanding cellular processes at the metabolome level. Metabolomics plays an important role in pathophysiological studies. Metabolomic studies in the fields of cancer (Araújo et al., 2020; Pandey et al., 2017), diabetes (Arneth et al., 2019), toxicology (Pohanka, 2020), and nutrition (Di Renzo et al., 2019) are among these studies. The use of metabolomics in clinical studies has focused on discovering new biomarkers to detect the initial stage of any disease, determine treatment and drug efficacy, and evaluate drug toxicity. With the rapid progress in the field of health and technology and the ease of access to information, personalized approaches are being developed in the diagnosis of diseases and in the illumination of the treatment mechanisms. For these reasons, the importance of metabolic profiling has increased tremendously.

In the future, in order to expand the scope of metabolites and improve data quality, it is necessary to develop new technologies with higher resolution, selectivity and flexibility, and lower detection limits, where more sensitive and sensitive measurements can be made (Ren et al., 2018). Mass spectrometry-based studies are particularly promising in metabolomic studies. More exciting technologies are expected in the near future.

Conclusion

As a result, metabolomic studies, personalized medicine applications, disease diagnosis, and process review, clinical studies on diet, drug research, etc., find their place in many fields. In the near future, a scientific infrastructure will be established that will enable people to access instantaneous information about their health status at the metabolome level with routine blood tests that can be applied to a drop of the blood sample. Thanks to the advance in analytical device technology with the developing software and computer technology, new ones are added to our knowledge about the metabolome and metabolites every day. With the developments in metabolomic studies, living metabolism is better understood every day.

References

Alseekh, S., Aharoni, A., Brotman, Y., Contrepois, K., D'Auria, J., Ewald, J., C Ewald, J., Fraser, P. D., Giavalisco, P., Hall, R. D., Heinemann, M., Link, H., Luo, J., Neumann, S., Nielsen, J., Perez de Souza, L., Saito, K., Sauer, U., Schroeder, F. C., Schuster, S., Siuzdak, G., Skirycz, A., Sumner, L. W., Snyder, M. P., Tang, H., Tohge, T., Wang, Y., Wen, W., Wu, S., Xu, G., Zamboni, N. and Fernie, A. R. (2021). Mass spectrometry-based metabolomics: a guide for annotation, quantification and best reporting practices. *Nature Methods*, 18(7), 747-756. https://doi.org/10.1038/s41592-021-01197-1.

Araújo, R., Bispo, D., Helguero, L. A. and Gil, A. M. (2020). Metabolomic studies of breast cancer in murine models: A review. Biochimica et biophysica acta. *Molecular Basis of Disease*, 1866(5), 165713. https://doi.org/10.1016/j.bbadis.2020.165713.

Arneth, B., Arneth, R. and Shams, M. (2019). Metabolomics of Type 1 and Type 2 Diabetes. *International Journal of Molecular Sciences*, 20(10), 2467. https://doi.org/10.3390/ijms20102467.

Becker, S., Kortz, L., Helmschrodt, C., Thiery, J. and Ceglarek, U. (2012). LC-MS-based metabolomics in the clinical laboratory. *Journal of chromatography. B, Analytical Technologies in The Biomedical and Life Sciences*, 883-884, 68-75. https://doi.org/10.1016/j.jchromb.2011.10.018.

Beltran, A., Suarez, M., Rodríguez, M. A., Vinaixa, M., Samino, S., Arola, L., Correig, X., and Yanes, O. (2012). Assessment of compatibility between extraction methods for NMR- and LC/MS-based metabolomics. *Analytical Chemistry*, 84(14), 5838-5844. https://doi.org/10.1021/ac3005567.

Bentley, D. R. (2000). The Human Genome Project--an overview. *Medicinal Research Reviews*, 20(3), 189-196. https://doi.org/10.1002/(sici)1098-1128(200005)20:3<189::aid-med2>3.0.co;2-#.

Di Renzo, L., Gualtieri, P., Romano, L., Marrone, G., Noce, A., Pujia, A., Perrone, M. A., Aiello, V., Colica, C. and De Lorenzo, A. (2019). Role of Personalized Nutrition in Chronic-Degenerative Diseases. *Nutrients*, 11(8), 1707. https://doi.org/10.3390/nu11081707.

Games, D,E., Alcock, N,J., van der, Greef, J., Nyssen, L,M., Maarse, H., Ten, M,C., and de Brauw, N.(1984) Analysis of pepper and capsicum oleoresins by high-performance liquid chromatography--mass spectrometry and field desorption mass spectrometry]. *Journal of Chromatography A*. 294,269-79. https://doi.org/10.1016/S0021-9673(01)96133-3.

Gu, H., Pan, Z., Xi, B., Asiago, V., Musselman, B. and Raftery, D. (2011). Principal component directed partial least squares analysis for combining nuclear magnetic resonance and mass spectrometry data in metabolomics: application to the detection of breast cancer. *Analytica Chimica Acta*, 686(1-2), 57–63. https://doi.org/10.1016/j.aca.2010.11.040.

Haggarty, J. and Burgess, K. E. (2017). Recent advances in liquid and gas chromatography methodology for extending coverage of the metabolome. *Current Opinion in Biotechnology*, 43, 77–85. https://doi.org/10.1016/j.copbio.2016.09.006.

Han, J., Danell, R. M., Patel, J. R., Gumerov, D. R., Scarlett, C. O., Speir, J. P., Parker, C. E., Rusyn, I., Zeisel, S. and Borchers, C. H. (2008). Towards high-throughput metabolomics using ultrahigh-field Fourier transform ion cyclotron resonance mass spectrometry. *Metabolomics,* 4(2), 128-140. https://doi.org/10.1007/s11306-008-0104-8.

Hastings, J., de Matos, P., Dekker, A., Ennis, M., Harsha, B., Kale, N., Muthukrishnan, V., Owen, G., Turner, S., Williams, M. and Steinbeck, C. (2013). The ChEBI reference database and ontology for biologically relevant chemistry: enhancements for 2013. *Nucleic Acids Research*, 41(Database issue), D456–D463. https://doi.org/10.1093/nar/gks1146.

HMDB (2022). HMDB Metabolite Statistics. Retrieved from https://hmdb.ca/statistics

Kaplan O. and Çelebier, M. (2020) Evaluation of Recent Data Processing Strategies on Q-TOF LC/MS Based Untargeted Metabolomics. *Mass Spectrometry Letters*, 11(1) https://doi.org/10.5478/MSL.2020.11.1.1.

Kaplan, O., Öncül, S., Ercan, A. and Çelebier, M. (2020) Comparison of Cell Lysis Techniques via Q-TOF LC/MS. *Mass Spectrometry Letters*, 11 (2) https://doi.org/10.5478/MSL.2020.11.2.36.

Kawai T. Recent Advances in Trace Bioanalysis by Capillary Electrophoresis. *Analytical Science*, 2021, 10;37(1):27-36. https://doi.org/10.2116/analsci.20SAR12.

Knox, C., Law, V., Jewison, T., Liu, P., Ly, S., Frolkis, A., Pon, A., Banco, K., Mak, C., Neveu, V., Djoumbou, Y., Eisner, R., Guo, A. C. and Wishart, D. S. (2011). DrugBank 3.0: a comprehensive resource for 'omics' research on drugs. *Nucleic Acids Research*, 39, D1035–D1041. https://doi.org/10.1093/nar/gkq1126.

Koçak, E., Kaplan, O. and Çelebier, M. (2020) Liquid-liquid extraction and ultrafiltration based sample preparation technique for Q-TOF LC/MS analysis of nonpolar metabolites in human plasma samples. *Journal of Research in Pharmacy*, 24(1), 38-43. https://doi.org/10.35333/jrp.2020.111.

Kopka, J., Schauer, N., Krueger, S., Birkemeyer, C., Usadel, B., Bergmüller, E., Dörmann, P., Weckwerth, W., Gibon, Y., Stitt, M., Willmitzer, L., Fernie, A. R. and Steinhauser, D. (2005). GMD@CSB.DB: The Golm Metabolome Database. *Bioinformatics* (Oxford, England), 21(8), 1635–1638. https://doi.org/10.1093/bioinformatics/bti236.

Kostal, V., Katzenmeyer, J. and Arriaga, E,Z. (2008). Capillary Electrophoresis in Bioanalysis. *Analytical Chemistry*, 15, 80(12), 4533-4550. https://doi.org/10.1021/ac8007384.

Kuhn, M., Szklarczyk, D., Franceschini, A., Campillos, M., von Mering, C., Jensen, L. J., Beyer, A. and Bork, P. (2010). STITCH 2: an interaction network database for small molecules and proteins. *Nucleic Acids Research*, 38, D552-D556. https://doi.org/10.1093/nar/gkp937.

Lei, Z., Huhman, D.V. and Sumner, L.W. (2011). Mass spectrometry strategies in metabolomics. *The Journal of Biological Chemistry* 286: 25435-25442. https://doi.org/10.1074/jbc.R111.238691.

Madsen, R., Lundstedt, T. and Trygg, J. (2010). Chemometrics in metabolomics--a review in human disease diagnosis. *Analytica Chimica Acta*, 659(1-2), 23–33. https://doi.org/10.1016/j.aca.2009.11.042.

Nenni, M., Doğan, A., Çelebier, M., Soyseven, M. and Kaynak, M,S. (2022) Ultrafiltration-based sample preparation and HPLC-UV determination of diclofenac in human plasma samples. *Turkish Journal of Chemistry*, 46(3), 777-785 https://doi.org/10.55730/1300-0527.3367.

Pandey, R., Caflisch, L., Lodi, A., Brenner, A. J. and Tiziani, S. (2017). Metabolomic signature of brain cancer. *Molecular Carcinogenesis*, 56(11), 2355–2371. https://doi.org/10.1002/mc.22694.

Patti, G. J., Yanes, O. and Siuzdak, G. (2012). Innovation: Metabolomics: the apogee of the omics trilogy. *Nature Reviews. Molecular Cell Biology*, 13(4), 263–269. https://doi.org/10.1038/nrm3314.

Plumb, R., Castro-Perez, J., Granger, J., Beattie, I., Joncour, K. and Wright, A. (2004). Ultra-performance liquid chromatography coupled to quadrupole-orthogonal time-of-flight mass spectrometry. *Rapid Communications in Mass Spectrometry,* 18(19), 2331-2337. https://doi.org/10.1002/rcm.1627.

Pohanka M. (2020). D-Lactic Acid as a Metabolite: Toxicology, Diagnosis, and Detection. *BioMed Research International*, 2020, 3419034. https://doi.org/10.1155/2020/3419034.

Ramautar, R., Somsen, G. W. and de Jong, G. J. (2009). CE-MS in metabolomics. *Electrophoresis,* 30(1), 276-291. https://doi.org/10.1002/elps.200800512.

Ren, J. L., Zhang, A. H., Kong, L. and Wang, X. J. (2018). Advances in mass spectrometry-based metabolomics for investigation of metabolites. *RSC Advances,* 8(40), 22335-22350. https://doi.org/10.1039/c8ra01574k.

Smith, C. A., O'Maille, G., Want, E. J., Qin, C., Trauger, S. A., Brandon, T. R., Custodio, D. E., Abagyan, R. and Siuzdak, G. (2005). METLIN: a metabolite mass spectral database. *Therapeutic Drug Monitoring*, 27(6), 747–751. https://doi.org/10.1097/01.ftd.0000179845.53213.39.

Solmaz, I., Kaplan, O., Çelebier, M., Lay, I. and Anlar, B. (2022) A combination of Q-TOF LC/MS and LC-MS/MS based metabolomics in pediatric-onset multiple sclerosis demonstrates potential biomarkers for unclassified patients. *Turkish Journal of Medical Sciences*, 52, 1299-1310. https://doi.org/10.55730/1300-0144.5436.

Tolstikov, V., Moser, A. J., Sarangarajan, R., Narain, N. R. and Kiebish, M. A. (2020). Current Status of Metabolomic Biomarker Discovery: Impact of Study Design and Demographic Characteristics. *Metabolites*, 10(6), 224. https://doi.org/10.3390/metabo10060224.

Trifonova, O., Lokhov, P. and Archakov, A. (2013). Postgenomics diagnostics: metabolomics approaches to human blood profiling. *Omics: A Journal of Integrative Biology*, 17(11), 550-559. https://doi.org/10.1089/omi.2012.0121.

Tsoka, S. and Ouzounis, C. A. (2003). Metabolic database systems for the analysis of genome-wide function. *Biotechnology and Bioengineering*, 84(7), 750-755. https://doi.org/10.1002/bit.10881.

Van der Greef, J. and Smilde, A,K. (2005) Symbiosis of chemometrics and metabolomics: past, present, and future. *Journal of Chemometrics*, 19: 376-386. https://doi.org/10.1002/cem.941.

Wang, Y., Xiao, J., Suzek, T. O., Zhang, J., Wang, J., Zhou, Z., Han, L., Karapetyan, K., Dracheva, S., Shoemaker, B. A., Bolton, E., Gindulyte, A. and Bryant, S. H. (2012). PubChem's BioAssay Database. *Nucleic Acids Research*, 40, D400-D412. https://doi.org/10.1093/nar/gkr1132.

Wishart, D. S., Jewison, T., Guo, A. C., Wilson, M., Knox, C., Liu, Y., Djoumbou, Y., Mandal, R., Aziat, F., Dong, E., Bouatra, S., Sinelnikov, I., Arndt, D., Xia, J., Liu, P., Yallou, F., Bjorndahl, T., Perez-Pineiro, R., Eisner, R., Allen, F., Neveu, V., Greiner, R. and Scalbert, A. (2013). HMDB 3.0--The Human Metabolome Database in 2013. *Nucleic Acids Research*, 41, D801-D807. https://doi.org/10.1093/nar/gks1065.

Wishart, D. S., Feunang, Y. D., Marcu, A., Guo, A. C., Liang, K., Vázquez-Fresno, R., Sajed, T., Johnson, D., Li, C., Karu, N., Sayeeda, Z., Lo, E., Assempour, N., Berjanskii, M., Singhal, S., Arndt, D., Liang, Y., Badran, H., Grant, J., Serra-Cayuela, A., Liu, Y., Mandal, R., Neveu, V., Pon, A., Knox, C., Wilson, M., Manach, C. and Scalbert, A. (2018). HMDB 4.0: the human metabolome database for 2018. *Nucleic Acids Research*, 46 (D1), D608-D617. https://doi.org/10.1093/nar/gkx1089.

Yoshida, M., Hatano, N., Nishiumi, S., Irino, Y., Izumi, Y., Takenawa, T. and Azuma, T. (2012). Diagnosis of gastroenterological diseases by metabolome analysis using gas chromatography-mass spectrometry. *Journal of Gastroenterology*, 47(1), 9-20. https://doi.org/10.1007/s00535-011-0493-8.

Zhou, B., Xiao, J. F., Tuli, L. and Ressom, H. W. (2012). LC-MS-based metabolomics. *Molecular BioSystems*, 8(2), 470-481. https://doi.org/10.1039/c1mb05350g.

Zhang, A., Sun, H., Wu, X. and Wang, X. (2012). Urine metabolomics. Clinica Chimica Acta, 414, 65-69. https://doi.org/10.1016/j.cca.2012.08.016.

Zhang, A., Sun, H., Yan, G., Wang, P. and Wang, X. (2015). Metabolomics for Biomarker Discovery: Moving to the Clinic. *BioMed Research International*, 354671. https://doi.org/10.1155/2015/354671.

Zhu, F., Han, B., Kumar, P., Liu, X., Ma, X., Wei, X., Huang, L., Guo, Y., Han, L., Zheng, C. and Chen, Y. (2010). Update of TTD: Therapeutic Target Database. *Nucleic Acids Research*, 38, D787-D791. https://doi.org/10.1093/nar/gkp1014.

Ziarek, J. J., Baptista, D. and Wagner, G. (2018). Recent developments in solution nuclear magnetic resonance (NMR)-based molecular biology. *Journal of Molecular Medicine (Berlin, Germany),* 96(1), 1-8. https://doi.org/10.1007/s00109-017-1560-2.

Chapter 10

Metabolomics in Traumatic Brain Injuries

Mustafa Karademir*, MD
Department of Neurosurgery, Sivas Cumhuriyet University, Faculty of Medicine, Sivas, Turkey

Abstract

Traumatic brain injury (TBI) is an important pathology that can cause severe disability and unexpected sudden death. In the pathogenesis of TBI, many biochemical reactions develop at the cellular level and these mechanisms can cause significant changes in some of the body's metabolites. Clinical, radiological, and biochemical data are used in the evaluation of traumatic brain injuries due to the complex physiology of the brain. For the classification of trauma, clinicians often use the Glasgow Coma Scale (GCS). In addition, radiologically taken MR Spectroscopy evaluations and biochemical markers made from samples such as blood and cerebrospinal fluid provide enlightening information about TBI. Metabolomics can be biochemically detected in body fluids such as blood, cerebrospinal fluid, etc., in sudden traumatic brain injury and can give important information about the course of the disease and the severity of the trauma and the mortality and morbidity of the patient.

Keywords: Metabolomics, traumatic brain injury, head trauma

Introduction

Traumatic brain injury (TBI) is linked to long-term neurological and mental weakness due to abnormal external mechanical forces. It is an important health

* Corresponding Author's E-mail: krdmr58@gmail.com.

In: Metabolomics and Clinical Approach
Editors: Sevgi Durna Daştan and Taner Daştan
ISBN: 979-8-89113-095-1

problem that requires hospitalization and prolonged intensive care. TBI can occur among people of all ages and different economic stages and can cause decisively large monetary and social impacts decisively in the public sphere. Due to the complex structure and multifunctional design of the human brain, head injuries can cause very different neurological and systemic pathologies depending on the severity of the impact. The number of head injuries that do not require surgical intervention but cause significant neurological sequelae has increased significantly today showing the importance of this issue. Timely and carefull intervention of these problems, which may arise at unexpected times in every moment of life, can increase the success of the treatment procedures. Secondary injury after a primary head injury is monitored after metabolic changes and causes high morbidity and mortality. The main goal of current medical treatment is to prevent the further progression of the existing pathological condition and to take measures to prevent the development of new undesirable physiopathological changes, that may cause the worsening of the patient's neurological condition (Banoei et al., 2018).

TBI may be classified according to severity (mild, moderate, and severe), physiological alterations after trauma (primary and secondary damage), and structural changes (focal or global) for better identification. To classify the severity of TBI, clinicians most commonly use the Glasgow Coma Scale (GCS), which is based on simple and non-specific clinical measurements and allows for the use of an internationally common language (Cook, 2021).

Brain tissue makes up approximately 2% of the body, it takes up 15% of the global cardiac output and takes 20% oxygen and 25% glucose. The only fuel for the healthy maintenance of brain metabolism, which has high energy requirements, is glucose, which has very limited storage in brain tissue. 60% of the energy produced is used for cellular activities, while 40% is used for homeostasis. Under normal conditions, oxidative phosphorylation is used for energy supply in the brain. In the absence of oxygen (hypoxia, hypoperfusion), the anaerobic respiratory system is immediately activated (Magistretti & Allaman, 2015).

The first mechanism that occurs after TBI is tissue destruction and disruption of the blood flow. This situation reduces ATP production and then creates an ischemic area that depletes energy stores. The non-oxidative phosphorylation step is immediately activated. After the energy decreases, excessive release of excitatory neurotransmitters (N-methyl D-aspartate, Glutamate, Aspartate, etc.) occurs. As a result of this oscillation, terminal membrane depolarization occurs in neurons. Therefore, intracellular sodium-calcium balance is disturbed, and an enhancement in free radicals and fatty acids and deterioration in cell homeostasis are observed. The basis of mechanism of cytotoxic edema formation is based on it. Free oxygen radicals in the cell also destroy the blood-brain barrier (BBB) and form the metabolic basis of the mechanism of vasogenic edema. Secondary brain injury includes many different factors. Also, changing brain blood flow, cell death after membrane depolarization, hypoxia, and cytotoxic and vasogenic brain edema. Clinicians often want to prevent secondary damage initially. To minimize the irreversible damage, improving the regeneration period is of great importance in treatment. Hypoxic ischemia is the main factor of secondary injury after TBI. Hypoxic ischemia exerts intense pressure on the cell. ATP deficiency occurs in brain tissue with a high need for oxidative phosphorylation. Disruptions in the cell membrane ion channels cause a disturbance in the intracellular ion and water balance. After cytotoxic edema, intracellular stimulating amino acids accumulate. As a result of activating the receptors of these amino acids, sodium membrane channels are opened, and there is an intense flow of sodium to the cell. The increase in sodium causes cell depolarization. Hence the increased cell density, an increase in intracellular fluid develops under the influence of oncotic pressure, and the amount of cerebral edema increases. In normal brain tissue, there are stimulating and suppressing agents and receptors in signal transduction. Due to tissue damage and overstimulation after TBI, excitatory agents such as glutamate and aspartate are increasingly released directly from these astrocytes and presynaptic neurons (Dem, 2020).

When all molecular mechanisms of TBI can be adequately elucidated, more effective and targeted therapies can be easily developed, reducing the length of hospitalization and intensive care unit stay due to TBI and the associated mortality rates. Molecular activities such as neuroinflammation, tauopathy, BBB disorders, and brain edema are the mechanisms that occur after acute TBI. Either way, the full understanding of the molecular mechanisms of acute TB is currently limited. Today's technologies do not allow for a complete and powerful elucidation of molecular mechanisms and post-traumatic changes in the brain. In addition to the complex respondents of brain tissue to trauma, new biomarkers have been needed to guide us on the physiopathological processes in body fluids. The great efforts of scientists worldwide are focused on the molecular mechanisms that are moving towards ideal and timely intervention in head injuries and discovering recovery strategies. Medical diagnosis of head injuries in any case and biomarkers that can be brain edema is caused by changes in cerebral blood flow and metabolic changes. The development and changes in the metabolic level in the body result in changes in metabolite concentrations. The portrayal of the arrival of these particular metabolites during the time spent in metabolic changes will be conceivable by looking at and explaining the pathophysiology from top to bottom. To assess and classify intense TBI in the examinations led; various metabolic biomarkers have been proposed, including S100 calcium-restricting protein B (S100B), glial fibrillar acidic protein (GFAP), neuron-specific enolase (NSE), sphingolipid (SPL), and medium-chain unsaturated fats. Notwithstanding, a solitary biomarker has restricted application to reveal the system and promote helpful techniques in treating of TBI. To overcome this issue, many of biomarker metabolites were required to have been distinguished to profoundly inspect the qualities of intense under. In the writing, the biomarker profile provides more point-by-point information on the surmised metabolic strategy compared to the utilization of a solitary metabolic variable during the intense TBI period compared to standard evaluations (Zheng et al., 2017).

Metabolomics may be useful in the management of patients with mild to severe brain injury, especially in mild TBI, where diagnosis is based entirely on clinical history. The resulting metabolic biomarkers can be used in conjunction with the GCS and neuroimaging findings. It is very difficult to diagnose mild and moderate TBI because contemporary imaging methods lack the sensitivity to reliably determine neurological damage. Biomarkers can be used in medical evaluation and treatment arrangement together with the demographic and clinical findings of the patient to contribute to the correct diagnosis. Thus, there are so many factors, including age, gender, and genetic factors that influence a patient's trauma-related neurological injury and disorder, the use of new metabolic biomarkers to predict TBI outcomes can also help predict the long-term consequences of TBI by measuring metabolic modifications. These small molecules can help focus on accurately identifying patients at risk of long-term sequelae exposure and arranging personalized rehabilitation therapy (Banoei et al., 2018).

There are various examinations that have applied a metabolomics strategy in TBI studies, and the metabolites which have been related to TBI in this exploration are distinguished. Viant and colleagues concentrated on brain tissue examples and plasma of rodents presented to liquid percussion injury. The examples were obtained one hour after injury. They found decreased phases of ascorbate in the cortex and hippocampus, glutamate inside the cortex and hippocampus, phosphocholine and glycerophospho-choline inside the cortex and hippocampus, and N-acetyl aspartate inside the cortex and hippocampus. Indeed, even though they had an effect at the not entirely settled in brain tissue, no spotless results have been recognized in plasma tests (Viant et al., 2005).

Radiologically, spectroscopic investigation of Proton Nuclear Magnetic Resonance (H-NMR) cerebrospinal liquid (CSF) is a fast and non-invasive technique for the assessment of digestion. Studies have shown that the metabolomic examination of CSF in TBI patients might open a novel window into the pathophysiology of this illness and lead to the disclosure of new biomarkers. After CSF examination, the connections between different metabolites might be viewed as a better approach to analyzing TBI metabolically. Glenn and associates inspected the cerebrospinal fluid tests of 44 patients affected by severe TBI and 13 control patients with hydrocephalus or intracranial aneurysms. H-NMR spectra tracked down a critical expansion in lactate, acetic acid derivation, beta-glucose, general creatine, pyruvate, glutamine, alanine, creatinine, alpha-glucose, and propylene glycol levels. In the review, higher propylene glycol levels and lower creatinine levels were seen in patients with severe TBI contrasted with controls. The planning of cerebrospinal liquid withdrawals in the review was not planned for neurological ailments, but rather in the multivariate rendition, the profile containing propylene glycol, glutamine, alpha glucose, and creatinine was related to cerebral oxygen metabolic rate, ICP, and final results (Glenn et al., 2013).

Orešič et al., analyzed a broad metabolic profiling of serum tests from TBI patients and controls, assessing 144 patients. According to the metabolite fixations in the brain micro dialysates of TBI patients during hospitalization, a calculation has been created that precisely predicts patient results. The expansion of metabolites to the laid out clinical model (CRASH), which incorporates clinical and registered tomography information, has altogether worked on the assessment of patient results. In this review, two medium-chain unsaturated fats have been demonstrated to be raised in Decanoic and octanoic acid (DA and OA) TBI and are related with unfortunate results in TBI patients. There is proof that medium-chain unsaturated fatty acids can without much of a stretch enter the blood-brain barrier (BBB), and free unsaturated fatty acids can be shipped in the two headings through the BBB. In this serum, it has been described as a 'TBI metabotype' that might be characteristic of impeded BBB and defensive physiology (Orešič et al., 2016).

Conclusion

In TBI's, a series of biochemical changes occur very soon after the injury, both due to the primary impact received by the brain tissue and caused by other unwanted physiopathological damage to other systemic organs that may accompany the head injury. In these changes, a series of reactions that are followed, especially on a cellular basis, is noteworthy. Stress and oxidation-reduction reactions at the neuronal level adversely affect ion transport mechanisms in neuronal membranes, leading to cell death with apoptosis or necrosis and causing the extracellular fluid to increase. Initially, cytotoxic edema and disruption of the BBB and the development of vasogenic edema led to herniations and death with increase in intracranial pressure. Knowing the metabolomics well in the treatment process of cranial traumas will contribute to the meticulous planning of the treatment modalities to be applied and to predict the mortality and long-term morbidity of the patient after trauma. However, current studies do not provide sufficient information about metabolomics in TBI's. Metabolomics profiles to be determined by radiological methods such as brain tissue, body fluids, and non-invasive MR spectroscopy alone cannot be sufficient. Supporting the laboratory data obtained from metabolomics with clinical and radiological scales will allow for detailed treatment planning and predictingof trauma-related death and disability rates.

References

Adibhatla, R. M., Hatcher, J. F., & Dempsey, R. J. (2006). Lipids and lipidomics in brain injury and diseases. *The AAPS journal, 8*(2), E314-E321. https://doi.org/10.1007/BF02854902.

Banoei, M. M., Casault, C., Metwaly, S. M., & Winston, B. W. (2018). Metabolomics and Biomarker Discovery in Traumatic Brain Injury. *Journal of Neurotrauma, 35*(16), 1831–1848. https://doi.org/10.1089/neu.2017.5326.

Cook, N. F. (2021). The Glasgow Coma Scale: A European and Global Perspective on Enhancing Practice. *Critical Care Nursing Clinics of North America*, *33*(1), 89–99. https://doi.org/10.1016/j.cnc.2020.10.005.

Dem, H. (2020). Travmatik Beyin Hasarında Beyin Metabolizması [Brain Metabolism in Traumatic Brain Injury], *Türk Nöroşir Journal*, *30*(2), 173–177.

Fernandis, A. Z., & Wenk, M. R. (2007). Membrane lipids as signaling molecules. *Current opinion in lipidology*, *18*(2), 121-128. https://www.doi.org/10.1097/MOL.0b013e328082e4d5.

Fonteh, A. N., Harrington, R. J., Huhmer, A. F., Biringer, R. G., Riggins, J. N., & Harrington, M. G. (2006). Identification of disease markers in human cerebrospinal fluid using lipidomic and proteomic methods. *Disease markers*, *22*(1-2), 39-64.

Glenn, T. C., Hirt, D., Mendez, G., McArthur, D. L., Sturtevant, R., Wolahan, S., Fazlollahi, F., Ordon, M., Bilgin-Freiert, A., Ellingson, B., Vespa, P., Hovda, D. A., & Martin, N. A. (2013). Metabolomic analysis of cerebral spinal fluid from patients with severe brain injury. *Acta Neurochirurgica. Supplement*, *118*, 115–119. https://doi.org/10.1007/978-3-7091-1434-6_20.

Magistretti, P. J., & Allaman, I. (2015). A Cellular Perspective on Brain Energy Metabolism and Functional Imaging. *Neuron*, *86*(4), 883–901. https://doi.org/10.1016/j.neuron.2015.03.035.

Orešič, M., Posti, J. P., Kamstrup-Nielsen, M. H., Takala, R. S. K., Lingsma, H. F., Mattila, I., Jäntti, S., Katila, A. J., Carpenter, K. L. H., Ala-Seppälä, H., Kyllönen, A., Maanpää, H. R., Tallus, J., Coles, J. P., Heino, I., Frantzén, J., Hutchinson, P. J., Menon, D. K., Tenovuo, O., & Hyötyläinen, T. (2016). Human Serum Metabolites Associate With Severity and Patient Outcomes in Traumatic Brain Injury. *EBioMedicine*, *12*, 118–126. https://doi.org/10.1016/j.ebiom.2016.07.015.

Viant, M. R., Lyeth, B. G., Miller, M. G., & Berman, R. F. (2005). An NMR metabolomic investigation of early metabolic disturbances following traumatic brain injury in a mammalian model. *NMR in Biomedicine*, *18*(8), 507–516. https://doi.org/10.1002/nbm.980.

Yi, L., Shi, S., Wang, Y., Huang, W., Xia, Z., Xing, Z., & Peng, W. (2016). Serum Metabolic Profiling Reveals Altered Metabolic Pathways in Patients with Post-traumatic Cognitive Impairments. *Nature Publishing Group, January*, 1–11. https://doi.org/10.1038/srep21320.

Zheng, F., Xia, Z. A., Zeng, Y. F., Luo, J. K., Sun, P., Cui, H. J., Wang, Y., Tang, T., & Zhou, Y. T. (2017). Plasma metabolomics profiles in rats with acute traumatic brain injury. *PLoS ONE*, *12*(8), 1–21. https://doi.org/10.1371/journal.pone.0182025.

Chapter 11

The Clinical Impact and Use of Metabolomics in Diabetes Research

Melike Mercan Başpinar*, MD
Department of Family Medicine, University of Health Sciences Gaziosmanpaşa Training and Research Hospital, Istanbul, Turkey

Abstract

Diabetes mellitus is a chronic metabolic disease in which hyperglycemia results from insulin resistance and reduced insulin, as in type 2 diabetes (T2D), or destruction of insulin-producing pancreatic β-cells as in type 1 diabetes (T1D). The mortality rate is higher in the diabetes population than in the general population, largely owing to cardiovascular and renal complications. Recent studies have shown that the only essential factor is the patient, not the disease. The genomic structure of each patient shapes the disease in its unique way. In this determination, an -omic identity emerges. The application of metabolomics in diabetes has simplified the identification of metabolites that can serve as screening and prognostic biomarkers. Metabolomic studies on diabetic subjects demonstrated many altered metabolic pathways and variations. Identifying predictive biomarkers involved in the pathogenesis of diabetes is essential, and avoiding complications related to personalized phenotyping and individualized drug response are recent study subjects. So, it is aimed to review the use of metabolomics and its impacts on diabetes research in this chapter.

Keywords: biomarkers; cardiovascular disease; chronic kidney disease; metabolomics; type 2 diabetes

---

* Corresponding Author's E-mail: drmelikemercan@gmail.com.

In: Metabolomics and Clinical Approach
Editors: Sevgi Durna Daştan and Taner Daştan
ISBN: 979-8-89113-095-1

Introduction

Type 2 diabetes mellitus (T2D) has reached the fourth position among the global health problem (James et al., 2018). The prevalences of microvascular complications of T2D (neuropathy, retinopathy, nephropathy) and macrovascular complications (stroke, diabetic foot, myocardial infarction, peripheral vascular disease) were reported as 50% and 30%, respectively (Jin & Ma, 2021). Metabolomics, emerging as a tool for biomarker discovery in diabetes and diabetic complications, provides a comprehensive molecular profile (Jin & Ma, 2021). The metabolome is related to genes in which a protein-coding gene can result in a 10,000-fold change in the level of a metabolite (Jin & Ma, 2021). Metabolomics attempts to systemically capture smaller biochemical compounds, including simple amino acids, as well as lipids, sugars, nucleotides, and other intermediary metabolites. Proteomics and metabolomics offer information on the complexity of a disease. Thus, genetic variation and transcriptional changes depend on proteins and metabolites which provide instantaneous "snapshots" of the state of a cell or organism. The response to environmental stressors such as exercise or directly the ingestion of foods or other compounds change the ingestion of foods or other compounds (Bonow et al., 2022). The last technological developments have supplied the profiling of many metabolites in biological samples (Shah et al., 2012).

Metabolites are the intermediary products of metabolism and provide molecular components of living systems. Identifying the metabolome can be done by nuclear magnetic resonance or mass spectrometry (Burks et al., 2019). The Di@bet.es study has described a metabolomic analysis based on 1 H-Nuclear Magnetic Resonance (1 H-NMR) spectroscopy of the patients with diabetes and showed a specific DM-associated profile related to inflammation and cardiometabolic disturbances (Ozcariz et al., 2020).

In light of advances in analytical techniques, metabolomics can further identify diabetes progression mechanisms by providing information on the underlying metabolic pathways.

Metabolomics in Diabetes

Subheading groups of metabolomics in diabetes research are presented in Figure 1.

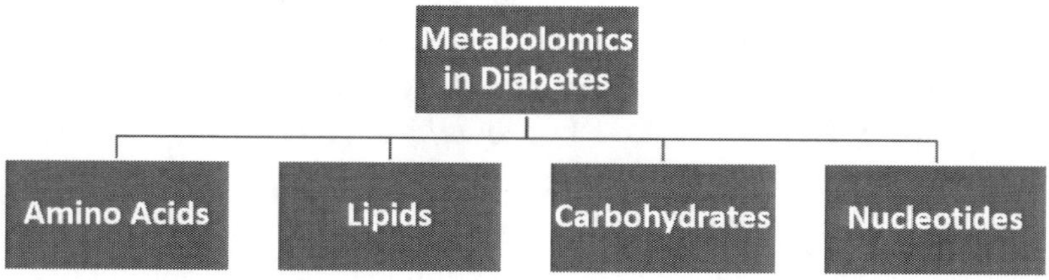

Figure 1. Subheading groups of metabolomics in diabetes research.

Amino Acids

- *Branched-Chain Amino Acids (BCAAs; isoleucine, leucine, and valine) and Aromatic Amino Acids (AAAs; phenylalanine and tyrosine)*

Insulin resistance is the first detectable defect of metabolic dysregulation before T2D development (DeFronzo & Tripathy, 2009). High fasting amounts of BCAAs obtained related to obesity, insulin resistance, and low serum insulin levels (Park et al., 2015). It depends on the variation which makes BCAA impact related to insulin resistance. The rs9637599 variant associated with circulating BCAA levels is located 2 kb upstream of the PPM1K gene that encodes a mitochondrial phosphatase in BCAA metabolism (Wynn et al., 2012).

Tyrosine and phenylalanine are two anti-incretin AAA precursors of dopamine, decreasing cell uptake of glucose (Floegel et al., 2013). The 3-(4-hydroxyphenyl) lactate (a phenylalanine product) has been found related to decreased insulin secretion and diabetes in the Metabolic Syndrome in Men study (Vangipurapu et al., 2020). Higher phenylalanine caused an increase in the macrovascular outcome and all-cause mortality in the ADVANCE trial (Welsh et al., 2018).

High amino acid levels can improve insulin secretion from primary islet β-cells (Brennan et al., 2002; Park et al., 2015). It was suggested that higher BCAA levels do not drive insulin resistance, while increased insulin resistance causes higher circulating fasting BCAA levels (Mahendran et al., 2017). In prospective studies, increased concentrations of fasting isoleucine, leucine, valine, tyrosine, and phenylalanine were associated with future diabetes (Chen et al., 2016; Newgard et al., 2009; Suhre et al., 2010). Also, five BCAA-related metabolites (2-hydroxyisocaproate, 3-hydroxy-2-ethylpropionate, 3-hydroxyisobutyrate, 2-hydroxy-3-methylbutyrate, and 3-hydrooxyvalerate) are associated with higher T2D risk (Morze et al., 2022).

Increased amino acids in diabetes are cysteine, pantothenic acid, creatine, acetylcarnitine, and butyryl carnitine. On the contrary, the decreased amino acids are arginine, glycine, asparagine, methionine, betaine, citrulline, aspartic acid, benzoic acid, sarcosine, 4-hydroxyproline, and 5-hydroxykynurenine (Bentley-Lewis et al., 2014; Park et al., 2015). BCAAs and glutamate are also found to increase in T1DM (Oresic et al., 2008). In addition, creatinine concentrations of the diabetes group versus the control were found to increase by more than 16%. The association of the cysteine to creatinine ratio with diabetes increased by a factor of 289.5. Cysteine concentrations were found to decrease in the diabetes group and creatinine values increased (Suhre et al., 2010). BCAAs level may be increased as early as a decade before overt diabetes. So then, BCAAs may be accepted as predictive biomarkers, especially be measured as early as a decade before overt diabetes (Jin & Ma, 2021).

BCAAs (valine, isoleucine, leucine) must be obtained from the diet cause they cannot be biologically synthesized. Few studies have explored lifestyle intervention effect on T2D or insulin resistance and it has been thought that lifestyle change may modify the relationship between T2D risk and circulating BCAAs (Kivelä et al., 2022). In a study of diabet and diet intervention, the elevation during one year in baseline BCAA was related to a higher T2D risk. After the intervention with Mediterranean diet at the end of the first year of, a significant reductions in leucine and isoleucine related to a low risk of diabetes have been demonstrated due to the Mediterranean diet (Ruiz-Canela et al., 2018).

Determining the metabolomic profile has replaced the missing one and paved the way for disease prevention studies. Could it prevent diabetes by finding and replacing amino acids? Arginine is a decreased amino acid in the metabolic profile of diabetes. Citrulline and nitric oxide(NO) are derivated from arginine in the endothelial cells. NO is a potent vasodilator in vessels, but vessels of diabetics have endothelial dysfunction resulting a reduced generation of NO. Prior searches indicate that intravenous administration of ascorbate or L-arginine can improve endothelial dysfunction, but the effect of the oral route is unknown (Huynh & Tayek, 2002). Mirmiran et al., showed an independent role on an increased risk of T2DM related to higher dietary L-arginine levels (Mirmiran et al., 2021).

On the other hand, it has been shown that oral arginine may increase endothelial nitric oxide synthase (NOS) and lead to increased vascular NO resulting in reduced blood pressure in mildly hypertensive T2D patients (Huynh & Tayek, 2002). In long-term use, L-arginine may also improve glucose intolerance and even reduce the risk of diabetes (Szlas et al., 2022). In conclusion, due to contradictory findings, oral arginine intake is still unclear in terms of T2D risk and complications, and new studies are needed.

Evodiamine (EVO) is an alkaloid with anti-infective, anti-inflammatory, hypolipidemic, and antitumor effects. Metabolomics analysis demonstrated that the EVO treatment affected the levels of 26 metabolites, such as cholesterol, methionine, and other metabolites. Additionally, EVO treatment improved oxidative stress and decreased the serum levels of pro-inflammatory cytokines in T2DM model rats (Yu et al., 2022).

Levels of sulfur amino acids (methionine (Met) and cysteine (Cys) are other risks for diabetes. During follow-up 16.9 years with 4636 deaths in the United States, diabetes-caused mortality rates were three times higher versus the low SAA intake (methionine, 2.45 cysteine, 2.91 times). The study demonstrates that high-SAA diets have a higher mortality risk in diabetes and that lowering intake towards Recommended Dietary Allowance levels could lead to reductions in lifetime risk (Dong et al., 2022).

Lipids

Lipoproteins and free fatty acids (FFAs) are lipid components of metabolomics in diabetes research. The relationship between dyslipidemia, cardiovascular organ damage, and inflammation is difficult to understand in T2D. Insulin resistance has an unintended effect on inflammatory cytokines interleukins (ILs) and increases plasma triglycerides (TG). ILs and TGs regulate the expression of matrix-metalloproteinases leading to a decrease high-density lipoprotein cholesterol (HDL) levels. High TG, low HDL, increased ILs, and matrix-metalloproteinases negatively affect the structure and function of the cardiovascular system (Kozakova et al., 2019). The METSIM study showed an increased T2D risk related to saturated FAAs versus the inverse association between unsaturated FAAs and T2D risk (Mahendran et al., 2013).

Obesity and T2D are like two inseparable siblings. Because obesity leads to T2D by triggering insulin resistance with increased β-oxidation and it is associated with elevated plasma FFAs. Carnitine is an indispensable key metabolite linked to obesity due to its metabolic pathways. FFAs can transfer energy only by β-oxidation after esterification and give to the mitochondrion requiring carnitine (Randle, 1998; Shah et al., 2012).

More carnitine for β-oxidation may be required for high-level plasma FFAs in obesity. Dyslipidemias make diabetic patients susceptible to complications related to atherosclerosis, such as heart disease and others. A number of factors, such as peripheral events of insulin on adipose tissue and muscle, the effects of insulin on apoprotein production by the liver, the function of cholesteryl ester transfer protein, and the regulation of lipoprotein lipase, are likely to be responsible for dyslipidemia in T2D (Park et al., 2015).

Decreased lipid metabolites related to obesity/T2D are found as sphingomyelin, ethanolamine, lysophosphatidylcholine, and increased lipid metabolites; stearic acid, oleic acid, phosphatidylcholine, 2-hydroxybutanoic acid, 3-hydroxybutanoic acid, palmitic acid, and palmitoleic acid (Park et al., 2015).

In a Finnish study, indole propionic acid, which is beside a reduced likelihood of progression to diabetes, was the metabolite most significantly and consistently related to both total carbohydrate and fiber intake. Lipid metabolites and indole propionic acid were also associated with high sensitive level of C-reactive protein (hsCRP) levels (De Mello et al., 2017).

Other studies have related T1D development with lipidomic changes in the metabolomic profiles of lipid classes(cholesterol esters, plasma phospholipids, triglycerides, glycerophospholipids, and sphingolipids) have been addressed. Stearic acid, palmitic, or mystic acid are low-carbon-number saturated lipid classes, and their low levels tend to be higher in individuals with T1D than those without diabetes. Especially, some researchers have reported reduced levels of glycerophospholipids and sphingomyelins in T1D patients (Arneth et al., 2019).

Carbohydrates

The glucose concentration of the blood is a marker of whether carbohydrate metabolism is healthy. Reduction in carbohydrate intake of a diabetic patient is the first and most important step (Franz, 2000; Park et al., 2015). It has been found that the levels of fructose, glucose, glycerol, sorbitol, mannose, xylose, inositol, 2,6-anhydrogalactose, 3,6-anhydrogalactose, gluconic acid, glucuronic acid, fumaric acid, isopropanol, malic acid, and cis-aconitic acid increase whereas those of deoxygalactose, pyruvic acid, glycerol-3-phosphate, and 1,5-anhydroglucitol are decreased in diabetes (Diao et al., 2014; Drogan et al., 2015; Gogna et al., 2015).

Nucleotides

Nucleotides are derived from tissues and then secreted to blood circulation and other extracellular fluids. High nucleotide levels and purinergic signaling may have a pathophysiological metabolic role in disorders (Sparks & Chatterjee, 2012). Compounds related to diabetes involved in nucleotide metabolism pathways, including AMP, IMP, GTP, GMP, inosine, guanosine, adenosine, are increased in both T1DM and T2DM (Dudzinska, 2014; Park et al., 2015). Additionally, uridine trimethylamine, and glyoxylic acid were found increased in T2DM (Dudzinska, 2014; Nikiforova et al., 2014; Park et al., 2015).

Is The Development of Diabetes Treatment or Prevention Possible with Metabolics Profile?

Fu-Zhu-Jiang-Tang tablet, which has beneficial clinical effects on patients with T2D, is a six-herb preparation, including Pueraria lobata, Morus alba, Lycium chinense, Panax notoginseng, Astragalus membranaceus, and Momordica charantia (Tao et al., 2017). A metabolomic approach was developed to search for the anti-diabetic effect of FZJT tablets. Untargeted serum metabolomics reveals that the FZJT tablet impaired glucose metabolism, down-regulate the high glucose level, and correct abnormal levels of metabolites in the serum of T2D rats (Tao et al., 2017).

Conclusion

Over the past two decades, metabolomics has been utilized and has provided novel approaches to understanding diabetes, thus attracting worldwide attention. Biomarkers indicating clinical risk profiles can help identify individuals who may benefit from early prevention and therapies compared to those who have no risk. Even though there are no miracle drugs to eliminate diabetes, there will always be a search for a miracle drug for diabetics. Drug and gene studies see metabolomes as our savior codes and offer hope for the future. Although it is still in the experimental stage of animal, the studies give hope for the development of new studies.

References

Arneth, B., Arneth, R., & Shams, M. (2019). Metabolomics of type 1 and type 2 diabetes. *International journal of molecular sciences, 20*(10), 2467. https://doi.org/10.3390/ijms20102467.

Bean, F. Brown, S. and J. Bachmeier. (2015). *Parents Without Papers: The Progress and PItfalls of the Mexican-American Middle Class.* New York: Russell Sage.

Bentley-Lewis, R., Xiong, G., Lee, H., Yang, A., Huynh, J., & Kim, C. (2014). Metabolomic analysis reveals amino-acid responses to an oral glucose tolerance test in women with prior history of gestational diabetes mellitus. *Journal of clinical & translational endocrinology, 1*(2), 38-43. https://doi.org/10.1016/j.jcte.2014.03.003.

Bonow, R. O., Mann, D. L., Zipes, D. P., & Libby, P. (2022). Proteomics and Metabolomics in Cardiovascular Medicine. In P. Libby (Ed.), *Braunwald's heart disease: a textbook of cardiovascular medicine* (pp. 87-91). Elsevier Health Sciences.

Brennan, L., Shine, A., Hewage, C., Malthouse, J. P. G., Brindle, K. M., McClenaghan, N., Flatt, P. R., & Newsholme, P. (2002). A nuclear magnetic resonance-based demonstration of substantial oxidative l-alanine metabolism and l-alanine-enhanced glucose metabolism in a clonal pancreatic β-cell line: metabolism of l-alanine is important to the regulation of insulin secretion. *Diabetes, 51*(6), 1714-1721. https://doi.org/10.2337/diabetes.51.6.1714.

Burks, A. W., Holgate, S. T., O'Hehir, R. E., Bacharier, L. B., Broide, D. H., Hershey, G. K., & Peebles, S. (2019). *Middleton's allergy E-Book: principles and practice* (9th ed.). Elsevier Health Sciences.

Chen, T., Ni, Y., Ma, X., Bao, Y., Liu, J., Huang, F., Hu, C., Xie, G., Zhao, A., & Jia, W. (2016). Branched-chain and aromatic amino acid profiles and diabetes risk in Chinese populations. *Scientific reports, 6*(1), 1-8. https://doi.org/10.1038/srep20594.

De Mello, V. D., Paananen, J., Lindström, J., Lankinen, M. A., Shi, L., Kuusisto, J., Pihlajamäki, J., Auriola, S., Lehtonen, M., & Rolandsson, O. (2017). Indolepropionic acid and novel lipid metabolites are associated with a lower risk of type 2 diabetes in the Finnish Diabetes Prevention Study. *Scientific reports, 7*(1), 1-12. https://doi.org/10.1038/srep46337.

DeFronzo, R. A., & Tripathy, D. (2009). Skeletal muscle insulin resistance is the primary defect in type 2 diabetes. *Diabetes Care, 32*(suppl_2), S157-S163. https://doi.org/10.2337/dc09-S302.

Diao, C., Zhao, L., Guan, M., Zheng, Y., Chen, M., Yang, Y., Lin, L., Chen, W., & Gao, H. (2014). Systemic and characteristic metabolites in the serum of streptozotocin-induced diabetic rats at different stages as revealed by a 1 H-NMR based metabonomic approach. *Molecular BioSystems, 10*(3), 686-693. https://doi.org/10.1039/C3MB70609E.

Dong, Z., Gao, X., Chinchilli, V. M., Sinha, R., Muscat, J., Winkels, R., & Richie, J. P. (2022). Association of dietary sulfur amino acid intake with mortality from diabetes and other causes. *European Journal of Nutrition, 61*(1), 289-298. https://doi.org/10.1007/s00394-021-02641-w.

Drogan, D., Dunn, W. B., Lin, W., Buijsse, B., Schulze, M. B., Langenberg, C., Brown, M., Floegel, A., Dietrich, S., & Rolandsson, O. (2015). Untargeted metabolic profiling identifies altered serum metabolites of type 2 diabetes mellitus in a prospective, nested case control study. *Clinical chemistry, 61*(3), 487-497. https://doi.org/10.1373/clinchem.2014.228965.

Dudzinska, W. (2014). Purine nucleotides and their metabolites in patients with type 1 and 2 diabetes mellitus. *Journal of biomedical science and engineering, 2014*, 38-44. https://doi.org/10.4236/jbise.2014.71006.

Floegel, A., Stefan, N., Yu, Z., Mühlenbruch, K., Drogan, D., Joost, H.-G., Fritsche, A., Häring, H.-U., Hrabě de Angelis, M., & Peters, A. (2013). Identification of serum metabolites associated with risk of type 2 diabetes using a targeted metabolomic approach. *Diabetes, 62*(2), 639-648. https://doi.org/10.2337/db12-0495.

Franz, M. (2000). Medical nutrition therapy for diabetes mellitus and hypoglycemia of nondiabetic origin In: Mahan LK, Escott-Stump S (eds). *Krause's Food, Nutritional and Diet Therapy*. Philadelphia: WB, Saunders Company.

Gogna, N., Krishna, M., Oommen, A. M., & Dorai, K. (2015). Investigating correlations in the altered metabolic profiles of obese and diabetic subjects in a South Indian Asian population using an NMR-based metabolomic approach. Molecular BioSystems, 11(2), 595-606. https://doi.org/10.1039/C4MB00507D.

Huynh, N. T., & Tayek, J. A. (2002). Oral arginine reduces systemic blood pressure in type 2 diabetes: its potential role in nitric oxide generation. *Journal of the American College of Nutrition, 21*(5), 422-427. https://doi.org/10.1080/07315724.2002.10719245.

James, S. L., Abate, D., Abate, K. H., Abay, S. M., Abbafati, C., Abbasi, N., Abbastabar, H., Abd-Allah, F., Abdela, J., & Abdelalim, A. (2018). Global, regional, and national incidence, prevalence, and years lived with disability for 354 diseases and injuries for 195 countries and territories, 1990-2017: a systematic analysis for the Global Burden of Disease Study 2017. *The Lancet, 392*(10159), 1789-1858. https://doi.org/10.1016/S0140-6736(18)32279-7.

Jin, Q., & Ma, R. C. W. (2021). Metabolomics in diabetes and diabetic complications: Insights from epidemiological studies. Cells, 10(11), 2832. https://doi.org/10.3390/cells10112832.

Kivelä, J., Meinilä, J., Uusitupa, M., Tuomilehto, J., & Lindström, J. (2022). Longitudinal Branched-Chain Amino Acids, Lifestyle Intervention, and Type 2 Diabetes in the Finnish Diabetes Prevention Study. *The Journal of Clinical Endocrinology & Metabolism, 107*(10), 2844-2853. https://doi.org/10.1210/clinem/dgac463.

Kozakova, M., Morizzo, C., Goncalves, I., Natali, A., Nilsson, J., & Palombo, C. (2019). Cardiovascular organ damage in type 2 diabetes mellitus: the role of lipids and inflammation. *Cardiovascular diabetology, 18*(1), 1-11. https://doi.org/10.1186/s12933-019-0865-6.

Mahendran, Y., Cederberg, H., Vangipurapu, J., Kangas, A. J., Soininen, P., Kuusisto, J., Uusitupa, M., Ala-Korpela, M., & Laakso, M. (2013). Glycerol and fatty acids in serum predict the development of hyperglycemia and type 2 diabetes in Finnish men. *Diabetes Care, 36*(11), 3732-3738. https://doi.org/10.2337/dc13-0800.

Mahendran, Y., Jonsson, A., Have, C. T., Allin, K. H., Witte, D. R., Jørgensen, M. E., Grarup, N., Pedersen, O., Kilpeläinen, T. O., & Hansen, T. (2017). Genetic evidence of a causal effect of insulin resistance on branched-chain amino acid levels. *Diabetologia, 60*(5), 873-878. https://doi.org/10.1007/s00125-017-4222-6.

Mirmiran, P., Bahadoran, Z., Gaeini, Z., & Azizi, F. (2021). Habitual intake of dietary L-arginine in relation to risk of type 2 diabetes: a prospective study. *BMC Endocrine Disorders, 21*(1), 1-7. https://doi.org/10.1186/s12902-021-00774-x.

Morze, J., Wittenbecher, C., Schwingshackl, L., Danielewicz, A., Rynkiewicz, A., Hu, F. B., & Guasch-Ferré, M. (2022). Metabolomics and Type 2 Diabetes Risk: An Updated Systematic Review and Meta-analysis of Prospective Cohort Studies. *Diabetes Care, 45*(4), 1013-1024. https://doi.org/10.2337/dc21-1705.

Newgard, C. B., An, J., Bain, J. R., Muehlbauer, M. J., Stevens, R. D., Lien, L. F., Haqq, A. M., Shah, S. H., Arlotto, M., & Slentz, C. A. (2009). A branched-chain amino acid-related metabolic signature that differentiates obese and lean humans and contributes to insulin resistance. *Cell metabolism, 9*(4), 311-326. https://doi.org/10.1016/j.cmet. 2009.02.002.

Nikiforova, V. J., Giesbertz, P., Wiemer, J., Bethan, B., Looser, R., Liebenberg, V., Ruiz Noppinger, P., Daniel, H., & Rein, D. (2014). Glyoxylate, a new marker metabolite of type 2 diabetes. *Journal of diabetes research, 2014,* 1-9. https://doi.org/10.1155/ 2014/685204.

Oresic, M., Simell, S., Sysi-Aho, M., Nanto-Salonen, K., Seppanen-Laakso, T., Parikka, V., Katajamaa, M., Hekkala, A., Mattila, I., & Keskinen, P. (2008). Dysregulation of lipid and amino acid metabolism precedes islet autoimmunity in children who later progress to type 1 diabetes. *The Journal of experimental medicine, 205*(13), 2975-2984. https://doi.org/10.1084/jem.20081800.

Ozcariz, E., Rojo, G., Gil, M., Guardiola, M., Amigo, N., & Ribalta, J. (2020). Characterization of the metabolomic profile by 1H-nuclear magnetic resonance spectroscopy in the DI@ BET. ES study. *Atherosclerosis, 315*, e71. https://doi.org/ 10.1016/j.atherosclerosis.2020.10.219.

Park, S., Sadanala, K. C., & Kim, E.-K. (2015). A metabolomic approach to understanding the metabolic link between obesity and diabetes. *Molecules and cells, 38*(7), 587. https://doi.org/10.14348/molcells.2015.0126.

Randle, P. J. (1998). Regulatory interactions between lipids and carbohydrates: the glucose fatty acid cycle after 35 years. *Diabetes/metabolism reviews, 14*(4), 263-283. https://doi.org/10.1002/(SICI)1099-0895(199812)14:4<263::AID-DMR233>3.0. CO;2-C.

Ruiz-Canela, M., Guasch-Ferré, M., Toledo, E., Clish, C. B., Razquin, C., Liang, L., Wang, D. D., Corella, D., Estruch, R., & Hernáez, Á. (2018). Plasma branched chain/aromatic amino acids, enriched Mediterranean diet and risk of type 2 diabetes: case-cohort study within the PREDIMED *Trial. Diabetologia, 61*(7), 1560-1571. https://doi.org/ 10.1007/s00125-018-4611-5.

Shah, S. H., Kraus, W. E., & Newgard, C. B. (2012). Metabolomic profiling for the identification of novel biomarkers and mechanisms related to common cardiovascular diseases: form and function. *Circulation, 126*(9), 1110-1120. https://doi.org/10.1161/CIRCULATIONAHA.111.060368.

Sparks, D. L., & Chatterjee, C. (2012). Purinergic signaling, dyslipidemia and inflammatory disease. *Cellular physiology and biochemistry, 30*(6), 1333-1339. https://doi.org/10.1159/000343322.

Suhre, K., Meisinger, C., Döring, A., Altmaier, E., Belcredi, P., Gieger, C., Chang, D., Milburn, M. V., Gall, W. E., & Weinberger, K. M. (2010). Metabolic footprint of diabetes: a multiplatform metabolomics study in an epidemiological setting. *PLoS One, 5*(11), e13953. https://doi.org/10.1371/journal.pone.0013953.

Szlas, A., Kurek, J. M., & Krejpcio, Z. (2022). The Potential of L-Arginine in Prevention and Treatment of Disturbed Carbohydrate and Lipid Metabolism-A Review. *Nutrients, 14*(5), 961. https://doi.org/10.3390/nu14050961.

Tao, Y., Chen, X., Cai, H., Li, W., Cai, B., Chai, C., Di, L., Shi, L., & Hu, L. (2017). Untargeted serum metabolomics reveals Fu-Zhu-Jiang-Tang tablet and its optimal combination improve an impaired glucose and lipid metabolism in type II diabetic rats. *Journal of Chromatography B, 1040*, 222-232. https://doi.org/10.1016/j.jchromb.2016.11.012.

Vangipurapu, J., Fernandes Silva, L., Kuulasmaa, T., Smith, U., & Laakso, M. (2020). Microbiota-related metabolites and the risk of type 2 diabetes. *Diabetes Care, 43*(6), 1319-1325. https://doi.org/10.2337/dc19-2533.

Welsh, P., Rankin, N., Li, Q., Mark, P. B., Würtz, P., Ala-Korpela, M., Marre, M., Poulter, N., Hamet, P., & Chalmers, J. (2018). Circulating amino acids and the risk of macrovascular, microvascular and mortality outcomes in individuals with type 2 diabetes: results from the ADVANCE trial. *Diabetologia, 61*(7), 1581-1591. https://doi.org/10.1007/s00125-018-4619-x.

Wynn, R. M., Li, J., Brautigam, C. A., Chuang, J. L., & Chuang, D. T. (2012). Structural and biochemical characterization of human mitochondrial branched-chain α-ketoacid dehydrogenase phosphatase. *Journal of Biological Chemistry, 287*(12), 9178-9192. https://doi.org/10.1074/jbc.M111.314963.

Yu, Y., Lu, Q., Chen, F., Wang, S., Niu, C., Liao, J., Wang, H., & Chen, F. (2022). Serum untargeted metabolomics analysis of the mechanisms of evodiamine on type 2 diabetes mellitus model rats. *Food & Function*, *13*(12), 6623-6635. https://doi.org/10.1039/D1FO04396J.

Chapter 12

The Current State and Future Perspectives of Metabolomics in Orthopedics

Anıl Aydin[*], MD
Department of Orthopedics and Traumatology, Erciyes University, Kayseri, Turkey

Abstract

Metabolomics is the process of detecting, quantifying, and recognizing metabolites present in the whole organism over a period of time as biomarkers or by using technologies to study disease pathogenesis. Many platforms are used for these procedures, including NMR and several MS technologies (Idle & Gonzales, 2007). Recently, metabolites have been used in many areas of orthopedics. Metabolite markers have been identified in many orthopedic diseases. An understanding of the pathogenesis of diseases was achieved. First, a metabolomic study of osteoarthritis was conducted. Additionally, metabolites show us an important way in many cases such as the diagnosis of diseases,treatment, fusion of bone fractures, and biomaterials used in orthopedics (Sun et al., 2015; Fan et al., 2021).

Keywords: metabolics, orthopedics

Introduction

In orthopedics, metabolic studies are found by examining many different samples, including serum, plasma, urine synovial tissue, and metabolic

[*] Corresponding Author's Email: Dr.Anil.Aydin@outlook.com.

In: Metabolomics and Clinical Approach
Editors: Sevgi Durna Daştan and Taner Daştan
ISBN: 979-8-89113-095-1

pathways are found (Kohlstadt & Cintron, 2018). Today, metabolic markers of many orthopedic diseases have been found (Sun et al., 2015). In the following, I will talk about the metabolic effect of the biomaterial used by metabolomic pathways in the main orthopedic diseases.

Osteoarthritis

Osteoarthritis is a degenerative joint disease characterized by cartilage destruction, synovitis, which is the formation of bone around the joint called osteophyte, and subchondral bone an increase in (Martel-Pelletier et al., 2016). Inthe blood of OA patients there are numerous metabolomic changes in the synovial fluid, in the idyll. In the examinations of the synovial fluid, differences in lipid, amino acid and glucose metabolomic pathways were found in the synovial fluids of healthy people and people with osteoarthritis. We canalso evaluate septic (Kosinska et al., 2014; Mickiewicz et al., 2015a; Jaggard et al., 2019) and non-septic states with various metabolomics measured proton nuclear magnetic resonance (1H-NMR) in synovial fluid. Metabolomics such as acetate, alanine, citrate, creatine phosphate, creatinine, glucose, glutamate, glutamine, glycine, phenylalanine, pyruvate, and valine were found to be high in the non-septic group, and glycylprolinein the sepsis group. In the study, it was seen that (Anderson et al., 2018) 6 metabolomic markers such as isobutyrate, glucose, hydroxyproline, asparagine, serine, and uridine could be used as a result of degenerativechanges seen after early knee joint injuries. This situation guides us in cases such as diagnosisand prognosis from the early stage of osteoarthritis (Mickiewicz et al., 2015b). In another study, it was shown that 28 metabolomics, such as malanate, ethanolamine, squalene, glycerol, etc., can be used for differentiation in radiologically early and late osteoarthritis cases (Kim et al., 2017).

In the case of osteoarthritis, metabolomic differences due to some amino acid metabolism was measured in the administration (H. Jiang et al., 2018). In serum-based studies of osteoarthritis, increased plasma ratiosof d allocated chain amino acids to histidine were associated with knee osteoarthritis. An elevated phosphatidylcholine ratio of lysophosphatidylcholines has been associated with osteoarthritis (Zhang et al., 2016).

Osteoporosis

Osteoporosis is a common bone disease with low bone mass and an increased risk of fracture in older age. Today, metabolics in osteoporosis offer an approach to the clinical diagnosis, understanding, and treatment of the pathology of the disease (Lv et al., 2016). The accuracy and robustness of the metabolomic measurements are better than traditional immunoanalysis and chemical measurements (Qi et al., 2016).

Today, the metabolomic pathway of osteoporosis is examined using animal models. Mice whose ovaries were removed had their estrogen and progesterone levels decreased, resulting in high bone loss, similar to postmenopausal women (Lv et al., 2016). Decreases in estrogen have an effect on lipid metabolism, arachidonic acid metabolism, and lineoic acid metabolism. (Y. C. Jiang et al., 2020). This estrogen reduction in postmenopausal women reveals an increase in lipid metabolic. These accumulated lipid metabolics inhibit osteoblastic activity (Ma et al., 2013; Qi et al., 2016). The exposed pubas activate the PPARy receptor and differentiate the mesenchymal cells from the adipocyte cells rather than to the osteoblasts (Kawai & Rosen, 2010). The increase in arachidonic fatty acid (AA) increases bone destruction and increases adipogenesis by increasing RANK-L, which allows osteoclasts to be activated. This explains bone loss in those who follow a high-fat diet (Casado-Díaz et al., 2013; Kasonga et al., 2015).

Metabolomics is used in the development of treatment methods for osteoporosis. Molecules suchas icariin act on bone metabolism and increase metabolites such as uridine, taurine, palmitic acid, adrenic acid, phexofenadine and have a positive effect on BMD (Huang et al., 2020). Sambucus Williamsii Ramulus, a folk herb in China, had a positive effect on bone healing by increasing 26 metabolics related to lipids, amino acids, and tryptophan metabolisms in a study conducted in ovariectomius squips (Xiao et al., 2018). It is being investigated that molecules such as osthole may be useful in the treatment of postmenopasal osteoporosis by acting on metabolic pathways (Si et al., 2020).

Rheumatoid Arthritis

Rheumatoid arthritis (RA) is a chronic autoimmune joint disease characterized by hyperplasia in the synovium, which is inflammation in the synovial region that causes the destruction of articular cartilage. The pathogenesis of rheumatoid arthritis is increased abnormal osteoclast activation (McInnes & Schett, 2011). In the studies conducted, it was seen that changes in glucose, lipid, and amino acid metabolism of synovitis in the metabolomic results of RA patients that led to synovial hyperplasia and inflammation. The levels of about 35 metabolites belonging to the class of amines, fatty acids, phosphates, and organic acids were found to be higher than osteoarthritis (Ahn et al., 2016). Additionally, the presence of mitochondrial damage to t cells is a cause that increases inflammation (Weyand et al., 2020). Some studies have shown that short-chain fatty acids (SCFAs) are reduced when RA mice are compared with healthy mice, and short-chain fatty acids (SCFAs) supplementation reduces arthritis (Rosser et al., 2020). n-6 polyunsaturated fatty acid (PUFA) has been shown to increase RA cartilage loss and inflammation, and n-3 polyunsaturated fatty acids have been shown to inhibit the anti-inflammatory effect (Miles & Calder, 2012).

Osteosarcoma

It is the most common malignant tumor of bone after multiple myeloma. The indication of metabolomics (Mirra, 1989) in osteosarcomas helps with early diagnosis and analysis of the clinical course of the tumor. In studies conducted from the blood serum of patients with osteosarcoma, differences in lipids, aromatic amino acids (phenylalanine and tyrosine), and histidine concentrations were found in healthy individuals (Quintero Escobar et al., 2020). In cells with osteosarcoma, like other tumor tissue cells, it is inthe first place in obtaining energy with glycolysis. Therefore, in the studies conducted in stem cellswith osteosarcoma, it was seen that there was a decrease in the metabolites of the TCA cycle and the metabolites in the glycolysis pathway were high when mitochondrial activity decreased. Metabolomic markers of osteosarcoma are important not only for diagnosis but also for the course of the disease (Zhong et al., 2019). It also contributes to the development of therapies targeting these metabolomic pathways. For example, new therapies targeting the amino acid metabolomic pathway of stem cells with osteosarcoma have been presented (Zhong et al., 2019).

Biomaterials

There is much metabolomic research on the cell-material relationship related to biomaterials used in orthopaedics.

It has a long history of use of Poly-L-lactic acid (PLLA) in implants used in fracture fixation (Middleton & Tipton, 2000). In studies on the metabolic effect of PLLA on osteoblasts, it is seen that PLLA triggers an anti-oxidative mechanism on osteoblasts and increases cellular growth (Araújo et al., 2019). Alginate hydrogels are a biomaterial that is used as a diffuse in tissue engineering. Metabolomic analyses and osteogenesis relationships of Glycine-Histidine-Lysine (GHK) modified alginate hydrogels were investigated (Klontzas et al., 2019). It has been investigated how biomaterials commonly used in orthopedics, such as titanium, affect metabolism by material surface topography (Moerke et al., 2016).

Conclusion

Metabolomics is a technique that has developed in the orthopaedic fields. It provides us with an important clue in understanding cell structure at the molecular level. In this way, it provides important information on diseases at the textural and cellular levels.

Many studies have been carried out to determine metabolomic pathways and metabolic markers and are still being done. Thanks to these studies, awareness of metabolic changes in diseases and early diagnosis of orthopaedic diseases are provided. We can learn about its clinical course by monitoring a decrease or increase in an effective metabolic biomarker in an orthopaedic disease. Thanks to these identified metabolic pathways and markers, we can develop the appropriate treatment approach to the disease. In addition, many drugs have been developed in the orthopaedicfield thanks to metabolomic studies, and these studies have been used to predict the therapeutic and side effects of drugs. Newer drug designs are still being developed and advanced metabolic studiesare required for the effectiveness of these drugs.

Metabolomic studies are carried out in the application and development of biomaterials used in the field of orthopaedics. The metabolic effects of biomaterials on cells are still an area that has not yet been fully resolved. Studies are carried out on the effect of the physical and chemical propertiesof these materials on cells.

As a result, metabolomic studies are being carried out in the field of orthopaedics, and there are many metabolomic conditions that have not yet been discovered. These metabolomic studies are promising for biomedical engineers, biologists, and clinicians.

References

Ahn, J. K., Kim, S., Hwang, J., Kim, J., Kim, K. H., & Cha, H. S. (2016). GC/TOF-MS-based metabolomic profiling in cultured fibroblast-like synoviocytes from rheumatoid arthritis. *Joint Bone Spine*, *83*(6), 707-713. https://doi.org/10.1016/j.jbspin.2015.11.009.

Anderson, J. R., Phelan, M. M., Clegg, P. D., Peffers, M. J., & Rubio-Martinez, L. M. (2018). Synovial fluid metabolites differentiate between septic and nonseptic joint pathologies. *Journal of proteome research*, *17*(8), 2735-2743. https://doi.org/10.1021/acs.jproteome.8b00190.

Araújo, R., Carneiro, T. J., Marinho, P., da Costa, M. M., Roque, A., da Cruz e Silva, O. A., Fernandes, M. H., Vilarinho, P. M., & Gil, A. M. (2019). NMR metabolomics to study the metabolic response of human osteoblasts to non-poled and poled poly (L-lactic) acid. *Magnetic Resonance in Chemistry*, *57*(11), 919-933. https://doi.org/10.1002/mrc.4883.

Casado-Díaz, A., Santiago-Mora, R., Dorado, G., & Quesada-Gómez, J. M. (2013). The omega-6 arachidonic fatty acid, but not the omega-3 fatty acids, inhibits osteoblastogenesis and induces adipogenesis of human mesenchymal stem cells: potential implication in osteoporosis. *Osteoporosis International*, *24*(5), 1647-1661. https://doi.org/10.1007/s00198-012-2138-z.

Fan, J., Jahed, V., & Klavins, K. (2021). Metabolomics in bone research. *Metabolites*, *11*(7), 434. https://doi.org/10.3390/metabo11070434.

Huang, J., Hu, Y., Tong, X., Zhang, L., Yu, Z., & Zhou, Z. (2020). Untargeted metabolomics revealed therapeutic mechanisms of icariin on low bone mineral density in older caged laying hens. *Food & function*, *11*(4), 3201-3212. https://doi.org/10.1039/C9FO02882J.

Idle, J. R., & Gonzalez, F. J. (2007). Metabolomics. *Cell metabolism*, *6*(5), 348-351. https://doi.org/10.1016/j.cmet.2007.10.005.

Jaggard, M. K. J., Boulangé, C. L., Akhbari, P., Vaghela, U., Bhattacharya, R., Williams, H. R. T., & Gupte, C. M. (2019). A systematic review of the small molecule studies of osteoarthritis using nuclear magnetic resonance and mass spectroscopy. *Osteoarthritis and Cartilage*, *27*(4), 560-570. https://doi.org/10.1016/j.joca.2018.08.024.

Jiang, H., Liu, J., Qin, X. J., Chen, Y. Y., Gao, J. R., Meng, M., Wang, Y., & Wang, T. (2018). Gas chromatography-time of flight/mass spectrometry-based metabonomics of changes in the urinary metabolic profile in osteoarthritic rats. *Experimental and therapeutic medicine*, *15*(3), 2777-2785. https://doi.org/10.3892/etm.2018.5788.

Jiang, Y. C., Li, Y. F., Zhou, L., & Zhang, D. P. (2020). UPLC-MS metabolomics method provides valuable insights into the effect and underlying mechanisms of Rhizoma Drynariae protecting osteoporosis. *Journal of Chromatography B*, *1152*, 122262. https://doi.org/10.1016/j.jchromb.2020.122262.

Kasonga, A. E., Deepak, V., Kruger, M. C., & Coetzee, M. (2015). Arachidonic acid and docosahexaenoic acid suppress osteoclast formation and activity in human CD14+ monocytes, in vitro. *PloS one*, *10*(4), e0125145. https://doi.org/10.1371/journal.pone.0125145.

Kawai, M., & Rosen, C. J. (2010). PPARγ: a circadian transcription factor in adipogenesis and osteogenesis. *Nature Reviews Endocrinology*, *6*(11), 629-636. https://doi.org/10.1038/nrendo.2010.155.

Kim, S., Hwang, J., Kim, J., Ahn, J. K., Cha, H. S., & Kim, K. H. (2017). Metabolite profiles of synovial fluid change with the radiographic severity of knee osteoarthritis. *Joint Bone Spine*, *84*(5), 605-610. https://doi.org/10.1016/j.jbspin.2016.05.018.

Klontzas, M. E., Reakasame, S., Silva, R., Morais, J. C., Vernardis, S., MacFarlane, R. J., Heliotis, M., Tsiridis, E., Panoltkaltsis, N., Boccaccini, A. R., & Mantalaris, A. (2019). Oxidized alginate hydrogels with the GHK peptide enhance cord blood mesenchymal stem cell osteogenesis: A paradigm for metabolomics-based evaluation of biomaterial design. *Acta biomaterialia*, *88*, 224-240. https://doi.org/10.1016/j.actbio.2019.02.017.

Kohlstadt, I., & Cintron, K. (Eds.). (2018). *Metabolic Therapies in Orthopedics*. Chapman and Hall/CRC.

Kosinska, M. K., Liebisch, G., Lochnit, G., Wilhelm, J., Klein, H., Kaesser, U., Lasczkowski, G., Rickert, M., Schmitz, G. & Steinmeyer, J. (2014). Sphingolipids in human synovial fluid-a lipidomic study. *PloS one*, *9*(3), e91769. https://doi.org/10.1371/journal.pone.0091769.

Lv, H., Jiang, F., Guan, D., Lu, C., Guo, B., Chan, C., Peng, S., Liu, B., Guo, W., Zho, H., Xu, X., Lu, A., & Zhang, G. (2016). Metabolomics and its application in the development of discovering biomarkers for osteoporosis research. *International journal of molecular sciences*, *17*(12), 2018. https://doi.org/10.3390/ijms17122018.

Ma, B., Liu, J., Zhang, Q., Ying, H., Sun, J., Wu, D., Wang, Y., Li, J., & Liu, Y. (2013). Metabolomic profiles delineate signature metabolic shifts during estrogen deficiency-induced bone loss in rat by GC-TOF/MS. *PLoS One*, *8*(2), e54965. https://doi.org/10.1371/journal.pone.0054965.

Martel-Pelletier, J., Barr, A. J., Cicuttini, F. M., Conaghan, P. G., Cooper, C., Goldring, M. B., Goldring, S. R., Jones, G., Teichtahl, A. J., & Pelletier, J. P. (2016). Osteoarthritis (Primer). *Nature Reviews: Disease Primers*, *2*(1). https://doi.org/10.1038/nrdp.2016.72.

McInnes, I. B., & Schett, G. (2011). The pathogenesis of rheumatoid arthritis. *New England Journal of Medicine*, *365*(23), 2205-2219. https://doi.org/10.1056/NEJMra1004965.

Mickiewicz, B., Heard, B. J., Chau, J. K., Chung, M., Hart, D. A., Shrive, N. G., Frank, C. B., & Vogel, H. J. (2015b). Metabolic profiling of synovial fluid in a unilateral ovine model of anterior cruciate ligament reconstruction of the knee suggests biomarkers for early osteoarthritis. *Journal of Orthopaedic Research*, *33*(1), 71-77. https://doi.org/10.1002/jor.22743.

Mickiewicz, B., Kelly, J. J., Ludwig, T. E., Weljie, A. M., Wiley, J. P., Schmidt, T. A., & Vogel, H. J. (2015a). Metabolic analysis of knee synovial fluid as a potential diagnostic approach for osteoarthritis. *Journal of Orthopaedic Research®*, *33*(11), 1631-1638. https://doi.org/10.1002/jor.22949.

Middleton, J. C., & Tipton, A. J. (2000). Synthetic biodegradable polymers as orthopedic devices. *Biomaterials*, *21*(23), 2335-2346. https://doi.org/10.1016/S0142-9612(00)00 101-0.

Miles, E. A., & Calder, P. C. (2012). Influence of marine n-3 polyunsaturated fatty acids on immune function and a systematic review of their effects on clinical outcomes in rheumatoid arthritis. *British Journal of Nutrition*, *107*(S2), S171-S184. https://doi.org/ 10.1017/S0007114512001560.

Mirra, J. M. (1989). Malignant Bone Tumours. In: Mirra, J. M., Picci, P., Gold, R. H. (eds.) *Bone Tumours: Clinical, Radiologic, and Pathologic Correlations* (pp. 248-389). Philadelphia, Lea and Febiger.

Moerke, C., Mueller, P., & Nebe, B. (2016). Attempted caveolae-mediated phagocytosis of surface-fixed micro-pillars by human osteoblasts. *Biomaterials*, *76*, 102-114. https://doi.org/10.1016/j.biomaterials.2015.10.030.

Qi, H., Bao, J., An, G., Ouyang, G., Zhang, P., Wang, C., Ying, H., Quyang, P., Ma, B., & Zhang, Q. (2016). Association between the metabolome and bone mineral density in pre-and post-menopausal Chinese women using GC-MS. *Molecular BioSystems*, *12*(7), 2265-2275. https://doi.org/10.1039/C6MB00181E.

Quintero Escobar, M., Costa, T. B. B. C., Martins, L. G., Costa, S. S., vanHelvoort Lengert, A., Boldrini, É., da Silva, S. R. M., Lopes, L. F., Vidal, D. O., Krepischi, A. C. V., Maschietto, M., & Tasic, L. (2020). Insights in Osteosarcoma by Proton Nuclear Magnetic Resonance Serum Metabonomics. *Frontiers in Oncology*, *10*, 506959. https://doi.org/10.3389/fonc.2020.506959.

Rosser, E. C., Piper, C. J., Matei, D. E., Blair, P. A., Rendeiro, A. F., Orford, M., Alber, D. G., Krausgruber, T., Catalan, D., Klein, N., Manson, J. J., Drozdov, I., Bock, C., Wedderburn, L. R., Eaton, S., & Mauri, C. (2020). Microbiota-derived metabolites suppress arthritis by amplifying aryl-hydrocarbon receptor activation in regulatory B cells. *Cell metabolism*, *31*(4), 837-851. https://doi.org/10.1016/j.cmet.2020.03.003.

Si, Z., Zhou, S., Shen, Z., & Luan, F. (2020). High-throughput metabolomics discovers metabolic biomarkers and pathways to evaluating the efficacy and exploring potential mechanisms of osthole against osteoporosis based on UPLC/Q-TOF-MS coupled with multivariate data analysis. *Frontiers in pharmacology*, *11*, 741. https://doi.org/10.33 89/fphar.2020.00741.

Sun, Z., Qiu, G., & Zhao, Y. (2015). Application and research advances of metabolomics in the field of orthopedics. *Zhonghua wai ke za zhi [Chinese Journal of Surgery]*, *53*(6), 476-480.

Weyand, C. M., Wu, B., & Goronzy, J. J. (2020). The metabolic signature of T cells in rheumatoid arthritis. *Current opinion in rheumatology*, *32*(2), 159. https://doi.org10. 1097/BOR.0000000000000683.

Xiao, H. H., Sham, T. T., Chan, C. O., Li, M. H., Chen, X., Wu, Q. C., Mok, D. K. W., Yao, X. S., & Wong, M. S. (2018). A metabolomics study on the bone protective effects of a lignan-rich fraction from Sambucus williamsii Ramulus in aged rats. *Frontiers in pharmacology*, *9*, 932. https://doi.org/10.3389/fphar.2018.00932.

Zhang, W., Sun, G., Aitken, D., Likhodii, S., Liu, M., Martin, G., Furey, A., Randell, E., Rahman, P., Jones, G., & Zhai, G. (2016). Lysophosphatidylcholines to phosphatidylcholines ratio predicts advanced knee osteoarthritis. *Rheumatology*, *55*(9), 1566-1574. https://doi.org/10.1093/rheumatology/kew207.

Zhong, Z., Mao, S., Lin, H., Li, H., Lin, J., & Lin, J. M. (2019). Alteration of intracellular metabolome in osteosarcoma stem cells revealed by liquid chromatography-tandem mass spectrometry. *Talanta*, *204*, 6-12. https://doi.org/10.1016/j.talanta.2019.05.088.

Chapter 13

Metabolomics and Metabolic Profiling in Embryos for Viability Assessment

Savaş Karakuş*, MD

Department of Obstetrics and Gynecology, Cumhuriyet University School of Medicine, Turkey

Abstract

It is essential to select the best embryos to transfer in any *in vitro* fertilization (IVF) treatment. Human embryos could only be assessed morphologically in the clinical setting until recent times. However, since this assessment is observation-based, it is open to both interpersonal and variability between observations made by the same person at different times. Preimplantation embryo metabolism demonstrates distinctive features associated with the developmental potential of embryos. On this basis, it has been assumed that the metabolite content of the culture medium reflects the implantation potential of individual embryos. The need for a non-invasive, reliable, and rapid embryo assessment strategy has promoted IVF metabolomic studies to increase the success rates of single embryo transfers. It is crucial to assess glucose, protein, or oxygen utilization according to the metabolism of human embryos.

Metabolomic profiling is an analysis of cell-free DNA released by the embryo into the culture medium. Although it is the most promising technologies developed to date for embryo selection, it is currently not suitable for clinical use.

Keywords: embryo, morphology, metabolomics, metabolic

---

* Corresponding Author's E-mail: karakussavas@yahoo.com.

In: Metabolomics and Clinical Approach
Editors: Sevgi Durna Daştan and Taner Daştan
ISBN: 979-8-89113-095-1

Introduction

In *in vitro* fertilization (IVF) treatment, the embryo with the highest quality and the highest probability of attachment to the uterus is selected according to the methodologies for assessing the embryo to transfer under the microscope, morphological observation, timing and speed of division, the development pattern of embryos, including the number of cells and fragmentation, their division patterns, and shape characteristics (Yang et al., 2022; Meseguer et al., 2012; Nadal-Desbarats et al., 2012).

However, the good image quality of the embryo does not indicate that the genetic and metabolic activities of the embryos are normal.

It is only possible to assess whether embryos are genetically normal by examining them using the pre-implantation genetic diagnosis (PGD) method. Among the technologies that are suitable for PGD are fluorescent in situ hybridization (FISH), single nucleotide polymorphism (SNP) array, or comparative genomic hybridization (CGH) array. To apply the PGD method, there must be advanced maternal age, a carrier of a genetic disease, recurrent pregnancy losses, repeated unsuccessful applications, severe male factor, etc. (Roche et al., 2021).

It is essential to select the best embryo in IVF cycles. While selecting this, it is aimed to increase the chance of pregnancy using both methods together by studying the metabolism, while the classical methods are based on embryo division, shape, etc.

In the treatment of infertility, it is very important to select the best embryo to achieve pregnancy. Many studies have demonstrated that successful pregnancies are obtained by paying attention to the morphology of the embryo and transferring embryos with appropriate morphology in pregnancies resulting in childbirth (Awadalla et al., 2022; Racowsky et al., 2010).

Of course, embryo morphology contributes to identifying the embryo to be transferred. However, publications have shown that even embryos with the best morphology can be genetically problematic, indicating that morphology is not the only criterion in determining the best embryo. It is considered that selecting embryos to be transferred using other criteria will increase the chance of success. Alternative non-invasive approaches to embryo assessment currently rely on the analysis of the embryonic culture medium. Of these, the metabolism of cells is significant. Since some normal preimplantation embryo development requires key nutrients, changes in the levels and metabolites of these nutrients have been suggested as indicators of metabolic activity during *in vitro* embryo culture. It is thought to be possible to obtain information about the health status and comment on the ability to assess the possibility of pregnancy by examining the metabolism of embryos, as comments are made on the body organs and health status by assessing a person's blood and urine tests. This is called 'Metabolomics.'

Metabolomics is the determination and identification of waste small molecule metabolites resulting from the use of lipids, carbohydrates, vitamins, and hormones in tissues, cells, and physiological fluids (Başaran et al., 2010). Metabolomic results may be important findings to assess the genetic function of the cell. They are important components of systems biology. The biological data acquired due to metabolomics has become a good source of information to research the sum of the whole system. The acquired metabolic products emerge as a result of the dynamic interaction of all enzymes, carriers, and chemical substances in the environment at the cell level. Because metabolite levels are sensitive to changes in enzyme activity and reflect interactions between the cell's genome and its environment, they provide an unbiased assessment of cellular status in the context of specific conditions (Chubukov et al., 2014).

In embryo metabolism, the embryo interacts with its medium. The said medium is the culture liquid in which the embryo is present. The fact that the embryo receives the molecules needed metabolizes them, and releases the residual molecules into the medium differs according to the metabolism of each embryo. Using a special technique, called spectroscopy, the culture fluid consisting of metabolic wastes can pass a light and the graph of molecules can be obtained. As a result, with this method named 'metabolomics,' each embryo can be mapped according to its metabolism, and these data can be associated with the development and pregnancy capacity of the embryo, assisting with selecting the embryo independently of its morphology.

Metabolites are defined as biomarkers in the diagnosis of many diseases with the development of analytical technologies. This situation helps select cells with high pregnancy potential in the field of in vitro fertilization (IVF) (Tang 2011). Nevertheless, metabolomic studies have demonstrated that embryo metabolism does not always indicate the embryo with the highest pregnancy capacity morphologically. It does not have the advantage of increasing the attachment of the embryo and pregnancy rates and has not yet been used routinely.

Analysis Techniques in Metabolomics

A cell's metabolome is inherently dynamic due to metabolic activity that changes based on the stage of the cell cycle. Moreover, the metabolomic profile changes considerably in pathological conditions or in response to treatment. The comparative metabolomic profiling of biological samples under various conditions makes it possible to determine the phenotypic differences between the samples studied.

Metabolomics refers to the rapid and high-throughput characterization of metabolism and allows systematic analysis of condition-dependent metabolic controls.

It is possible to study the waste culture media released by embryos during IVF using various methods, such as spectroscopic and metabolite methods. Information about the metabolic state of the embryo can be acquired with these methods. Both infrared and Raman spectroscopy are vibrational spectroscopic techniques. They create a waste metabolite profile of embryos by examining the vibrational characteristics of the waste molecules in the culture. The two techniques are advantageous over each other in terms of defining the characteristics and specific components of the signal produced. Wastes in the embryo media are assessed by magnetic resonance spectroscopy (Botros et al., 2009).

Seli et al., revealed the metabolite differences of embryos in embryo transfers resulting from and without pregnancy using both techniques. This method has been demonstrated to facilitate the selection of successful embryos by creating viability indices useful in measuring the reproductive potential of embryos (Seli et al., 2007).

Using magnetic resonance spectroscopy to identify metabolites, Seli et al., who tried to identify changes in the metabolite profiles of embryos resulting in pregnancy, found alanine, pyruvate, and glucose despite detecting high glutamate concentrations in their waste in the embryo media (Seli et al., 2008).

In clinical practice, it can help to make more accurate decision-making by combining multiple tests, although it is not ideal for the metabolomic mapping of embryo culture media.

Clinical Practices

Although embryo morphology is still used in the first step to determine the embryo's quality, there is no effective standard for this assessment. Various classification systems have been developed for embryo quality, and embryos are divided into three categories: Good-quality, medium-quality, and low-quality (Awadalla et al., 2022). It is possible to acquire different results from different embryologists due to differences in interpretation at various stages of embryonic development (Guerif et al., 2007). Especially on the third day, when all embryos have the same appearance, it is highly difficult to choose a viable embryo with a high blastocyst development potential for transfer.

Although metabolomics is not used in embryo selection, it seems possible to use it in the future. Scott et al., found the reproductive potential of embryos on days 3 and 5 with a diagnostic sensitivity of 80.5% (Scott et al., 2008). While demonstrating the predictive value of metabolomic profiling, the researchers found no correlation between metabolomic viability indices and morphological classifications of embryos on day 2 or 3 (Vergouw et al., 2008). Seli et al., showed that they could predict the reproductive potential of the embryo without seeing the results of pregnancy (20).

In Vitro Maturation

In *in vitro* maturation (IVM), oocytes containing unstimulated antral follicles are collected in meiosis I stage of prophase, and oocytes kept in the *in vitro* culture for 24-48 hours until meiosis II stage of metaphase are fertilized by the insemination or intracytoplasmic sperm injection method (Loutradis et al., 2006).

Serum in the culture environment is a source of albumin and a precursor of steroids. It is required for cell growth and proliferation (Picton et al., 2008). In the selected media, pyruvate has been demonstrated to be an energy source for cells (Roberts et al., 2002).

Carbohydrate Metabolism

The capacity to metabolize glucose increases greatly during the transition from morale to the blastocyst stage and reflects the development potential and viability of the embryo (Fangtao et al., 2020).

Various studies have indicated metabolic differences between viable and non-viable embryos. The metabolism of carbohydrates in human embryos prior to implantation has been studied, mainly in terms of private absorption and glucose and lactate production. Researchers have found that using pyruvate and glucose up to day 4 in embryos reaching the blastocyst stage is significantly higher than in embryos not progressing in culture and is related to the morphological grade.

These results in the study by Gardner et al., (2001) indicate a relationship between pyruvate uptake and blastocyst development. Furthermore, other studies have not been able to demonstrate any association between glucose intake and blastocyst development in human embryos. It should be noted that the environment used to evaluate embryo metabolism in these studies was lacking lactate, amino acids, and vitamins. Hence, it is possible that embryos are under significant stress in these culture conditions (Gardner et al., 2001; Lane et al., 1998), and the results obtained may be limited by this factor.

Amino Acid Turnover

In the same study, analysis of amino acid metabolism in eight-cell and morula-stage embryos was demonstrated that lower release of asparagine and alanine by embryos on days 2 and 3 and a lower intake of methionine, arginine, and glutamine were associated with lower serine uptake and lower alanine and glycine release and blastocyst development. The depletion of the amino acids examined was demonstrated to be lower in developing embryos compared to non-developing embryos (Leese et al., 2008).

Brison et al., studied the correlation between amino acid turnover and implantation and pregnancy outcomes when embryos were selected using routine morphological criteria and transferred on day 2. They suggested that glycine and leucine levels decreased in the embryo culture environment and were related to increased clinical pregnancy and live birth rates when asparagine levels were ensured (Brison et al., 2004).

Seli et al. (2008) Demonstrated higher rates of clinical pregnancy and live births in cases with elevated levels of glutamate in cultural settings. Brison et al., (2004) used the same approach to examine changes in the concentration of amino acids secreted from single-cultured human embryos. They reported an association between a decrease in blood sugar and leucine and an increase in asparagus levels in culture media with an increase in clinical pregnancy and live birthrates. In addition, the researchers noted that embryos with high viability had lower or quieter amino acid metabolism than those arrested.

Zivi et al., (2014) argued that a reduction in serine and possibly proline uptake in embryo culture was related to pregnancy and could be useful for embryo selection.

Conclusion

Studies have used numerous technologies and have not yet determined the exact criteria for selecting embryos with higher reproductive potential among embryos. Alternative or additional non-invasive techniques that can detect changes in the culture medium surrounding embryos have been suggested because it is not sufficient alone to obtain them using the morphology assessment approach determined by the current microscopy. Measuring physiological metabolomic changes in the culture medium of embryos and oocytes is one of the recent approaches. The embryo viability index created by metabolomic tests may be a better predictor of implantation potential than the traditional morphological evaluation. All of these data reveal the potential benefits of incorporating metabolomic assessment into the embryo selection process. As indicated by researchers, especially in single embryo transfer, the embryo to be transferred can be selected by assessing metabolomics between two embryos with the same morphological appearance. Nevertheless, none of the embryo selection methods used has been prospectively validated as a method that shows a relationship with the implantation potential of the transferred embryos. Therefore, a validated technology that non-invasively predicts the viability of embryos through rapid, in-situ evaluation of multiple methods is needed to select embryos with high reproductive potential.

References

Awadalla, M. S., Ho, J. R., McGinnis, L. K., Ahmady, A., Cortessis, V. K., & Paulson, R. J. (2022). Embryo morphology and live birth in the United States. *F&S Reports*, *3*(2), 131-137. https://doi.org/10.1016/j.xfre.2022.02.006.

Başaran, E., Aras, S., & Cansaran-Duman, D. (2010). General outlook and applications of genomics, proteomics and metabolomics. *Turkish Bulletin of Hygiene and Experimental Biology*, *67*(2), 85-96.

Botros, L., Sakkas, D., & Seli, E. (2008). Metabolomics and its application for non-invasive embryo assessment in IVF. *Molecular human reproduction*, *14*(12), 679-690. https://doi.org/10.1093/molehr/gan066.

Brison, D. R., Houghton, F. D., Falconer, D., Roberts, S. A., Hawkhead, J., Humpherson, P. G., Lieberman, B. A.,& Leese, H. J. (2004). Identification of viable embryos in IVF by non-invasive measurement of amino acid turnover. *Human reproduction*, *19*(10), 2319-2324. https://doi.org/10.1093/humrep/deh409.

Chi, F., Sharpley, M. S., Nagaraj, R., Roy, S. S., & Banerjee, U. (2020). Glycolysis-independent glucose metabolism distinguishes TE from ICM fate during mammalian embryogenesis. *Developmental cell*, *53*(1), 9-26. https://doi.org/10.1016/j.devcel.2020.02.015.

Chubukov, V., Gerosa, L., Kochanowski, K., & Sauer, U. (2014). Coordination of microbial metabolism. *Nature Reviews Microbiology*, *12*(5), 327-340. https://doi.org/10.1038/nrmicro3238.

Gardner, D. K., Lane, M., Stevens, J., & Schoolcraft, W. B. (2001). Noninvasive assessment of human embryo nutrient consumption as a measure of developmental potential. *Fertility and sterility*, *76*(6), 1175-1180. https://doi.org/10.1016/S0015-0282(01)02888-6.

Guerif, F., Le Gouge, A., Giraudeau, B., Poindron, J., Bidault, R., Gasnier, O., & Royere, D. (2007). Limited value of morphological assessment at days 1 and 2 to predict blastocyst development potential: a prospective study based on 4042 embryos. *Human reproduction*, *22*(7), 1973-1981. https://doi.org/10.1093/humrep/dem100.

Lane, M., & Gardner, D. K. (1998). Amino acids and vitamins prevent culture-induced metabolic perturbations and associated loss of viability of mouse blastocysts. *Human reproduction (Oxford, England)*, *13*(4), 991-997. https://doi.org/10.1093/humrep/13.4.991.

Leese, H. J., Baumann, C. G., Brison, D. R., McEvoy, T. G., & Sturmey, R. G. (2008). Metabolism of the viable mammalian embryo: quietness revisited. *Molecular human reproduction*, *14*(12), 667-672. https://doi.org/10.1093/molehr/gan065

Loutradis, D., Kiapekou, E., Zapanti, E., & Antsaklis, A. (2006). Oocyte maturation in assisted reproductive techniques. *Annals of the New York Academy of Sciences*, *1092*(1), 235-246. https://doi.org/10.1196/annals.1365.020.

Meseguer, M., Rubio, I., Cruz, M., Basile, N., Marcos, J., & Requena, A. (2012). Embryo incubation and selection in a time-lapse monitoring system improves pregnancy outcome compared with a standard incubator: a retrospective cohort study. *Fertility and sterility*, *98*(6), 1481-1489. https://doi.org/10.1016/j.fertnstert.2012.08.016.

Nadal-Desbarats, L., Veau, S., Blasco, H., Emond, P., Royere, D., Andres, C. R., & Guérif, F. (2013). Is NMR metabolic profiling of spent embryo culture media useful to assist in vitro human embryo selection?. *Magnetic Resonance Materials in Physics, Biology and Medicine*, *26*, 193-202. https://doi.org/10.1007/s10334-012-0331-x.

Picton, H. M., Harris, S. E., Muruvi, W., & Chambers, E. L. (2008). The in vitro growth and maturation of follicles. *Reproduction*, *136*(6), 703-715. https://doi.org/10.1530/REP-08-0290.

Racowsky, C., Vernon, M., Mayer, J., Ball, G. D., Behr, B., Pomeroy, K. O., Wininger, D., Gibbons, W., Conaghan, J., & Stern, J. E. (2010). Standardization of grading embryo morphology. *Journal of Assisted Reproduction and Genetics*, *27*, 437-439. https://doi.org/10.1007/s10815-010-9443-2.

Roberts, R., Franks, S., & Hardy, K. (2002). Culture environment modulates maturation and metabolism of human oocytes. *Human Reproduction*, *17*(11), 2950-2956. https://doi.org/10.1093/humrep/17.11.2950.

Roche, K., Racowsky, C., & Harper, J. (2021). Utilization of preimplantation genetic testing in the USA. *Journal of Assisted Reproduction and Genetics*, *38*, 1045-1053. https://doi.org/10.1007/s10815-021-02078-4.

Scott, R., Seli, E., Miller, K., Sakkas, D., Scott, K., & Burns, D. H. (2008). Noninvasive metabolomic profiling of human embryo culture media using Raman spectroscopy predicts embryonic reproductive potential: a prospective blinded pilot study. *Fertility and Sterility*, *90*(1), 77-83. https://doi.org/10.1016/j.fertnstert.2007.11.058.

Seli, E., Botros, L., Sakkas, D., & Burns, D. H. (2008). Noninvasive metabolomic profiling of embryo culture media using proton nuclear magnetic resonance correlates with reproductive potential of embryos in women undergoing in vitro fertilization. *Fertility and Sterility*, *90*(6), 2183-2189. https://doi.org/10.1016/j.fertnstert.2008.07.1739.

Seli, E., Sakkas, D., Scott, R., Kwok, S. C., Rosendahl, S. M., & Burns, D. H. (2007). Noninvasive metabolomic profiling of embryo culture media using Raman and near-infrared spectroscopy correlates with reproductive potential of embryos in women undergoing in vitro fertilization. *Fertility and sterility*, *88*(5), 1350-1357. https://doi.org/10.1016/j.fertnstert.2007.07.1390.

Tang, J. (2011). Microbial metabolomics. *Current genomics*, *12*(6), 391-403. https://doi.org/10.2174/138920211797248619.

Vergouw, C. G., Botros, L. L., Roos, P., Lens, J. W., Schats, R., Hompes, P. G. A., Burns, D. H., & Lambalk, C. B. (2008). Metabolomic profiling by near-infrared spectroscopy as a tool to assess embryo viability: a novel, non-invasive method for embryo selection. *Human reproduction*, *23*(7), 1499-1504. https://doi.org/10.1093/humrep/den111.

Yang, L., Peavey, M., Kaskar, K., Chappell, N., Zhu, L., Devlin, D., Valdes, C., Schutt, A., Woodard, T., Zarutskie, P., Cochran, R., Gibbons, W. E. (2022). Development of a dynamic machine learning algorithm to predict clinical pregnancy and live birth rate with embryo morphokinetics. *F&S Reports*, *3*(2), 116-123. https://doi.org/10.1016/j.xfre.2022.04.004.

Zivi, E., Barash, D., Aizenman, E., Gibson, D., & Shufaro, Y. (2014). Zygote serine decreased uptake from the fertilization medium is associated with implantation and pregnancy. *Journal of assisted reproduction and genetics*, *31*, 889-897. https://doi.org/10.1007/s10815-014-0231-2.

Chapter 14

Metabolomics in the Diagnosis of Pregnancy Complications

Nazan Yurtcu*
and Dilay Karademir
Department of Obstetrics and Gynecology, Sivas Cumhuriyet University, Sivas, Turkey

Abstract

The pregnancy process is an intricate and unique period that requires control examinations to ensure the continuity of the well-being of the mother and the baby. The accompanying changes are also evident biologically, physiologically, psychologically, and socially. Several factors must be considered to determine when a woman's pregnancy is at risk and when unfavorable pregnancy outcomes will occur. Biomedical indicators are critical in medicine. Studies show that the variables in these indicators are vital in determining the risk status. Once the metabolic pathways are understood clearly in healthy and diseased conditions, we can gain more applicable information on disease mechanisms and precise treatment approaches. The prenatal medicine practices require the development of novel non-invasive approaches that cover diverse categories of diseases with lower rates of false-positives. Metabolomics for this purpose has the potential of great advantage. Metabolomic studies measure and analyze the biochemistry products of cells. As a biomarker, metabolomics may uncover new diagnostic and therapeutic approaches. This chapter reviews the idea and utilization of metabolomics for maternal health and perinatal medicine, emphasizing the latest developments in metabolomics studies and the research agenda. In addition, the existence of studies that will increase our knowledge

* Corresponding Author's Email: nyurtcu58@gmail.com.

In: Metabolomics and Clinical Approach
Editors: Sevgi Durna Daştan and Taner Daştan
ISBN: 979-8-89113-095-1

about the etiopathogenesis of maternal complications is exciting and promising.

Keywords: metabolomics, prediction, preeclamcia, fetal growth restriction, preterm birth, prenatal diagnosis

Introduction

During pregnancy, various adaptive physiological changes are required for the healthy continuation of both fetal and placental functions in the mother during pregnancy. Changes occur in circulating maternal metabolic products during pregnancy to meet the nutritional requirement for the development of the fetus and sufficient production of breast milk after birth.

Various concealed causes are known to be present in pregnancy complications, which include preeclampsia, fetal growth restriction, preterm birth, and gestational diabetes mellitus, and since these complications are complicated by their nature, their early diagnosis is a daunting task. New approaches to maternal and perinatal health have seen little advancement over the years, which points to omics fields as a new avenue. Metabolomics is the integrative study of sets of metabolites from a bio-specimen that portray the metabolism of a particular scene. Overall, metabolomics has inherent edges over other omics by studying the final products from interactions between DNA, transcripts, and proteins.

Protecting maternal and perinatal health and taking the necessary precautions worldwide will save women and children from a significant burden of disease in their later lives. For this purpose, metabolomic biomarkers are new promising tools to predict conditions that will cause adverse health conditions. Soon, metabolomics will be of particular interest because of its potentially important role in maintaining and managing perinatal and neonatal health. This section summarizes the information available on metabolomics, which is new in complicated pregnancies, and represents future diagnostic and screening tools.

Pregnancy and Amniotic Fluid

Soluble components of cellular nature, which contain carbohydrates, lipids, hormones, enzymes, proteins, and others (e.g., lactate, pyruvate, and other electrolytes) are present in amniotic fluid (Tarui et al., 2017). These components mostly function as a preliminary defense against antigens that might be present in the amniotic pocket (Clark et al., 2016; Tarui et al., 2017). The shed cells from the developing fetus, notably from tissues having a cavity, are present in the amniotic fluid. Certain components of innate immunity, particularly neutrophils, macrophages, and ILCs (innate lymphoid cells), are shown to be present in low amounts in the amniotic fluid when there is no infection, as is evident from cytological research (Espinoza et al., 2003; Maddipati et al., 2016). However, under conditions where fetal organs are pathologic e.g., neural tube defects, and gastroschisis, the amounts of macrophages and ILCs were found as elevated (Espinoza et al., 2003; Maddipati et al., 2016). Yet, the amount of amniotic fluid neutrophils is a valuable intra-amniotic inflammation indicator. However, the immunologic composition of amniotic fluid without infection, inflammation, or congenital disabilities is still poorly understood (Gomez-Lopez et al., 2017a; Gomez-Lopez et al., 2017b; Gomez et al., 1994; Martinez-Varea et al., 2017).

Preeclampsia

Preeclampsia (PE) can be defined as the development of hypertension, edema, and proteinuria symptoms roughly 20 weeks into gestation (Myatt et al., 2014; Sibai, 2003). It complicates 5 to 10% of pregnancies worldwide and is prominent in maternal mortality rates (Roberge et al., 2012). PE has clinical risk assets for the mother, which can be listed as age, clinical history of PE occurrence, nulliparity, multi-fetal pregnancy, chronic diseases such as diabetes mellitus, hypertension, and kidney diseases (Polsani et al., 2013; Poon et al., 2010). Two kinds of PE are known; one is early-onset PE, and the other is late-onset PE. While in early-onset PE, the clinical manifestation is seen before 34 weeks of pregnancy, symptoms become apparent after 34 weeks of late-onset (Poon et al., 2010). Early-onset PE is a disorder of the placenta, where exceeding maternal blood pressure leads to fetal incapability of taking oxygen and nutrients from the mother due to a decrease in spiral artery remodeling and an increase in trophoblast invasion (R. O. Bahado-Singh et al., 2012). Previously existing metabolic or vascular disorders present in the mother are considered as the causes of late-onset PE (Wikström et al., 2007).

Despite efforts, the exact reason for PE development remains a mystery, and the removal of the fetus along with the placenta is considered as the sole solution (Staff, 2011). If it is detected early, prophylactic measures can be taken. Currently, there are several indicators for clinical assessment of PE, which include clinical parameters for angiogenesis (e.g., sFlt-1, PIGF, and endoglin), laboratory results, and abnormal ultrasound readings (Austdal et al., 2014; Cnossen et al., 2009). Therefore, research on new and non-invasive diagnostic methods to predict PE before the onset of symptoms is critical and may enhance preventive clinical manipulations.

Since PE includes many complexities, high-throughput technologies containing multiple markers can be effective screening methods for the diagnosis of PE. In research conducted on the metabolomics approach to urinary samples from the first-trimester period to assess preeclampsia and gestational hypertension, it was shown that decreased urinary hippurate was associated with increased blood pressure (Holmes et al., 2008). Intestinal microflora impairment is speculated to be the cause, which might be affected by nutritional and circulatory factors (Holmes et al., 2008; Nicholson et al., 2012). Metabolites are products of diet, lifestyle, gut microbiota, and genetic interactions (Dumas et al., 2006; Nicholson et al., 2005; Sabeti et al., 2007).

A comparison of patients having a normal pregnancy and having PE or gestational hypertension revealed changes in the first-trimester clinical parameters of urinary hippurate (decrease), urinary creatinine (increase), and serum lipids (increase). These results were reported as the most striking metabolic difference detected in patients with PE or gestational hypertension (Austdal et al., 2015). Striking metabolic changes in patients at risk of PE or gestational hypertension were discovered by utilizing early metabolite profiling in urinary and serum samples (Austdal et al., 2015). Since urinary samples are easily obtained, early metabolite profiling of urinary samples is an intriguing aspect of clinical practice to deduct the risk of PE and gestational hypertension, which can be further improved by combining the maternal traits into metabolite profiles.

Late-onset PE is common but more challenging to predict. Slowly developing microvascular conditions e.g., obesity, diabetes, and hypertension are generally associated with late-onset PE (Kenneth et al., 2010). In a study in which the metabolomic and proteomic methods were used together, dimethyl-sulfone or methyl sulfonyl methane concentrations were significantly lower in pregnant women with late-onset PE compared to controls in both trimesters (R. Bahado-Singh et al., 2017). Methyl sulfonyl methane is a bio-organic compound and is a prominent antioxidant and anti-inflammatory agent. Therefore, it improves oxidative stress conditions

(Butawan et al., 2017; Mohammadi et al., 2012). A notable metabolic feature of PE is its potential for oxidative stress.

Between 8-to-10 weeks of pregnancy, urinary creatinine amounts were found to be elevated in a study for early PE deduction (Kuromoto et al., 2010). Alterations in BMI and mean arterial pressure can be attributed to increases in urinary creatinine, and it has the potential of being an indicator of early renal involvement (Kuromoto et al., 2010). Studies have shown that glomerular filtration rates increase in pre-hypertensive subjects (Palatini, 2012). Gestational hypertension was attributed to the decrease in urinary citrate, which is also associated with an increased in BMI. Again, there is an opposite relationship between urinary citrate and adiposity (Elliott et al., 2015).

Noteworthy research on prenatal diagnostics was used in normal and PE pregnancies for metabolite alterations in the early period. In one such example, serum metabolite profiles obtained from patients having early- and late-onset PE were contrasted to metabolite profiles from healthy individuals, and researchers discovered increases in certain metabolites (arginine, 3-hydroxyisovalate, and glycerol), which is coupled with uterine artery PI, particularly in early-onset PE patients (R. O. Bahado-Singh et al., 2015, 2017). For the prediction of PE, a combined approach that contains metabolomics, proteomics, and ultrasound reached over 90% sensitivity along with almost 90% specificity. Combining the clinical parameters of the mother with the data from emerging omics, particularly metabolomics and proteomics, for the early PE deduction can be considered as a striking achievement. The researchers revealed considerable alterations in the following aspects: glycosaminoglycan metabolism, serotonin amounts, and Gp-receptors (Koster et al., 2015).

There is a serious debate is on the changeability of the proposed metabolites found by different researchers, and some research even favors clinical factors over metabolites, dismissing the predictive potential of metabolites (Kuc et al., 2014). However, further studies can identify consistent factors that can be used to create prediction algorithms for PE with increased accuracy, sensitivity, and specificity (Koster et al., 2015).

Fetal Growth Restriction

Falling below the 10th percentile in fetal growth and failure to reach expected growth in a given gestational period are known as fetal growth restriction (FGR), which is observed in up to 10% of all pregnancies (Vedmedovska et al., 2011). It occurs for many reasons and is the reason for notable rates of morbidity and mortality during both the perinatal period and infancy (Vedmedovska et al., 2011). The application of metabolomics for the estimation of FGR is an engaging endeavor.

In many metabolomic studies conducted in pregnancies resulting in slow-growing newborns, it was emphasized that abnormal lipid metabolism was found (Bernard et al., 2017; Leite et al., 2018). Research has indicated a decline in the ratio of medium-length fatty acids in mother to baby, particularly in periods close to labor, that leads to an energetic imbalance occurring in the baby (Visentin et al., 2017). Fetuses with FGR contrasted with healthy fetuses and notable alterations in cholesterol synthesis were found (Clinton et al., 2020). Cholesterol levels were slightly increased in pregnant women with FGR, while they increased significantly in the pregnant control group with naturally developing fetuses. Myo-inositol, associated with the down-regulation of free fatty acid release from fats, is increased in the urine of newborns born with FGR pregnancies (Dessì et al., 2011, 2014).

Amino acid metabolism is critical for FGR occurrence. Ornithine obtained from serum samples of mothers with aberrant umbilical arteries helped the revelation of its involvement in fetal growth (Porter et al., 2020). Angiogenesis via the polyamine pathway may explain the relationship between ornithine and umbilical circulation. the placenta of FGR pregnancies shows reduced metabolite levels (R. O. Bahado-Singh et al., 2022). In cases of FGR, alterations in metabolite levels are evident in hair samples from mothers (Sulek et al., 2014).

Alterations in protein biosynthesis have been stated to cause growth failure (Sibley et al., 2005). A study has reported that the most notable pathways affected in FGR include arginine, proline, glycine, serine and threonine metabolism, ammonia recycling, and the urea cycle, which are involved in protein and amino acid metabolism (R. O. Bahado-Singh et al., 2022). It has been shown that FGR is accompanied by numerous metabolic impairments of amino acids, including the metabolism of tryptophan, aspartate, methionine, glutamate, and arginine. It has also been shown in the study that amino acids are associated with FGR-related growth, brain-vascular function, and antioxidant capacity and fulfil vital functions (R. O. Bahado-Singh et al., 2022).

Preterm Birth

In cases of preterm birth, approximately 10% of all births occur earlier than 37 weeks. The biggest reason for the increase in perinatal morbidity and mortality is preterm birth (Conde-Agudelo et al., 2018; Crump, 2020). Preterm birth is known to provide newborns particularly prone to later chronic conditions, which include cardiovascular and metabolic syndromes, neurological and cognitive impairments, stroke occurrence, and dyslipidemia (Behrman & Butler, 2007; Conde-Agudelo et al., 2018; Crump, 2020). Long-term studies have not been able to contribute enough to create a screening algorithm and develop effective treatments (Georgiou et al., 2015).

The omics may help in describing normal pregnancy mechanism and the pathophysiological preterm courses that lead to preterm labor and delivery (Georgiou et al., 2015). Metabolomics methods are suggested for the detailing of diverse obstetric syndromes that have placental and adaptive dysfunctions (Tsiartas et al., 2012).

Conclusion

Metabolomics has exciting potential for researchers to reveal new aspects of perinatal pathophysiology and generate clinically useful biomarkers. Metabolomics can transform into an easily available large-scale monitoring method with its high-throughput analysis capabilities for numerous metabolites. Nevertheless, complete metabolome analysis can be challenging to perform routinely in a clinical setting. To identify and validate biomarkers for clinical applications in a timely manner, technical limitations should be reduced. By overcoming the technical limitations, the utilization of spectroscopy would become routine in clinical environments, and metabolite screening would become a norm. Metabolomics could be made into a cost-effective technology advantageous for the identification and management of patients. In the sense of perinatology, the field of metabolomics proposes an auspicious future. Overall, metabolomics can be translated into a fully personalized medicine to cover all individual aspects of DNA to the metabolites. Both physiological and pathophysiological mechanisms can benefit from the research avenues provided by metabolomics, particularly for designing targeted treatment strategies.

Currently, large-scale, dedicated studies in combination with conventional methods are a necessity to reduce technical limitations and to provide validated results for clinical practice. Three of the most evident limitations for their use in routine clinical applications can be detailed as following:

1. Mass spectrometry interpretation: Distinguishing clinically relevant biomarkers from all the detected metabolites in a spectral dataset during the preclinical phase is the most daunting aspect of the clinical application of metabolomics due to the numerous overlapping correlations.
2. Clinical biomarker identification: Clinically relevant and disease-specific biomarkers are seeing a stagnant development in identification, which is further hindered by the inherent dynamism of the metabolism. Additionally, the need for rigorous validation of proposed biomarkers for their intended purposes slows down the already slow-moving field.
3. Standardization: Standard ranges for identified and validated biomarkers that contain acceptable variations caused by individual differences should be established in healthy individuals. Only after these ranges are established, routine clinical applications can utilize such metabolites in pathology.

References

Austdal, M., Skråstad, R. B., Gundersen, A. S., Austgulen, R., Iversen, A. C., and Bathen, T. F. (2014). Metabolomic biomarkers in serum and urine in women with preeclampsia. *PloS One*, 9(3), e91923. https://doi.org/10.1371/journal.pone.0091923.

Austdal, M., Tangerås, L. H., Skråstad, R. B., Salvesen, K., Austgulen, R., Iversen, A. C., and Bathen, T. F. (2015). First Trimester Urine and Serum Metabolomics for Prediction of Preeclampsia and Gestational Hypertension: A Prospective Screening Study. *International Journal of Molecular Sciences*, 16(9), 21520–21538. https://doi.org/10.3390/ijms160921520.

Bahado-Singh, R. O., Akolekar, R., Mandal, R., Dong, E., Xia, J., Kruger, M., Wishart, D. S., and Nicolaides, K. (2012). Metabolomics and first-trimester prediction of early-onset preeclampsia. *The Journal of Maternal-Fetal & Neonatal Medicine*, 25(10), 1840–1847. https://doi.org/10.3109/14767058.2012.680254.

Bahado-Singh, R. O., Syngelaki, A., Akolekar, R., Mandal, R., Bjondahl, T. C., Han, B., Dong, E., Bauer, S., Alpay-Savasan, Z., and Graham, S. (2015). Validation of metabolomic models for prediction of early-onset preeclampsia. *American Journal of Obstetrics and Gynecology*, 213(4), 530-e1. https://doi.org/10.1016/j.ajog.2015.06.044.

Bahado-Singh, R. O., Syngelaki, A., Mandal, R., Graham, S. F., Akolekar, R., Han, B., Bjondahl, T. C., Dong, E., Bauer, S., and Alpay-Savasan, Z. (2017). Metabolomic determination of pathogenesis of late-onset preeclampsia. *The Journal of Maternal-Fetal & Neonatal Medicine*, 30(6), 658–664. https://doi.org/10.1080/14767058.2016.1185411.

Bahado-Singh, R. O., Turkoglu, O., Yilmaz, A., Kumar, P., Zeb, A., Konda, S., Sherman, E., Kirma, J., Allos, M., Odibo, A., Maulik, D., and Graham, S. F. (2022). Metabolomic identification of placental alterations in fetal growth restriction. The Journal of Maternal-Fetal & Neonatal Medicine: *The Official Journal of the European Association of Perinatal Medicine, the Federation of Asia and Oceania Perinatal Societies, the International Society of Perinatal Obstetricians*, 35(3), 447–456. https://doi.org/10.1080/14767058.2020.1722632.

Bahado-Singh, R., Poon, L. C., Yilmaz, A., Syngelaki, A., Turkoglu, O., Kumar, P., Kirma, J., Allos, M., Accurti, V., Li, J., Zhao, P., Graham, S. F., Cool, D. R., and Nicolaides, K. (2017). *Integrated Proteomic and Metabolomic prediction of Term Preeclampsia. Scientific Reports*, 7(1), 16189. https://doi.org/10.1038/s41598-017-15882-9.

Behrman, R. E., and Butler, A. S. (2007). *Preterm birth: causes, consequences, and prevention*. Washington, DC: National Academies Press. ISBN: 0-309-65898-5.

Bernard, J. Y., Tint, M. T., Aris, I. M., Chen, L. W., Quah, P. L., Tan, K. H., Yeo, G. S. H., Fortier, M. V, Yap, F., and Shek, L. (2017). Maternal plasma phosphatidylcholine polyunsaturated fatty acids during pregnancy and offspring growth and adiposity. *Prostaglandins, Leukotrienes and Essential Fatty Acids*, 121, 21–29. https://doi.org/10.1016/j.plefa.2017.05.006.

Butawan, M., Benjamin, R. L., and Bloomer, R. J. (2017). Methylsulfonylmethane: Applications and Safety of a Novel Dietary Supplement. *Nutrients*, 9(3), 290. https://doi.org/10.3390/nu9030290.

Clark, S. L., Romero, R., Dildy, G. A., Callaghan, W. M., Smiley, R. M., Bracey, A. W., Hankins, G. D., D'Alton, M. E., Foley, M., Pacheco, L. D., Vadhera, R. B., Herlihy, J. P., Berkowitz, R. L., and Belfort, M. A. (2016). Proposed diagnostic criteria for the case definition of amniotic fluid embolism in research studies. *American Journal of Obstetrics and Gynecology*, 215(4), 408–412. https://doi.org/10.1016/j.ajog.2016.06.037.

Clinton, C. M., Bain, J. R., Muehlbauer, M. J., Li, Y., Li, L., O'Neal, S. K., Hughes, B. L., Cantonwine, D. E., Mcelrath, T. F., and Ferguson, K. K. (2020). Non-targeted urinary metabolomics in pregnancy and associations with fetal growth restriction. *Scientific Reports*, 10(1), 1–8. https://doi.org/10.1038/s41598-020-62131-7.

Cnossen, J. S., Riet, G. Ter, Mol, B. W., Van Der Post, J. A., Leeflang, M. M., Meads, C. A., Hyde, C., and Khan, K. S. (2009). Are tests for predicting pre-eclampsia good enough to make screening viable? A review of reviews and critical appraisal. *Acta Obstetricia et Gynecologica Scandinavica*, 88(7), 758–765. https://doi.org/10.1080/00016340903008953.

Conde-Agudelo, A., Romero, R., Da Fonseca, E., O'Brien, J. M., Cetingoz, E., Creasy, G. W., Hassan, S. S., Erez, O., Pacora, P., and Nicolaides, K. H. (2018). Vaginal progesterone is as effective as cervical cerclage to prevent preterm birth in women with a singleton gestation, previous spontaneous preterm birth, and a short cervix:

updated indirect comparison meta-analysis. *American Journal of Obstetrics and Gynecology*, 219(1), 10–25. https://doi.org/10.1016/j.ajog.2017.11.576.

Crump, C. (2020). Preterm birth and mortality in adulthood: a systematic review. *Journal of Perinatology*, 40(6), 833–843. https://doi.org/10.1038/s41372-019-0563-y.

Dessì, A., Atzori, L., Noto, A., Adriaan Visser, G. H., Gazzolo, D., Zanardo, V., Barberini, L., Puddu, M., Ottonello, G., and Atzei, A. (2011). Metabolomics in newborns with intrauterine growth retardation (IUGR): urine reveals markers of metabolic syndrome. *The Journal of Maternal-Fetal & Neonatal Medicine*, 24(sup2), 35–39. https://doi.org/10.1038/s41372-020-00893-8.

Dessì, A., Marincola, F. C., Pattumelli, M. G., Ciccarelli, S., Corbu, S., Ossicini, C., Fanos, V., and Agostino, R. (2014). Investigation of the 1H-NMR based urine metabolomic profiles of IUGR, LGA and AGA newborns on the first day of life. *The Journal of Maternal-Fetal & Neonatal Medicine*, 27(sup2), 13–19. https://doi.org/10.3109/14767058.2014.955674.

Dumas, M.-E., Maibaum, E. C., Teague, C., Ueshima, H., Zhou, B., Lindon, J. C., Nicholson, J. K., Stamler, J., Elliott, P., Chan, Q., and Holmes, E. (2006). Assessment of analytical reproducibility of 1H NMR spectroscopy based metabonomics for large-scale epidemiological research: the INTERMAP Study. *Analytical Chemistry*, 78(7), 2199–2208. https://doi.org/10.1021/ac0517085.

Elliott, P., Posma, J. M., Chan, Q., Garcia-Perez, I., Wijeyesekera, A., Bictash, M., Ebbels, T. M. D., Ueshima, H., Zhao, L., van Horn, L., Daviglus, M., Stamler, J., Holmes, E., and Nicholson, J. K. (2015). Urinary metabolic signatures of human adiposity. *Science Translational Medicine*, 7(285), 285ra62. https://doi.org/10.1126/scitranslmed.aaa5680.

Espinoza, J., Chaiworapongsa, T., Romero, R., Edwin, S., Rathnasabapathy, C., Gomez, R., Bujold, E., Camacho, N., Kim, Y. M., Hassan, S., Blackwell, S., Whitty, J., Berman, S., Redman, M., Yoon, B. H., and Sorokin, Y. (2003). Antimicrobial peptides in amniotic fluid: defensins, calprotectin and bacterial/permeability-increasing protein in patients with microbial invasion of the amniotic cavity, intra-amniotic inflammation, preterm labor and premature rupture of membranes. *The Journal of Maternal-Fetal & Neonatal Medicine*, 13(1), 2–21. https://doi.org/10.1080/jmf.13.1.2.21.

Georgiou, H. M., Di Quinzio, M. K. W., Permezel, M., and Brennecke, S. P. (2015). Predicting preterm labour: current status and future prospects. *Disease Markers*, 2015, 1-9. https://doi.org/10.1155/2015/435014.

Gomez-Lopez, N., Romero, R., Xu, Y., Leng, Y., Garcia-Flores, V., Miller, D., Jacques, S. M., Hassan, S. S., Faro, J., and Alsamsam, A. (2017a). Are amniotic fluid neutrophils in women with intraamniotic infection and/or inflammation of fetal or maternal origin? *American Journal of Obstetrics and Gynecology*, 217(6), 693-e1. https://doi.org/10.1016/j.ajog.2017.09.013.

Gomez-Lopez, N., Romero, R., Garcia-Flores, V., Xu, Y., Leng, Y., Alhousseini, A., Hassan, S. S., and Panaitescu, B. (2017b). Amniotic fluid neutrophils can phagocytize bacteria: A mechanism for microbial killing in the amniotic cavity. *American Journal of Reproductive Immunology*, 78(4), e12723. https://doi.org/10.1111/aji.12723.

Gomez, R., Romero, R., Galasso, M., Behnke, E., Insunza, A., and Cotton, D. B. (1994). The value of amniotic fluid interleukin-6, white blood cell count, and gram stain in the diagnosis of microbial invasion of the amniotic cavity in patients at term. *American Journal of Reproductive Immunology (New York, N.Y.: 1989)*, 32(3), 200–210. https://doi.org/10.1111/j.1600-0897.1994.tb01115.x.

Holmes, E., Loo, R. L., Stamler, J., Bictash, M., Yap, I. K. S., Chan, Q., Ebbels, T., De Iorio, M., Brown, I. J., Veselkov, K. A., Daviglus, M. L., Kesteloot, H., Ueshima, H., Zhao, L., Nicholson, J. K., and Elliott, P. (2008). Human metabolic phenotype diversity and its association with diet and blood pressure. *Nature*, 453(7193), 396–400. https://doi.org/10.1038/nature06882.

Kenneth, L., Hall, D. R., Gebhardt, S., and Grové, D. (2010). Late onset preeclampsia is not an innocuous condition. *Hypertension in Pregnancy*, 29(3), 262–270. https://doi.org/10.3109/10641950902777697.

Koster, M. P. H., Vreeken, R. J., Harms, A. C., Dane, A. D., Kuc, S., Schielen, P. C. J. I., Hankemeier, T., Berger, R., Visser, G. H. A., and Pennings, J. L. A. (2015). First-trimester serum acylcarnitine levels to predict preeclampsia: a metabolomics approach. *Disease Markers*, 2015, 1-8. https://doi.org/10.1155/2015/857108.

Kuc, S., Koster, M. P. H., Pennings, J. L. A., Hankemeier, T., Berger, R., Harms, A. C., Dane, A. D., Schielen, P. C. J. I., Visser, G. H. A., and Vreeken, R. J. (2014). Metabolomics profiling for identification of novel potential markers in early prediction of preeclampsia. *PloS One*, 9(5), e98540. https://doi.org/10.1371/journal.pone.0098540.

Kuromoto, K., Watanabe, M., Adachi, K., Ohashi, K., and Iwatani, Y. (2010). Increases in urinary creatinine and blood pressure during early pregnancy in pre-eclampsia. *Annals of Clinical Biochemistry*, 47(Pt 4), 336–342. https://doi.org/10.1258/acb.2010.090290.

Leite, D. F. B., Morillon, A. C., Júnior, E. F. M., Souza, R. T., Khashan, A. S., Baker, P. N., Kenny, L. C., and Cecatti, J. G. (2018). Metabolomics for predicting fetal growth restriction: protocol for a systematic review and meta-analysis. *BMJ Open*, 8(12), e022743. http://dx.doi.org/10.1136/bmjopen-2018-022743.

Maddipati, K. R., Romero, R., Chaiworapongsa, T., Chaemsaithong, P., Zhou, S. L., Xu, Z., Tarca, A. L., Kusanovic, J. P., Gomez, R., Docheva, N., and Honn, K. V. (2016). Clinical chorioamnionitis at term: the amniotic fluid fatty acyl lipidome. *Journal of Lipid Research*, 57(10), 1906–1916. https://doi.org/10.1194/jlr.P069096.

Martinez-Varea, A., Romero, R., Xu, Y., Miller, D., Ahmed, A. I., Chaemsaithong, P., Chaiyasit, N., Yeo, L., Shaman, M., Lannaman, K., Cher, B., Hassan, S. S., and Gomez-Lopez, N. (2017). Clinical chorioamnionitis at term VII: the amniotic fluid cellular immune response. *Journal of Perinatal Medicine*, 45(5), 523–538. https://doi.org/10.1515/jpm-2016-0225.

Mohammadi, S., Najafi, M., Hamzeiy, H., Maleki-Dizaji, N., Pezeshkian, M., Sadeghi-Bazargani, H., Darabi, M., Mostafalou, S., Bohlooli, S., and Garjani, A. (2012). Protective effects of methylsulfonylmethane on hemodynamics and oxidative stress in monocrotaline-induced pulmonary hypertensive rats. *Advances in Pharmacological Sciences*, 2012, 507278. https://doi.org/10.1155/2012/507278.

Myatt, L., Redman, C. W., Staff, A. C., Hansson, S., Wilson, M. L., Laivuori, H., Poston, L., and Roberts, J. M. (2014). Strategy for standardization of preeclampsia research study design. *Hypertension (Dallas, Tex.: 1979)*, 63(6), 1293–1301. https://doi.org/10.1161/HYPERTENSIONAHA.113.02664.

Nicholson, J. K., Holmes, E., Kinross, J., Burcelin, R., Gibson, G., Jia, W., and Pettersson, S. (2012). Host-gut microbiota metabolic interactions. *Science (New York, N.Y.)*, 336(6086), 1262–1267. https://doi.org/10.1126/science.1223813.

Nicholson, J. K., Holmes, E., and Wilson, I. D. (2005). Gut microorganisms, mammalian metabolism and personalized health care. *Nature Reviews. Microbiology*, 3(5), 431–438. https://doi.org/10.1038/nrmicro1152.

Palatini, P. (2012). Glomerular hyperfiltration: a marker of early renal damage in pre-diabetes and pre-hypertension. *Nephrology, dialysis, transplantation: official publication of the European Dialysis and Transplant Association - European Renal Association*, 27(5), 1708–1714). https://doi.org/10.1093/ndt/gfs037.

Polsani, S., Phipps, E., and Jim, B. (2013). Emerging new biomarkers of preeclampsia. *Advances in Chronic Kidney Disease*, 20(3), 271–279. https://doi.org/10.1053/j.ackd.2013.01.001.

Poon, L. C. Y., Stratieva, V., Piras, S., Piri, S., and Nicolaides, K. H. (2010). Hypertensive disorders in pregnancy: combined screening by uterine artery Doppler, blood pressure and serum PAPP-A at 11–13 weeks. *Prenatal Diagnosis: Published in Affiliation with the International Society for Prenatal Diagnosis*, 30(3), 216–223. https://doi.org/10.1002/pd.2440.

Porter, A. C., Gumina, D. L., Armstrong, M., Maclean, K. N., Reisdorph, N., Galan, H. L., Stabler, S. P., Bailey, B. A., Hobbins, J. C., and Hurt, K. J. (2020). Maternal amino acid profiles to distinguish constitutionally small versus growth-restricted fetuses defined by Doppler ultrasound: a pilot study. *American Journal of Perinatology*, 37(11), 1084–1093. https://doi.org/10.1055/s-0040-1701504.

Roberge, S., Villa, P., Nicolaides, K., Giguère, Y., Vainio, M., Bakthi, A., Ebrashy, A., and Bujold, E. (2012). Early administration of low-dose aspirin for the prevention of preterm and term preeclampsia: a systematic review and meta-analysis. *Fetal Diagnosis and Therapy*, 31(3), 141–146. https://doi.org/10.1159/000336662.

Sabeti, P. C., Varilly, P., Fry, B., Lohmueller, J., Hostetter, E., Cotsapas, C., Xie, X., Byrne, E. H., McCarroll, S. A., Gaudet, R., Schaffner, S. F., Lander, E. S., Frazer, K. A., Ballinger, D. G., Cox, D. R., Hinds, D. A., Stuve, L. L., Gibbs, R. A., Belmont, J. W., and Stewart, J. (2007). Genome-wide detection and characterization of positive selection in human populations. *Nature*, 449(7164), 913–918. https://doi.org/10.1038/nature06250.

Sibai, B. M. (2003). Diagnosis and management of gestational hypertension and preeclampsia. *Obstetrics and Gynecology*, 102(1), 181–192. https://doi.org/10.1016/s0029-7844(03)00475-7.

Sibley, C. P., Turner, M. A., Cetin, I., Ayuk, P., Boyd, C. A., D'Souza, S. W., Glazier, J. D., Greenwood, S. L., Jansson, T., and Powell, T. (2005). Placental phenotypes of intrauterine growth. *Pediatric Research*, 58(5), 827–832. https://doi.org/10.1203/01.PDR.0000181381.82856.23.

Staff, A. C. (2011). Circulating predictive biomarkers in preeclampsia. Pregnancy Hypertension: An International *Journal of Women's Cardiovascular Health*, 1(1), 28–42. https://doi.org/10.1016/j.preghy.2010.10.012.

Sulek, K., Han, T. L., Villas-Boas, S. G., Wishart, D. S., Soh, S. E., Kwek, K., Gluckman, P. D., Chong, Y. S., Kenny, L. C., and Baker, P. N. (2014). Hair metabolomics: identification of fetal compromise provides proof of concept for biomarker discovery. *Theranostics*, 4(9), 953. https://doi.org/10.7150/thno.9265.

Tarui, T., Kim, A., Flake, A., McClain, L., Stratigis, J. D., Fried, I., Newman, R., Slonim, D. K., and Bianchi, D. W. (2017). Amniotic fluid transcriptomics reflects novel disease mechanisms in fetuses with myelomeningocele. *American Journal of Obstetrics and Gynecology*, 217(5), 587-e1. https://doi.org/10.1016/j.ajog.2017.07.022.

Tsiartas, P., Holst, R. M., Wennerholm, U. B., Hagberg, H., Hougaard, D. M., Skogstrand, K., Pearce, B. D., Thorsen, P., Kacerovsky, M., and Jacobsson, B. (2012). Prediction of spontaneous preterm delivery in women with threatened preterm labour: a prospective cohort study of multiple proteins in maternal serum. *BJOG: An International Journal of Obstetrics & Gynaecology*, 119(7), 866–873. https://doi.org/10.1111/j.1471-0528.2012.03328.x.

Vedmedovska, N., Rezeberga, D., Teibe, U., Melderis, I., and Donders, G. G. G. (2011). Placental pathology in fetal growth restriction. *European Journal of Obstetrics & Gynecology and Reproductive Biology*, 155(1), 36–40. https://doi.org10.1016/j.ejogrb.2010.11.017.

Visentin, S., Crotti, S., Donazzolo, E., D'Aronco, S., Nitti, D., Cosmi, E., and Agostini, M. (2017). Medium chain fatty acids in intrauterine growth restricted and small for gestational age pregnancies. *Metabolomics*, 13(5), 1–9. https://doi.org/10.1007/s11306-017-1197-8.

Wikström, A. K., Larsson, A., Eriksson, U. J., Nash, P., Nordén-Lindeberg, S., and Olovsson, M. (2007). Placental growth factor and soluble FMS-like tyrosine kinase-1 in early-onset and late-onset preeclampsia. *Obstetrics & Gynecology*, 109(6), 1368–1374. https://doi.org/10.1097/01.AOG.0000264552.85436.a1.

Chapter 15

Metabolomic Markers and Their Clinical Uses in Neurology

Gülay Soykök*, MD
Department of Neurology, Kayseri City Hospital, Kayseri, Turkey

Abstract

Metabolomics has presented specific findings about metabolite variations in multi-biofluids and tissues and has provided countless potential biomarkers and therapeutic targets. Metabolomics is significant when considering the need for diagnostic biopsies of the central neural system tissues in neurological diseases and difficulties in clinical practice.

Additional metabolic pathways that show involvement in different disease steps are demonstrated despite the genetic and pathophysiological heterogeneity of neurological diseases. Metabolic pathways are variable dynamic systems that are controlled by endogenous circadian mechanisms. Experimental models on metabolic reprogramming are significantly informative about the molecular mechanisms underlying metabolic changes. These mechanisms and steps are essential in terms of defining the therapeutic window. Additionally, knowing the next step in the disease progress enables critical practices for treatment to be applied.

Keywords: neurological diseases, metabolomics, biomarker

---

* Corresponding Author's E-mail: drgulayuzun@gmail.com.

In: Metabolomics and Clinical Approach
Editors: Sevgi Durna Daştan and Taner Daştan
ISBN: 979-8-89113-095-1

Introduction

Metabolomics is a detailed and quantitative measurement of metabolites in tissues, cells, and body fluids (Coşkun, 2007). Metabolomics is the last fact in genomics, transcriptomics, and proteomics processes, and it enables us to understand the cellular and molecular basis of diseases. For compound analyses and metabolic profiles, mass spectrometry (MS) and nuclear magnetic resonance (NMR) are commonly used. The combined use of MS and chromatography separation technologies provides better results. Gas chromatography from chromatography methods has a two-stage approach and detects volatile and non-volatile metabolites. GC-MS (Gas chromatography-mass spectrometry), tricarboxylic acid (TCA) cycle, glycolysis, fatty acid, and amino acid cycle are significant in detecting metabolites. Liquid chromatography (LC) includes non-volatile metabolites. Capillary electrophoresis is used to detect carbon metabolites.

Energy is needed for signal mechanisms and cognitive functions in the brain. The brain needs approximately 25% of the glucose source in the body for energy usage. Generally, the production of ATP (adenosine triphosphate) is based on this glucose source. In the physiopathology of chronic neuronal damages, it has been thought that, generally, there are the decreased energy metabolism and mitochondrial dysfunctions. Pathologies (glycolysis, oxidative phosphorylation pentose phosphate pathway) in energy and central carbon metabolism have a crucial role in the formation of neurodegenerative and psychiatric diseases. Astroglial and neuronal oxidation is not only related to glucose, but also related to substrates that contain a combination of neuromediators such as fatty acid oxidation, pruvate, lactate, glutamate, and GABA (Gamma aminobutyric acid) (A. Panov et al., 2009; A. V. Panov et al., 2011). In fact, lipids are also essential in terms of their participation in cell membrane structure and signal transduction, in the central neural system hemostasis. Although the amino acid effect partially seems as in the second plan during gluconeogenesis and neuronal activity, protein proteolysis, ketoglutarate, and pyruvate transamination cycle are also active. The blood brain barrier is an important vascular structure that protects the neuronal area and has a role in biomolecule exchange. Intracellular and extracellular enzyme combinations also contribute to molecular transition by metabolizing and inactivating neuroactive and neurotoxic structures (Kasser et al., 1986; El-Bacha & Minn, 1999). Because these mechanisms are more active in the central neural system, it is more protected against toxins than the peripheral neural system. The blood brain barrier partially decreases the detection of brain metabolomics, and yet, it is not clear how much it reflected the tissue activity of the metabolite (Griffin & Salek, 2007). Additionally, knowing the next step in the disease progress enables critical practices for treatment to be applied (Bonomo et al., 2020).

Theoretical Perspectives

Metabolomics is significant when considering the need for diagnostic biopsies of the central neural system tissues in neurological diseases and difficulties in clinical practice. Metabolomics can track dynamic changes in biological systems by providing correct knowledge for clinical practices and translational medicine (Pagani et al., 2017). In many diseases, specific chemical and biochemical changes occur before clinical symptoms. In detecting potential biomarkers, the most accessible biofluids are cerebrospinal fluid (CSF), plasma, and urine. The CSF provides knowledge about neuropathology in the brain and the biochemical environment of the central neural system.

Alzheimer Disease

Alzheimer disease (AD) is characterize with abnormal ß-amyloid and Tau protein accumulation in the brain, and it generates the most common form of progressive dementia (Karran et al., 2011). The substructure of AD metabolic could not be understood completely, and the relation between systematic pathology and AD is unclear. Many metabolic network and glucose energy dysfunctions that involve lipids and amino acids have a role in AD in pathomechanism (Wilkins & Trushina, 2017). Changed levels of arginine and its metabolites were found in the superior frontal gyrus and the hippocampus, which are important areas affected by AD (Liu et al., 2014). Additionally, the amount of arginine in the temporal cortices of AD was found 25% less compared to the control group (Gueli & Taibi, 2013). In pre-clinical and clinical studies for AD, differences were detected in glutamine, glutamate, aspartate, N-(L-arginino) succinate, N-acetyl-aspartate, and alanine levels. The glutamate NMDA receptor antagonist memantine is one of the two types of medical treatment used in clinical practice in suppressing the increase in glutamate level.

In the stage of prodrome and pre-clinical, determining AD pathology is essential in terms of slowing the disease progress and treatment strategy. In AD autopsy studies, there are pathological findings of sphingolipid metabolism disorder (Varma et al., 2018). Especially, changes in eicosanoids, which are part of the arachidonic acid metabolism, have been observed and, this situation can be related to neuro inflammatory (Latta et al., 2015). CSF (cerebrospinal fluid) impaired citrate balance was detected in Alzheimer disease (Ghauri et al., 1993). In AD, the amounts of ethanolamine plasmalogens reduce in both the brain and plasma. Plasmalogens are important endogenous antioxidants that protect lipids and lipoproteins (Goodenowe et al., 2007). In AD, it is detected that there is a decrease in long-chain aliphatic sphingolipids and a decrease in the level of ceramide. It is thought that there is a relation between changed plasma ceramide levels and disease physiopathology (X. Han et al., 2011). In AD pathogenesis, there are data to support the involvement of an abnormal membrane metabolism.

The decrease in polyunsaturated fatty acids (PUFA) and phospholipid (PL) and the increase with the effect of phospholipase C and D, and diglycerides, which are by-products of phospholipid hydrolysis were found (González-Domínguez et al., 2014). There is a need for a comprehensive level of approach to understand the multi-directional pathophysiology of AD completely.

Parkinson's Disease

Parkinson's disease (PD) is a movement disorder characterized by resting tremor, bradykinesia, rigidity, and degeneration of dophaminergic neurons in the prominent basal ganglia in the substantia nigra. In PD, the plasma amount of uric acid with antioxidant featured, which is the end product of purine metabolism, is low and it has been shown that PD increases as the uric acid level decreases (Johansen et al., 2009). Significant decreases in tryptophan, creatinine, and 3-hydroxyvalerate levels have been reported in PD (Trupp et al., 2014).

There is an opinion that protein misfolding and aggregation, mitochondrial damage, oxidative stress, and inflammation are involved in the PD pathogenesis (Sommer et al., 2017). PD α-synuclein aggregation forms the beginning of neurodegenerative processes, and the TCA cycle is regulated downward besides the metabolism of glycine, serine, and threonine (Graham et al., 2018). This situation is a marker of insufficient energy and mitochondrial dysfunction. There has not yet been a successful response yet from treatment protocols that are based on the mechanism of preventing or removing the α-synuclein aggregation. It can provide comprehensive biochemical bases to resolve the molecular mechanism of PD pathogenesis.

Significant decreases in catecholamines including homovanilic acid (HVA), dihydroxyphenylacetic acid (DOPAC), L-dopa and dihydroxyphenylglycol have been reported in PD (Goldstein et al., 2012). DOPAC levels are not specific for PD and a significant decrease is observed in catechols in patients with other synucleinopathies such as pure autonomic failure and multiple system atrophy (MSA). Amino acids, fatty acids, acylcarnitines, lipids, purines, organic acids, and sugars, which are parts of PD branched-chain amino acids metabolism, have been determined differently compared to the control groups. Additionally, kynurenine metabolites changes in PD can be accepted as a potential biomarker and provide new treatment opportunities (W. Han et al., 2017).

Huntington Disease

Huntington disease (HD) is a progressive autosomal dominant inherited neurodegenerative disease with chorea, dystonia, coordination disorders, cognitive, and behavioral disorders. Increased glucose amount in plasma has been associated with diabetes (Farrer, 1985). Increased lactate and glucose concentrations have been found in the CSF metabolism in HD (Verwaest et al., 2011). The observed increase is the result of an increase in glucose concentration with closure of the neuronal-glial, glutamate-glutamine cycle. All of these metabolites support energy metabolism dysfunction. Additionally, increased lipid β-oxidation markers such as glycerol and diethylene glycol and variable lactate levels are likely to be associated with cachexia (Underwood et al., 2006).

Motor Neuron Disease

Motor neuron disease (MND) is a heterogeneous neurodegenerative disease that affects upper and lower motor neurons. It has clinical findings such as wide muscle weakness, swallowing difficulty, and respiratory difficulty. The most common form is amyotrophic lateral sclerosis. Changed glutamate metabolism is important in MND.

There are studies showing that branched-chain amino acid metabolites such as phenylalanine and tyrosine can be used in differential diagnosis (Blasco et al., 2014). Plasma acetate, acetone and ß-hydroxybutyrate levels are increased in ALS, supporting the systemic energy metabolism disorder (Graham et al., 2018).

Cerebrovascular Disease

A part of the brain is deprived of oxygen and nutrients depending on cerebral malnutrition with blood vessel occlusion by the reason of a thrombus or embolism during cerebrovascular disease (CVD) and is severely damaged by the induction of metabolic and cellular disturbances. In the serum and plasma of patients with cerebral ischemia, changes in metabolite levels, including organic acids, amino acids, free fatty acids, lipids, and low-density lipoproteins, have been reported. In its metabolomic analyses with CVD, glycine, isoleucine, and lysine levels, which are associated with inflammation, have been decreased compared to the control groups. While changes in membrane lipid metabolism are observed in serum of patients with middle cerebral artery occlusion, changes in the branched-chain amino acids leucine, isoleucine, and valine have been observed in cardioembolic stroke (Kimberly et al., 2013). Basically, glucose metabolic pathways are highly affected by cerebral ischemia based on reduced oxygen and nutrient availability (Rink & Khanna 2011). In the glycolysis process, the anaerobic pathways are activated instead of the aerobic pathway in cerebral ischemia. Additionally, suppression of the tricarboxylic acid (TCA) cycle with oxidative radicals also activates anaerobic glycolysis (Sahni et al., 2018). The pentose-phosphate pathway is activated as an endogenous antioxidant mechanism by increasing the nicotinamide adenine dinucleotide phosphate (NADPH)/nicotinamide adenine dinucleotide (NAD)+ ratio. Lactate is produced as the end product and the cytosolic environment becomes acidic. As a reflection of these metabolic changes in the brain, increased formate, glycolate, lactate, and pyruvate levels have been reported in patients with cerebral ischemia. Additionally, it is suggested that increased formate and glycolate levels and decreased dimethylamine, glycine, hippurate, and methanol levels in CVD are related to hyperhomocysteinemia, which is an important risk factor in CVD (Jung et al.,

2011). Serum betaine levels were found to be low in CVD, and the occurrence of this situation is quite surprising because high levels of betaine, which is a methyl donor, decrease the level of homocysteine, which is a risk factor for stroke (Spence, 2006). Impaired insulin sensitivity and increased glucose levels are also known risk factors for CVD. Lactate levels are high in CVD.

Idiopathic Intracranial Hypertension (IIH)

Idiopathic intracranial hypertension (IIH) is a disease characterized by high intracranial pressure, which mostly affects overweight young women, with clinical findings ranging from headache, visual impairment, and blindness in which the imaging findings are mostly normal (Friedman & Jacobson 2002). Because of the high cranial pressure and compressed vascular system of IHH, the anaerobic respiration mechanisms are activated, and oxaloacetate levels rise. Furthermore, citrate levels decrease with impaired of the citrate synthase effect in the citric acid cycle. Thus, ketone bodies such as 3-hydroxybutyrate rise and anaerobic environment controls because there is a carbohydrate substrate deficit (Hassan-Smith et al., 2012).

Multiple Sclerosis

Multiple sclerosis (MS) is an inflammatory demyelinating disease of the central neural system of unknown etiology, and is progressive and causes a high rate of disability even though some of its subtypes may progress with relative remissions.

Peripheral myelin-like antigen-activated T cells are transported through the blood and cross the blood brain barrier and infiltrate the central neural system. The special formed cytokinins affect the oligodendrocytes and axons and cause demyelination and axonal damage. At the end of these damages, the neurodegeneration process begins, and the rate of disability increases. The complexity of physiological and pathological processes also complicates the evaluation of central neural system damages. N-acetyl aspartate produced by neurons is a biomarker that indicates axonal damage. In the previous study conducted with in vivo proton magnetic resonance spectroscopy (^{1}H-MRS) in MS, it was determined that lactate and fructose increased and creatinine decreased. In another study, an unidentified N-methyl compound and increased acetate, lactate were found (Simone et al., 1996). The different prognostic subgroups of MS disease and heterogeneous patient groups in the studies may have caused different results. In a comprehensive study with a homogeneous patient group, increased lactate, creatinine, ß glucose, glutamine, β-hydroxyisobutyrate (BHIB), fructose, and decreased phenylalanine levels have been found in MS (Lutz et al., 2007). It has been reported that the hypoxia-like damage mechanism in MS is related to plaque formation (Lassmann, 2003). It has activated the anaerobic mechanism to tolerate the decreased oxidative metabolism in and around plaque in MS. Mitochondrial dysfunction is important in the pathogenesis and progression of MS. CSF sorbitol, fructose, and lactate amounts have been found as increased in MS patients compared to healthy control groups (Regenold et al., 2008). These findings contribute to mitochondrial dysfunction in MS where glycolysis dependency increases and mitochondrial energy production decreases. Additionally, the findings of mitochondrial dysfunction are available not only in the lesions but also in the normal brain area.

Neuromyelitis Optica (NMO) is an inflammatory and demyelinating central nervous system disease similar to MS with severe optic neuritis and myelitis attacks. For that reason, more specific metabolomic markers contribute to differential diagnosis in diseases with similar characteristics. In the 1H-NMR spectral analyzes performed in MS patients, it has been shown that the amount of sycllоinositol is 0.15 to 3 times higher than the control groups (Moussallieh et al., 2014). The amount of myo-inositol, which is a stereoisomer of syclloinositol, has also been found to increase in MS patients. The amounts acetate have been found to be higher in NMO patients compared to the control group and MS patients.

Epilepsy

Epilepsy is a clinical case with a sudden involuntary repetitive contraction and changes in consciousness that occur after abnormal and excessive electrical discharge in cortical neurons. The diagnosis of epilepsy is currently based on symptomatology and EEG (electroencephalography). During the seizure, there is an increase related to dysregulation of the base components of energy, amino acid, phospholipid, and purine metabolism. In the studies on patients with focal epilepsy and animal form, it was determined that the extracellular concentrations of endogenous components such as glutamate, isolosine,

GABA (Gamma aminobutyric acid), lactate, and adenosine changed related to seizures (Ong et al., 2021; Dhaher et al., 2021; Varma et al., 2018; During et al., 1994; During & Spencer, 1992). It was also suggested that epilepsy pathogenesis may be related to the citrate cycle (Bainbridge et al., 2017). It has been found that the metabolism or transport disorder of glycine, which is an inhibitory neurotransmitter, may be related to the pathogenesis of epilepsy and cognitive impairment in patients with epilepsy (Shen et al., 2015). Alpha-ketoisocaproic acid, xylose, and glycine are expressed in a different way in the cerebrospinal fluid of patients and are related to epilepsy and convulsive symptoms (Niu et al., 2022).

Migraine

Migraine is an episodic neurological disease that causes severe headaches and significant loss of workforce. Hypoglycemia, dehydration, hypoxia, and insomnia are essential triggering factors. Because of increased ADP and decreased organophosphate levels, mitochondrial oxidative phosphorylation is effective in the pathogenesis of the disease. High brain lactate levels were observed in migraine patients with aura; however, they were not detected in those without aura (Prescot et al., 2009). The metabolic abnormalities observed during migraine attacks are not pathogenic changes, but moderator effects.

Peripheral Neuropathies

Peripheral neuropathies are diseases with metabolic, toxic, and genetic causes and peripheral nerve damage. Mitochondrial dysfunction is effective in etiology. Mutations causing mitochondrial dysfunction form the etiological causes in hereditary neuropathies (Niemann et al., 2006). In a metabolomic study with Charcot-Marie-Tooth-2D (CMT2D), it demonstrated that the amounts of ascorbic acid and carnitine decreased, while glycine increased moderately in the spinal cord and sciatic nerve (Bais et al., 2016). The early decrease in TCA metabolites and the increase in valine, isoleucine, and leucine indicate a shift towards alternative energy pathways in the diabetic modeling study for peripheral nerve injury. Additionally, an increase in sorbitol levels has also been observed in advanced diabetic conditions. At the end of progressive changes on energy usage, caused tissue-specific dysfunction has been found (Rojas et al., 2019). In acute polyneuropathy variants, decreased acetate and increased monoglycerols, such as monopalmitate and monostearin, cause abnormality in myelin lipid biosynthesis.

Conclusion

Genomic, epigenomic, proteineomic, and fundamentally metabolomic approaches will provide a comprehensive view of system biology. Metabolomics has provided a general "fingerprint" in metabolite variations in multi-biofluids and tissues and has provided countless potential biomarkers and therapeutic targets.

Genetic, stem cell, and immunomodulatory treatments have gained importance in neurological diseases. The use of metabolic markers is important in the development and conventionalization of these treatments. Additionally, metabolic profiling will provide information on the cell-specific secondary effects of drugs and will assist in the development of treatments. Differences in models of up- or down-regulation of metabolites have been observed because of limitations in standardizing disease severity, when it started, race, diet, age, and other patient characteristics in metabolic analyzes involving patients.

Metabolomics should be optimized and evaluated on a large scale. Also, a detailed etiological evaluation and examination of clinical variables are required for standardization. The potential biomarkers and metabolic pathways that occurred in current studies should be confirmed by large-scale independent populations.

References

Bainbridge, M. N., Cooney, E., Miller, M., Kennedy, A. D., Wulff, J. E., Donti, T., Jhangiani, S. N., Gibbs, R. A., Elsea, S. H., Porter, B. E., & Graham, B. H. (2017). Analyses of SLC13A5-epilepsy patients reveal perturbations of TCA cycle. *Molecular genetics and metabolism*, *121*(4), 314–319. https://doi.org/10.1016/j.ymgme.2017.06.009

Bais, P., Beebe, K., Morelli, K. H., Currie, M. E., Norberg, S. N., Evsikov, A. V., Miers, K. E., Seburn, K. L., Guergueltcheva, V., Kremensky, I., Jordanova, A., Bult, C. J., & Burgess, R. W. (2016). Metabolite profile of a mouse model of Charcot-Marie-Tooth type 2D neuropathy: implications for disease mechanisms and interventions. *Biology Open*, *5*(7), 908–920. https://doi.org/10.1242/BIO.019273

Blasco, H., Nadal-Desbarats, L., Pradat, P. F., Gordon, P. H., Antar, C., Veyrat-Durebex, C., Moreau, C., Devos, D., Mavel, S., Emond, P., Andres, C. R., & Corcia, P. (2014). Untargeted 1H-NMR metabolomics in CSF: Toward a diagnostic biomarker for motor neuron disease. *Neurology*, *82*(13), 1167–1174. https://doi.org/10.1212/WNL.0000000000000274

Bonomo, R., Cavaletti, G., & Skene, D. J. (2020). Metabolomics markers in Neurology: current knowledge and future perspectives for therapeutic targeting. *Expert Review of Neurotherapeutics*, *20*(7), 725–738. https://doi.org/10.1080/14737175.2020.1782746

Coşkun, T. (2007). Nütrisyonel genomik [Nutritional genomics]. *Çocuk Sağlığı ve Hastalıkları Dergisi [Journal of Pediatric Health and Diseases], 50,* 47-66.

Dhaher, R., Gruenbaum, S. E., Sandhu, M. R. S., Ottestad-Hansen, S., Tu, N., Wang, Y., Lee, T. W., Deshpande, K., Spencer, D. D., Danbolt, N. C., Zaveri, H. P., & Eid, T. (2021). Network-Related Changes in Neurotransmitters and Seizure Propagation During Rodent Epileptogenesis. *Neurology*, *96*(18), e2261–e2271. https://doi.org/10.1212/WNL.0000000000011846

During, M. J., Fried, I., Leone, P., Katz, A., & Spencer, D. D. (1994). Direct Measurement of Extracellular Lactate in the Human Hippocampus During Spontaneous Seizures. *Journal of Neurochemistry*, *62*(6), 2356–2361. https://doi.org/10.1046/J.1471-4159.1994.62062356.X

During, M. J., & Spencer, D. D. (1992). Adenosine: A potential mediator of seizure arrest and postictal refractoriness. *Annals of Neurology*, *32*(5), 618–624. https://doi.org/10.1002/ANA.410320504

El-Bacha, R. S., & Minn, A. (1999). Drug metabolizing enzymes in cerebrovascular endothelial cells afford a metabolic protection to the brain. *Cellular and molecular biology (Noisy-le-Grand, France)*, *45*(1), 15–23. PMID: 10099836

Farrer, L. A. (1985). Diabetes mellitus in Huntington disease. *Clinical Genetics*, *27*(1), 62–67. https://doi.org/10.1111/J.1399-0004.1985.TB00185.X

Friedman, D. I., & Jacobson, D. M. (2002). Diagnostic criteria for idiopathic intracranial hypertension. *Neurology*, *59*(10), 1492–1495. https://doi.org/10.1212/01.wnl.0000029570.69134.1b

Ghauri, F. Y., Nicholson, J. K., Sweatman, B. C., Wood, J., Beddell, C. R., Lindon, J. C., & Cairns, N. J. (1993). NMR spectroscopy of human post mortem cerebrospinal fluid: distinction of Alzheimer's disease from control using pattern recognition and statistics. *NMR in Biomedicine*, *6*(2), 163–167. https://doi.org/10.1002/nbm.1940060210

Goldstein, D. S., Holmes, C., & Sharabi, Y. (2012). Cerebrospinal fluid biomarkers of central catecholamine deficiency in Parkinson's disease and other synucleinopathies. *Brain*, *135*(6), 1900–1913. https://doi.org/10.1093/BRAIN/AWS055

González-Domínguez, R., García-Barrera, T., & Gómez-Ariza, J. L. (2014). Metabolomic study of lipids in serum for biomarker discovery in Alzheimer's disease using direct infusion mass spectrometry. *Journal of Pharmaceutical and Biomedical Analysis*, *98*, 321–326. https://doi.org/10.1016/j.jpba.2014.05.023

Goodenowe, D. B., Cook, L. L., Liu, J., Lu, Y., Jayasinghe, D. A., Ahiahonu, P. W. K., Heath, D., Yamazaki, Y., Flax, J., Krenitsky, K. F., Sparks, D. L., Lerner, A., Friedland, R. P., Kudo, T., Kamino, K., Morihara, T., Takeda, M., & Wood, P. L. (2007). Peripheral ethanolamine plasmalogen deficiency: a logical causative factor in Alzheimer's disease and dementia. *Journal of Lipid Research*, *48*(11), 2485–2498. https://doi.org/10.1194/jlr.P700023-JLR200

Graham, S. F., Rey, N. L., Yilmaz, A., Kumar, P., Madaj, Z., Maddens, M., Bahado-Singh, R. O., Becker, K., Schulz, E., Meyerdirk, L. K., Steiner, J. A., Ma, J., & Brundin, P. (2018). Biochemical Profiling of the Brain and Blood Metabolome in a Mouse Model of Prodromal Parkinson's Disease Reveals Distinct Metabolic Profiles. *Journal of Proteome Research*, *17*(7), 2460–2469. https://doi.org/10.1021/ACS.JPROTEOME.8B00224

Griffin, J. L., & Salek, R. M. (2007). Metabolomic applications to neuroscience: More challenges than chances? *Expert Review of Proteomics*, *4*(4), 435–437. https://doi.org/10.1586/14789450.4.4.435

Gueli, M. C., & Taibi, G. (2013). Alzheimer's disease: amino acid levels and brain metabolic status. Neurological Sciences : Official Journal of the Italian Neurological Society and of the Italian Society of Clinical Neurophysiology, 34(9), 1575–1579. https://doi.org/10.1007/s10072-013-1289-9

Han, W., Sapkota, S., Camicioli, R., Dixon, R. A., & Li, L. (2017). Profiling novel metabolic biomarkers for Parkinson's disease using in-depth metabolomic analysis. *Movement Disorders*, *32*(12), 1720–1728. https://doi.org/10.1002/MDS.27173

Han, X., Rozen, S., Boyle, S. H., Hellegers, C., Cheng, H., Burke, J. R., Welsh-Bohmer, K. A., Doraiswamy, P. M., & Kaddurah-Daouk, R. (2011). Metabolomics in early Alzheimer's disease: identification of altered plasma sphingolipidome using shotgun lipidomics. *PloS One*, *6*(7), e21643. https://doi.org/10.1371/journal.pone.0021643

Hassan-Smith, G., Wallace, G. R., Douglas, M. R., & Sinclair, A. J. (2012). The role of metabolomics in neurological disease. *Journal of Neuroimmunology*, *248*(1–2), 48–52. https://doi.org/10.1016/J.JNEUROIM.2012.01.009

Johansen, K. K., Wang, L., Aasly, J. O., White, L. R., Matson, W. R., Henchcliffe, C., Beal, M. F., & Bogdanov, M. (2009). Metabolomic profiling in LRRK2-related Parkinson's disease. *PloS One*, *4*(10), e7551. https://doi.org/10.1371/journal.pone.0007551

Jung, J. Y., Lee, H. S., Kang, D. G., Kim, N. S., Cha, M. H., Bang, O. S., Ryu, D. H., & Hwang, G. S. (2011). 1 H-NMR-based metabolomics study of cerebral infarction. *Stroke*, *42*(5), 1282–1288. https://doi.org/10.1161/STROKEAHA.110.598789

Karran, E., Mercken, M., & De Strooper, B. (2011). The amyloid cascade hypothesis for Alzheimer's disease: an appraisal for the development of therapeutics. *Nature Reviews. Drug Discovery*, *10*(9), 698–712. https://doi.org/10.1038/nrd3505

Kasser, T. R., Deutch, A., & Martin, R. J. (1986). Uptake and utilization of metabolites in specific brain sites relative to feeding status. *Physiology & behavior*, *36*(6), 1161-1165. https://doi.org/10.1016/0031-9384(86)90494-4

Kimberly, W. T., Wang, Y., Pham, L., Furie, K. L., & Gerszten, R. E. (2013). Metabolite profiling identifies a branched chain amino acid signature in acute cardioembolic stroke. *Stroke*, *44*(5), 1389–1395. https://doi.org/10.1161/STROKEAHA.111.000397

Lassmann, H. (2003). Hypoxia-like tissue injury as a component of multiple sclerosis lesions. *Journal of the neurological sciences, 206*(2), 187–191. https://doi.org/10.1016/s0022-510x(02)00421-5

Latta, C. H., Brothers, H. M., & Wilcock, D. M. (2015). Neuroinflammation in Alzheimer's disease; A source of heterogeneity and target for personalized therapy. *Neuroscience, 302*, 103–111. https://doi.org/10.1016/j.neuroscience.2014.09.061

Liu, P., Fleete, M. S., Jing, Y., Collie, N. D., Curtis, M. A., Waldvogel, H. J., Faull, R. L. M., Abraham, W. C., & Zhang, H. (2014). Altered arginine metabolism in Alzheimer's disease brains. *Neurobiology of Aging, 35*(9), 1992–2003. https://doi.org/10.1016/j.neurobiolaging.2014.03.013

Lutz, N. W., Viola, A., Malikova, I., Confort-Gouny, S., Audoin, B., Ranjeva, J. P., Pelletier, J., & Cozzone, P. J. (2007). Inflammatory multiple-sclerosis plaques generate characteristic metabolic profiles in cerebrospinal fluid. *PLoS ONE, 2*(7). https://doi.org/10.1371/JOURNAL.PONE.0000595

Moussallieh, F. M., Elbayed, K., Chanson, J. B., Rudolf, G., Piotto, M., De Seze, J., & Namer, I. J. (2014). Serum analysis by 1H Nuclear Magnetic Resonance spectroscopy: a new tool for distinguishing neuromyelitis optica from multiple sclerosis. *Journals.Sagepub.Com, 20*(5), 558–565. https://doi.org/10.1177/1352458513504638

Niemann, A., Berger, P., & Suter, U. (2006). Pathomechanisms of mutant proteins in Charcot-Marie-Tooth disease. *Neuromolecular Medicine, 8*(1–2), 217–242. https://doi.org/10.1385/nmm:8:1-2:217

Niu, D., Sun, P., Zhang, F., & Song, F. (2022). Metabonomic analysis of cerebrospinal fluid in epilepsy. *Annals of Translational Medicine, 10*(8), 449–449. https://doi.org/10.21037/ATM-22-1219

Ong, C., Damisah, E. C., Gruenbaum, S. E., Dhaher, R., Deng, Y., Sandhu, M. R. S., Zaveri, H. P., Spencer, D. D., & Eid, T. (2021). Increased branched-chain amino acids at baseline and hours before a spontaneous seizure in the human epileptic brain. *Epilepsia, 62*(6), e88–e97. https://doi.org/10.1111/EPI.16920

Pagani, M., Nobili, F., Morbelli, S., Arnaldi, D., Giuliani, A., Öberg, J., Girtler, N., Brugnolo, A., Picco, A., Bauckneht, M., Piva, R., Chincarini, A., Sambuceti, G., Jonsson, C., & De Carli, F. (2017). Early identification of MCI converting to AD: a FDG PET study. *European Journal of Nuclear Medicine and Molecular Imaging, 44*(12), 2042–2052. https://doi.org/10.1007/S00259-017-3761-X

Panov, A., Schonfeld, P., Dikalov, S., Hemendinger, R., Bonkovsky, H. L., & Brooks, B. R. (2009). The neuromediator glutamate, through specific substrate interactions, enhances mitochondrial ATP production and reactive oxygen species generation in nonsynaptic brain mitochondria. *Journal of Biological Chemistry, 284*(21), 14448-14456. https://doi.org/10.1074/jbc.M900985200

Panov, A. V., Kubalik, N., Zinchenko, N., Ridings, D. M., Radoff, D. A., Hemendinger, R., Brooks, B. R., & Bonkovsky, H. L. (2011). Metabolic and functional differences between brain and spinal cord mitochondria underlie different predisposition to pathology. *American Journal of Physiology - Regulatory Integrative and Comparative Physiology, 300*(4), 844–854. https://doi.org/10.1152/AJPREGU.00528.2010

Prescot, A., Becerra, L., Pendse, G., Tully, S., Jensen, E., Hargreaves, R., Renshaw, P., Burstein, R., & Borsook, D. (2009). Excitatory neurotransmitters in brain regions in interictal migraine patients. *Molecular Pain*, *5*, 34. https://doi.org/10.1186/1744-8069-5-34

Regenold, W. T., Phatak, P., Makley, M. J., Stone, R. D., & Kling, M. A. (2008). Cerebrospinal fluid evidence of increased extra-mitochondrial glucose metabolism implicates mitochondrial dysfunction in multiple sclerosis disease progression. *Journal of the neurological sciences*, *275*(1-2), 106–112. https://doi.org/10.1016/j.jns.2008.07.032

Rink, C., & Khanna, S. (2011). Significance of brain tissue oxygenation and the arachidonic acid cascade in stroke. *Antioxidants & redox signaling*, *14*(10), 1889–1903. https://doi.org/10.1089/ars.2010.3474

Rojas, D. R., Kuner, R., & Agarwal, N. (2019). Metabolomic signature of type 1 diabetes-induced sensory loss and nerve damage in diabetic neuropathy. *Journal of Molecular Medicine (Berlin, Germany)*, *97*(6), 845–854. https://doi.org/10.1007/S00109-019-01781-1

Sahni, P. V., Zhang, J., Sosunov, S., Galkin, A., Niatsetskaya, Z., Starkov, A., Brookes, P. S., & Ten, V. S. (2018). Krebs cycle metabolites and preferential succinate oxidation following neonatal hypoxic-ischemic brain injury in mice. *Pediatric Research*, *83*(2), 491–497. https://doi.org/10.1038/PR.2017.277

Shen, H. Y., van Vliet, E. A., Bright, K. A., Hanthorn, M., Lytle, N. K., Gorter, J., Aronica, E., & Boison, D. (2015). Glycine transporter 1 is a target for the treatment of epilepsy. *Neuropharmacology*, *99*, 554–565. https://doi.org/10.1016/j.neuropharm.2015.08.031

Simone, I. L., Federico, F., Trojano, M., Tortorella, C., Liguori, M., Giannini, P., Picciola, E., Natile, G., & Livrea, P. (1996). High resolution proton MR spectroscopy of cerebrospinal fluid in MS patients. Comparison with biochemical changes in demyelinating plaques. *Journal of the neurological sciences*, *144*(1-2), 182–190. https://doi.org/10.1016/s0022-510x(96)00224-9

Sommer, A., Winner, B., & Prots, I. (2017). The Trojan horse - Neuroinflammatory impact of T cells in neurodegenerative diseases. *Molecular Neurodegeneration*, *12*(1). https://doi.org/10.1186/S13024-017-0222-8

Spence, J. D. (2006). Homocysteine and stroke prevention: Have the trials settled the issue? *International Journal of Stroke*, *1*(4), 242–244. https://doi.org/10.1111/J.1747-4949.2006.00057.X

Trupp, M., Jonsson, P., Ohrfelt, A., Zetterberg, H., Obudulu, O., Malm, L., Wuolikainen, A., Linder, J., Moritz, T., Blennow, K., Antti, H., & Forsgren, L. (2014). Metabolite and peptide levels in plasma and CSF differentiating healthy controls from patients with newly diagnosed Parkinson's disease. *Journal of Parkinson's disease*, *4*(3), 549–560. https://doi.org/10.3233/JPD-140389

Underwood, B. R., Broadhurst, D., Dunn, W. B., Ellis, D. I., Michell, A. W., Vacher, C., Mosedale, D. E., Kell, D. B., Barker, R. A., Grainger, D. J., & Rubinsztein, D. C. (2006). Huntington disease patients and transgenic mice have similar pro-catabolic serum metabolite profiles. *Brain*, *129*(4), 877–886. https://doi.org/10.1093/BRAIN/AWL027

Varma, V. R., Oommen, A. M., Varma, S., Casanova, R., An, Y., Andrews, R. M., O'Brien, R., Pletnikova, O., Troncoso, J. C., Toledo, J., Baillie, R., Arnold, M., Kastenmueller, G., Nho, K., Doraiswamy, P. M., Saykin, A. J., Kaddurah-Daouk, R., Legido-Quigley,

C., & Thambisetty, M. (2018). Brain and blood metabolite signatures of pathology and progression in Alzheimer disease: A targeted metabolomics study. *PLoS Medicine*, *15*(1), e1002482. https://doi.org/10.1371/journal.pmed.1002482

Verwaest, K. A., Vu, T. N., Laukens, K., Clemens, L. E., Nguyen, H. P., Van Gasse, B., Martins, J. C., Van Der Linden, A., & Dommisse, R. (2011). (1)H NMR based metabolomics of CSF and blood serum: a metabolic profile for a transgenic rat model of Huntington disease. *Biochimica et biophysica acta*, *1812*(11), 1371–1379. https://doi.org/10.1016/j.bbadis.2011.08.001

Wilkins, J. M., & Trushina, E. (2017). Application of Metabolomics in Alzheimer's Disease. *Frontiers in Neurology*, *8*, 719. https://doi.org/10.3389/fneur.2017.00719

Chapter 16

Metabolomics in Immunology Research

Semih Dalkiliç*, PhD
and Lütfiye Kadioğlu Dalkiliç, PhD
Department of Molecular Biology, Firat University, Elazig, Turkey

Abstract

Metabolomics is the large-scale study of small molecules produced from the metabolic activities of the organism, and these molecules are generally called metabolites. The relationships of these metabolites with each other and with the biological system are called the metabolome. Unlike genomics, proteomics and transcriptomics, metabolomics is a field of study that examines in a broad spectrum of all metabolic activities in organisms. These metabolites are commonly divided into two groups, targeted and untargeted: targeted metabolites are based on quantitative methods that allow the metabolite concentration to be measured; and untargeted metabolites are those that envisage the simultaneous evaluation of large-scale metabolites without any prior sample information to form hypotheses. It is also suitable for describing changes in different pathophysiological conditions. There are many considerations about the functions of metabolic processes and individual metabolites, and important information has been recorded. They have important roles in immune cells. To identify metabolites that explain how the immune system works, the use of mass spectrometry and NMR spectroscopy-based platforms provides important biomarkers of how the immune system functions. This section gives important clues about how metabolomics is used in the immunology field. In particular, future roles of metabolomics in the immune system will be discussed.

---

* Corresponding Author's Email: sdalkilic@firat.edu.tr.

In: Metabolomics and Clinical Approach
Editors: Sevgi Durna Daştan and Taner Daştan
ISBN: 979-8-89113-095-1

Keywords: metabolomics, immune cells, biomarkers, mass spectrometry, immune system

Introduction

Metabolites are small molecules formed by cellular metabolism, which can reflect the results of biochemical reactions, thus allowing information about the physiology of the cell (Liu & Locasale, 2017). It covers the measurement of endogenous, exogenous molecules, and even small molecules at the substrate level in biological systems. Metabolome, on the other hand, is defined as the qualitative and quantitative combination of all low molecular weight molecules that are included in the general metabolic reactions of the cell and are necessary for the proliferation, growth, and normal functioning of the cell (Harrigan & Goodacre, 2003). The size of the metabolome varies according to the organism in which it is found. For example, Saccharomyces cerevisiae contains about 600 metabolites (Förster et al., 2003); however, plants have about 200,000 primary and secondary metabolites (Fiehn, 2002), while the human metabolome is estimated to be larger.

Today, Fourier transform infrared (FT-IR) spectroscopy, NMR, and liquid chromatography-mass spectrometry are used to identify metabolic biomarkers that may change in response to the presence of a disease or in response to drug intervention. Among them, the determination of the effect against biochemical or environmental stress on genetically modified (GM) organisms (Le Gall et al., 2003) and it is also used in bacterial identification and is important in this sense (Vaidyanathan et al., 2002). Recently, there have been new searches for cellular immunometabolism in immunological studies, as well as future prospects. It is in the direction that metabolomics will contribute to immunology research. The metabolome influences the cellular physiology of the genome, epigenome, transcriptome, and proteome through the modulation of omic levels (Rinschen et al., 2019). The mRNA and protein levels studies may not be used to directly determine cellular functions and interactions. In order to determine the response to an environmental stimulus of an organism or a cell, it is necessary to examine the biochemical parameters that constitute the metabolic response, in addition to analyzes at the gene and protein level. Omics provides answers to questions surrounding the biological effects of exposure to environmental factors (Lin et al., 2006).

Relationship of Metabolomics with Immune Diseases

Metabolites are known to be associated with immune diseases. Many studies have been conducted to show that the molecules formed as a result of the metabolic activities of the organism can affect the immune system's activity by affecting the immune system cells. It is important to reveal how these metabolites affect our health, and therefore our immune system, or the relationship of these metabolites with diseases. The determination of metabolites that play a role in the emergence of different diseases and their use as a biomarker that can be used in the diagnosis of diseases constitute the research areas of metabolomics. It has been determined that there is an absolute relationship between metabolites and type 1 diabetes (Galderisi et al., 2018; Sas et al., 2015; Wang et al., 2011). T1D is a chronic autoimmune disease that develops when the insulin-producing cells in the pancreas are damaged and the body cannot produce insulin. Studies have shown that some changes in metabolites are associated with an increased risk of T1D and, as a result of the analysis of metabolites, it has been determined that it facilitates the diagnosis of T1D (Orešič et al., 2013; Pflueger et al., 2011; Sysi-Aho et al., 2011). A study investigated the link between branched-chain amino acids and Type 2 diabetes in overweight children, targeting the total concentration of the three branched-chain amino acids, namely leucine, isoleucine, and valine (McCormack et al., 2013). It was recorded in a cross-sectional cohort study, with the identification of high concentrations of branched-chain amino acids associated with insulin resistance (Savolainen et al., 2017). After all, it is concluded that the density in these branched amino acids is an association among T2D patients. It is known that there is a relationship between chronic lung diseases and metabolites. Some studies using mass spectrometry (MS) have reported changes in the sphingolipid metabolism of chronic obstructive (COPD) patients (Nambiar et al., 2020). Metabolomics is used to investigate many sample types such as plasma, serum, and cerebrospinal fluid in order to obtain fast and efficient results in the use of biomarkers for cylinder purposes (Adamko et al., 2016; Kumar et al., 2017; Locasale et al., 2012). These sample types are very convenient as they are noninvasive. Studies show that diet and bacterial metabolites have an important role in the examination of intestinal and immune balance and immune pathways (Thorburn et al., 2014).

Short chain fatty acids (SCFAs) are among the metabolites with a protective role and have many functions (Thorburn et al., 2014). SCFA are important nutrient sources for intestinal epithelial cells (Martin-Gallausiaux et al., 2021). SFCAs are shown to be among the main metabolites produced in the intestine. The rate of SFCA increases in the dietary intake of fiber. In a study, the stool microbiota of African and European children was compared. *Prevotella* and *Xylanibacter* genera were found in large amounts in the feces of African children, but they were not seen in the feces of European children (De Filippo et al., 2010). Asthma is a heterogeneous and chromic airway disease (Diette et al., 2008; Ober & Hoffjan, 2006). Metabolomics profiles are associated with asthma (Xu et al., 2022). Metabolomics is also used to identify endotypes of asthma.

Methods Used to Determine Metabolomics

Metabolomics of a cell or organism is physiological, metabolic changes in genetic or environmental modulation, similar to the fields of genomics and proteomics, aims to investigate metabolites at certain levels for acquire biological information, and different mechanisms are used to model and determine biological processes (Stanley et al., 2005; Stentiford et al., 2005). Many methods are used for these purposes, such as high-performance liquid chromatography (HPLC), Fourier-converted infrared (FT-IR) spectroscopy, mass spectrometry, and nuclear magnetic resonance (NMR) techniques (Defernez et al., 2004; Gidman et al., 2003; Harrigan et al., 2004; Lenz et al., 2005; Viant et al., 2003; Wilson et al., 2005).

Mass Spectrometry (MS)

MS is the most commonly used technology in metabolomics and, with its selectivity and ability to identify metabolites immediately, it is an accessible analysis method for both qualitative and quantitative analysis. With this method, according to the mass/charge ratio of the ions, it allows them to be easily separated from each other and to work with the detected ions (Dunn & Ellis, 2005).

Nuclear Magnetic Resonance (NMR) Spectroscopy

NMR spectroscopy in metabolomics is a useful method that is very fast in terms of time, highly efficient, and requires minimal sample preparation (Lindon et al., 2003; Reo, 2002). NMR spectroscopy causes the nuclei to affect the nuclear spin of the nucleus in a magnetic field by acting on the nuclear charges of the atoms with strong magnetic fields and radio frequency. Then, the radiation oscillation will be determined by the transition from the low energy spin number to the high energy spin number. *S. cerevisiae* mutants were analyzed by the NMR method, although the enzyme flux was small due to changes in metabolite concentrations (Raamsdonk et al., 2001).

Metabolomics in Uncovering Biomarkers of Immune Responses

It is known that most diseases are caused by the immune system. Metabolomes are important biomarkers in this sense. Examining the metabolites resulting from the activities and interactions of the immune system and using these metabolites as biomarkers in the diagnosis or prognosis of the disease provide important advantages. Profiling metabolomics using NMR spectroscopy constitutes a very important perspective (Altonen et al., 2020; Saric, 2010). Developments in the field of metabolomics have revealed the connection between the cellular and immune systems of conditions that were previously thought to be unrelated to the immune system. Personalized metabolites are important biomarkers for immune parameters in both infectious and non-communicable diseases (Alonso et al., 2016).

Investigation of the Effects of Intracellular Signaling Metabolites on Immune Cell Function

The domain of immunometabolism depends on changes in intracellular metabolism that aid immune cell action and control immune cell functioning. Depending on the effect, immune cells are metabolically reprogrammed to support immune cell tasks such as cytokine production, proliferation, and transfer activities to increase energy demand (O'Neill et al., 2016). All cells that are mobile, immobile, proliferating, reproducing, or activated need to produce ATP and synthesize macromolecules in order to continue their life processes. Cells' needs are fulfilled by interconnected glycolysis, the tricarboxylic acid (TCA) cycle, and oxidative phosphorylation (OXPHOS) (Ganeshan & Chawla, 2014). In immunometabolism, it comprises an effective energy production process by forming a whole with OXPHOS that consumes mitochondrial TCA (Loftus & Finlay, 2016).

Extracellular Vesicles Untargeted Metabolomics Analysis

Extracellular vesicles (EV) are nano-vesicles that have a bilayer lipid layer (Guan et al., 2021). EVs are heterogeneous and are divided into 2 groups: exosomes and micro-vesicles. They also differ from each other in terms of functionality. This difference is also due to the metabolite difference in their composition (Guan et al., 2021). Exosomes, micro-vesicles, and apoptotic bodies play an important role in cell-to-cell signal transmission. They also control biological processes such as immunomodulation, carcinogenesis, and tissue regeneration (Dudzik et al., 2021).

Conclusion

Metabolomics, especially in cancer biology, was used to substantiate hypotheses and identify new avenues of treatments; was used in the study of untargeted LC-HRMS to discover that cancer cells with mutant IDH1 produce 2-hydroxyglutarate, a metabolite found in the spectrum of mutants using LC-HRMS. It has been stated that this metabolite provides a relationship between metabolism and epigenetics (Dang et al., 2009; Lu et al., 2012). Cell and tissue-based metabolomics aims to provide new targets for understanding and interpreting the pathogenesis of disease or disease. Immunometabolism; New therapeutic drug targets and biomarkers that interact with the link between metabolism and the immune system can reveal agents that may be hope for the future where biomarkers are needed (Maas et al., 2022). Amino acids, carbohydrates, lipids, and nucleotides are closely related to the immune system response and molecular mechanisms. Processes, such as diseases and infections, affect this response and the system. Metabolomics research is a promising field in evaluating the host response and determining the metabolites that make this interaction.

References

Adamko, D. J., Saude, E., Bear, M., Regush, S., & Robinson, J. L. (2016). Urine metabolomic profiling of children with respiratory tract infections in the emergency department: a pilot study. *BMC Infect Dis*, *16*(1), 439. https://doi.org/10.1186/s12879-016-1709-6.

Alonso, A., Julià, A., Vinaixa, M., Domènech, E., Fernández-Nebro, A., Cañete, J. D., Ferrándiz, C., Tornero, J., Gisbert, J. P., Nos, P., Casbas, A. G., Puig, L., González-Álvaro, I., Pinto-Tasende, J. A., Blanco, R., Rodríguez, M. A., Beltran, A., Correig, X., Marsal, S., for the IMID Consortium. (2016). Urine metabolome profiling of immune-mediated inflammatory diseases. *BMC Medicine*, *14*(1), 133. https://doi.org/10.1186/s12916-016-0681-8.

Altonen, B. L., Arreglado, T. M., Leroux, O., Murray-Ramcharan, M., & Engdahl, R. (2020). Characteristics, comorbidities and survival analysis of young adults hospitalized with COVID-19 in New York City. *PLOS ONE*, *15*(12), e0243343. https://doi.org/10.1371/journal.pone.0243343.

Dang, L., White, D. W., Gross, S., Bennett, B. D., Bittinger, M. A., Driggers, E. M., Fantin, V. R., Jang, H. G., Jin, S., Keenan, M. C., Marks, K. M., Prins, R. M., Ward, P. S., Yen, K. E., Liau, L. M., Rabinowitz, J. D., Cantley, L. C., Thompson, C. B., Vander Heiden, M. G., & Su, S. M. (2009). Cancer-associated IDH1 mutations produce 2-hydroxyglutarate. *Nature*, *462*(7274), Art. 7274. https://doi.org/10.1038/nature08617.

De Filippo, C., Cavalieri, D., Di Paola, M., Ramazzotti, M., Poullet, J. B., Massart, S., Collini, S., Pieraccini, G., & Lionetti, P. (2010). Impact of diet in shaping gut microbiota revealed by a comparative study in children from Europe and rural Africa. *Proceedings of the National Academy of Sciences*, *107*(33), 14691-14696. https://doi.org/10.1073/pnas.1005963107.

Defernez, M., Gunning, Y. M., Parr, A. J., Shepherd, L. V. T., Davies, H. V., & Colquhoun, I. J. (2004). NMR and HPLC-UV profiling of potatoes with genetic modifications to metabolic pathways. *Journal of Agricultural and Food Chemistry*, *52*(20), 6075-6085. https://doi.org/10.1021/jf049522e.

Diette, G. B., McCormack, M. C., Hansel, N. N., Breysse, P. N., & Matsui, E. C. (2008). Environmental issues in managing asthma. *Respir Care*, *53*(5), 602-615; discussion 616-607.

Dudzik, D., Macioszek, S., Struck-Lewicka, W., Kordalewska, M., Buszewska-Forajta, M., Waszczuk-Jankowska, M., Wawrzyniak, R., Artymowicz, M., Raczak-Gutknecht, J., Siluk, D., & Markuszewski, M. J. (2021). Perspectives and challenges in extracellular vesicles untargeted metabolomics analysis. *TrAC Trends in Analytical Chemistry*, *143*, 116382. https://doi.org/10.1016/j.trac.2021.116382.

Dunn, W. B., & Ellis, D. I. (2005). Metabolomics: current analytical platforms and methodologies. *TrAC Trends in Analytical Chemistry*, *24*(4), 285-294.

Fiehn, O. (2002). Metabolomics - the link between genotypes and phenotypes. *Functional genomics*, 155-171.

Förster, J., Famili, I., Fu, P., Palsson, B. Ø., & Nielsen, J. (2003). Genome-scale reconstruction of the Saccharomyces cerevisiae metabolic network. *Genome research*, *13*(2), 244-253.

Galderisi, A., Pirillo, P., Moret, V., Stocchero, M., Gucciardi, A., Perilongo, G., Moretti, C., Monciotti, C., Giordano, G., & Baraldi, E. (2018). Metabolomics reveals new metabolic perturbations in children with type 1 diabetes. *Pediatric Diabetes*, *19*(1), 59-67. https://doi.org/10.1111/pedi.12524.

Ganeshan, K., & Chawla, A. (2014). Metabolic Regulation of Immune Responses. *Annual Review of Immunology*, *32*(1), 609-634. https://doi.org/10.1146/annurev-immunol-032713-120236.

Gidman, E., Goodacre, R., Emmett, B., Smith, A. R., & Gwynn-Jones, D. (2003). Investigating plant-plant interference by metabolic fingerprinting. *Phytochemistry*, *63*(6), 705-710. https://doi.org/10.1016/s0031-9422(03)00288-7.

Guan, F., Xiang, X., Xie, Y., Li, H., Zhang, W., Shu, Y., Wang, J., & Qin, W. (2021). Simultaneous metabolomics and proteomics analysis of plasma-derived extracellular vesicles. *Analytical Methods*, *13*(16), 1930-1938. https://doi.org/10.1039/D1AY 00060H.

Harrigan, G. G., & Goodacre, R. (2003). *Metabolic profiling: its role in biomarker discovery and gene function analysis: its role in biomarker discovery and gene function analysis*. Springer Science & Business Media.

Harrigan, G. G., LaPlante, R. H., Cosma, G. N., Cockerell, G., Goodacre, R., Maddox, J. F., Luyendyk, J. P., Ganey, P. E., & Roth, R. A. (2004). Application of high-throughput Fourier-transform infrared spectroscopy in toxicology studies: Contribution to a study on the development of an animal model for idiosyncratic toxicity. *Toxicology Letters*, *146*(3), 197-205. https://doi.org/10.1016/j.toxlet.2003. 09.011.

Kumar, N., Shahjaman, M., Mollah, M. N. H., Islam, S. M. S., & Hoque, M. A. (2017). Serum and Plasma Metabolomic Biomarkers for Lung Cancer. *Bioinformation*, *13*(6), 202-208. https://doi.org/10.6026/97320630013202.

Le Gall, G., Colquhoun, I. J., Davis, A. L., Collins, G. J., & Verhoeyen, M. E. (2003). Metabolite Profiling of Tomato (Lycopersicon esculentum) Using 1H NMR Spectroscopy as a Tool To Detect Potential Unintended Effects Following a Genetic Modification. *Journal of Agricultural and Food Chemistry*, *51*(9), 2447-2456. https://doi.org/10.1021/jf0259967.

Lenz, E. M., Weeks, J. M., Lindon, J. C., Osborn, D., & Nicholson, J. K. (2005). Qualitative high field 1H-NMR spectroscopy for the characterization of endogenous metabolites in earthworms with biochemical biomarker potential. *Metabolomics*, *1*(2), 123-136. https://doi.org/10.1007/s11306-005-4435-4.

Lin, C. Y., Viant, M. R., & Tjeerdema, R. S. (2006). Metabolomics: Methodologies and applications in the environmental sciences. *Journal of Pesticide Science*, *31*(3), 245-251. https://doi.org/10.1584/jpestics.31.245.

Lindon, J. C., Holmes, E., & Nicholson, J. K. (2003). Peer reviewed: so what's the deal with metabonomics? *Analytical chemistry*, *75*(17), 384 A-391 A. https://doi.org/10. 1021/ac031386+.

Liu, X., & Locasale, J. W. (2017). Metabolomics: A Primer. *Trends in Biochemical Sciences*, *42*(4), 274-284. https://doi.org/10.1016/j.tibs.2017.01.004.

Locasale, J. W., Melman, T., Song, S., Yang, X., Swanson, K. D., Cantley, L. C., Wong, E. T., & Asara, J. M. (2012). Metabolomics of Human Cerebrospinal Fluid Identifies Signatures of Malignant Glioma. *Molecular & Cellular Proteomics : MCP*, *11*(6), M111.014688. https://doi.org/10.1074/mcp.M111.014688.

Loftus, R. M., & Finlay, D. K. (2016). Immunometabolism: Cellular Metabolism Turns Immune Regulator*. *Journal of Biological Chemistry*, *291*(1), 1-10. https://doi.org/10.1074/jbc.R115.693903.

Lu, C., Ward, P. S., Kapoor, G. S., Rohle, D., Turcan, S., Abdel-Wahab, O., Edwards, C. R., Khanin, R., Figueroa, M. E., Melnick, A., Wellen, K. E., O'Rourke, D. M., Berger, S. L., Chan, T. A., Levine, R. L., Mellinghoff, I. K., & Thompson, C. B. (2012). IDH mutation impairs histone demethylation and results in a block to cell differentiation. *Nature*, *483*(7390), Art. 7390. https://doi.org/10.1038/nature10860.

Maas, P., Hartog, I. den, Kindt, A., Boman, S., Hankemeier, T., & Hasselt, C. van. (2022). The Immunometabolic Atlas: A tool for design and interpretation of metabolomics studies in immunology. *PLOS ONE*, *17*(5), e0268408. https://doi.org/10.1371/journal.pone.0268408.

Martin-Gallausiaux, C., Marinelli, L., Blottière, H. M., Larraufie, P., & Lapaque, N. (2021). SCFA: mechanisms and functional importance in the gut. *Proc Nutr Soc*, *80*(1), 37-49. https://doi.org/10.1017/s0029665120006916.

McCormack, S. E., Shaham, O., McCarthy, M. A., Deik, A. A., Wang, T. J., Gerszten, R. E., Clish, C. B., Mootha, V. K., Grinspoon, S. K., & Fleischman, A. (2013). Circulating branched-chain amino acid concentrations are associated with obesity and future insulin resistance in children and adolescents. *Pediatric Obesity*, *8*(1), 52-61. https://doi.org/10.1111/j.2047-6310.2012.00087.x.

Nambiar, S., Bong How, S., Gummer, J., Trengove, R., & Moodley, Y. (2020). Metabolomics in chronic lung diseases. *Respirology*, *25*(2), 139-148. https://doi.org/10.1111/resp.13530.

O'Neill, L. A. J., Kishton, R. J., & Rathmell, J. (2016). A guide to immunometabolism for immunologists. *Nature Reviews Immunology*, *16*(9), Art. 9. https://doi.org/10.1038/nri.2016.70.

Ober, C., & Hoffjan, S. (2006). Asthma genetics 2006: The long and winding road to gene discovery. *Genes & Immunity*, *7*(2), Art. 2. https://doi.org/10.1038/sj.gene.6364284.

Orešič, M., Gopalacharyulu, P., Mykkänen, J., Lietzen, N., Mäkinen, M., Nygren, H., Simell, S., Simell, V., Hyöty, H., Veijola, R., Ilonen, J., Sysi-Aho, M., Knip, M., Hyötyläinen, T., & Simell, O. (2013). Cord Serum Lipidome in Prediction of Islet Autoimmunity and Type 1 Diabetes. *Diabetes*, *62*(9), 3268. https://doi.org/10.2337/db13-0159.

Pflueger, M., Seppänen-Laakso, T., Suortti, T., Hyötyläinen, T., Achenbach, P., Bonifacio, E., Orešič, M., & Ziegler, A.-G. (2011). Age- and Islet Autoimmunity–Associated Differences in Amino Acid and Lipid Metabolites in Children at Risk for Type 1 Diabetes. *Diabetes*, *60*(11), 2740-2747. https://doi.org/10.2337/db10-1652.

Raamsdonk, L. M., Teusink, B., Broadhurst, D., Zhang, N., Hayes, A., Walsh, M. C., Berden, J. A., Brindle, K. M., Kell, D. B., Rowland, J. J., Westerhoff, H. V., van Dam, K., & Oliver, S. G. (2001). A functional genomics strategy that uses metabolome data to reveal the phenotype of silent mutations. *Nature Biotechnology*, *19*(1), Art. 1. https://doi.org/10.1038/83496.

Reo, N. V. (2002). NMR-based metabolomics. *Drug and chemical toxicology*, *25*(4), 375-382.

Rinschen, M. M., Ivanisevic, J., Giera, M., & Siuzdak, G. (2019). Identification of bioactive metabolites using activity metabolomics. *Nat Rev Mol Cell Biol*, *20*(6), 353-367. https://doi.org/10.1038/s41580-019-0108-4.

Saric, J. (2010). Interactions between immunity and metabolism – contributions from the metabolic profiling of parasite-rodent models. *Parasitology*, *137*(9), 1451-1466. https://doi.org/10.1017/S0031182010000697.

Sas, K. M., Karnovsky, A., Michailidis, G., & Pennathur, S. (2015). Metabolomics and diabetes: analytical and computational approaches. *Diabetes*, *64*(3), 718-732. https://doi.org/10.2337/db14-0509.

Savolainen, O., Fagerberg, B., Vendelbo Lind, M., Sandberg, A. S., Ross, A. B., & Bergström, G. (2017). Biomarkers for predicting type 2 diabetes development-Can metabolomics improve on existing biomarkers? *PloS one*, *12*(7), e0177738. https://doi.org/10.1371/journal.pone.0177738.

Stanley, E. G., Bailey, N. J. C., Bollard, M. E., Haselden, J. N., Waterfield, C. J., Holmes, E., & Nicholson, J. K. (2005). Sexual dimorphism in urinary metabolite profiles of Han Wistar rats revealed by nuclear-magnetic-resonance-based metabonomics. *Analytical Biochemistry*, *343*(2), 195-202. https://doi.org/10.1016/j.ab.2005.01.024.

Stentiford, G. d., Viant, M. r., Ward, D. g., Johnson, P. j., Martin, A., Wenbin, W., Cooper, H. J., Lyons, B. P., & Feist, S. W. (2005). Liver Tumors in Wild Flatfish: A Histopathological, Proteomic, and Metabolomic Study. *OMICS: A Journal of Integrative Biology*, *9*(3), 281-299. https://doi.org/10.1089/omi.2005.9.281.

Sysi-Aho, M., Ermolov, A., Gopalacharyulu, P. V., Tripathi, A., Seppänen-Laakso, T., Maukonen, J., Mattila, I., Ruohonen, S. T., Vähätalo, L., Yetukuri, L., Härkönen, T., Lindfors, E., Nikkilä, J., Ilonen, J., Simell, O., Saarela, M., Knip, M., Kaski, S., Savontaus, E., & Orešič, M. (2011). Metabolic Regulation in Progression to Autoimmune Diabetes. *PLOS Computational Biology*, *7*(10), e1002257. https://doi.org/10.1371/journal.pcbi.1002257.

Thorburn, A. N., Macia, L., & Mackay, C. R. (2014). Diet, metabolites, and "western-lifestyle" inflammatory diseases. *Immunity*, *40*(6), 833-842. https://doi.org/10.1016/j.immuni.2014.05.014.

Vaidyanathan, S., Kell, D. B., & Goodacre, R. (2002). Flow-injection electrospray ionization mass spectrometry of crude cell extracts for high-throughput bacterial identification. *Journal of the American Society for Mass Spectrometry*, *13*(2), 118-128. https://doi.org/10.1016/S1044-0305(01)00339-7.

Viant, M. R., Rosenblum, E. S., & Tjeerdema, R. S. (2003). NMR-Based Metabolomics: A Powerful Approach for Characterizing the Effects of Environmental Stressors on Organism Health. *Environmental Science & Technology*, *37*(21), 4982-4989. https://doi.org/10.1021/es034281x.

Wang, T. J., Larson, M. G., Vasan, R. S., Cheng, S., Rhee, E. P., McCabe, E., Lewis, G. D., Fox, C. S., Jacques, P. F., Fernandez, C., O'Donnell, C. J., Carr, S. A., Mootha, V. K., Florez, J. C., Souza, A., Melander, O., Clish, C. B., & Gerszten, R. E. (2011). Metabolite profiles and the risk of developing diabetes. *Nature Medicine*, *17*(4), Art. 4. https://doi.org/10.1038/nm.2307.

Wilson, I. D., Plumb, R., Granger, J., Major, H., Williams, R., & Lenz, E. M. (2005). HPLC-MS-based methods for the study of metabonomics. *Journal of Chromatography B*, *817*(1), 67-76. https://doi.org/10.1016/j.jchromb.2004.07.045.

Xu, S., Panettieri, R. A., Jr., & Jude, J. (2022). Metabolomics in asthma: A platform for discovery. *Mol Aspects Med*, *85*, 100990. https://doi.org/10.1016/j.mam.2021.100990.

Chapter 17

The Clinical Uses of Mass Spectrometry-Based Approaches in Neurology and Psychiatry

Suna Dagli Atalay*, **MD**
Department of Neurology, Kayseri Training and Research Hospital, Kayseri, Turkey

Abstract

Neurological and psychiatric diseases and disorders remain great public health hazards. There is a need for research for their early diagnosis and for developing more effective treatment approaches. In neurological and psychiatric diseases, which are multifactorial conditions without a single gene mutation, metabolomics is important for a holistic assessment. Nuclear magnetic resonance (NMR)-based and chromatography/mass spectrometry-based approaches can be clinically applied to assess the metabolome. MS has become significantly important in biological and biomedical research in the last 20 years. Ionization sources, matrix-assisted laser desorption/ionization (MALDI), secondary ion mass spectrometry (SIMS), and desorption electrospray ionization (DESI), are now included in the most important mass spectrometry imaging (IMS) studies. The ability to identify the spatial distribution of hundreds of analytes in a single imaging study without needing a label or preliminary information is one of the main advantages of MALDI-IMS over other imaging methods. Studies using MALDI-IMS have been conducted to better understand the cellular pathology and/or severity of the disease in neurology and psychiatry. Moreover, MALDI-IMS has enabled the matching of specific classes of analytes with brain regions that may have been lost using more traditional methods. The clinical uses of mass spectrometry-based approaches in neurology and psychiatry will be addressed in this section.

* Corresponding Author's Email: suna33@gmail.com.

In: Metabolomics and Clinical Approach
Editors: Sevgi Durna Daştan and Taner Daştan
ISBN: 979-8-89113-095-1

Keywords: mass spectrometry; neurology; psychiatry

Introduction

Nowadays, it is reported that only genome or proteome analysis is inadequate to clarify the molecular mechanism of any disease; alternatively, more realistic results are obtained from a holistic assessment, which also involves metabolomic studies (Fiehn, 2001; Ibanez et al., 2012). Metabolomics has the potential to diagnose diseases, classify subjects in a heterogeneous patient population, monitor the effectiveness of treatment and the progression of disease, and identify novel therapeutic goals (Nordström and Lewensohn, 2010; Abu-Asab et al., 2011). Almost all of them are significant characteristics for psychiatric and neurological diseases, multifactorial circumstances without single gene mutation. Considering a high increase in diseases, it is urgently necessary to better understand the mechanisms related to endogenous metabolism. Untargeted and targeted metabolomics are two different approaches for measuring metabolites in biological materials.

Untargeted Metabolomics

It represents the detailed analysis of all measurable analytes in a sample, regardless of their identity. The fact that it is agnostic in metabolome measurement is one of the benefits of this approach. Thus, it allows discovery of new or unexpected molecules for further studies. Its biggest disadvantage is that it has a natural bias for detecting large amounts of molecules. There are difficulties in processing and interpreting data since each sample analysis produces large amounts of data that can be both complex and time-consuming. The identification of each metabolite measured requires database searching, and there is usually a need for more experimental studies to verify the full identity of a relevant signal.

Targeted Metabolomics

It involves measuring a predefined set of chemically characterized metabolites to cover a selected part of the metabolome. The metabolites measured represent only a subset of those to be measured with a non-targeted approach. Hence, a targeted approach generates a much smaller data series in which individual metabolites are detected with higher confidence. The metabolome is composed of a series of various biomolecules, the end products of transcription, translation, and protein activities, and mentions the complete set of small molecule metabolites (e.g., metabolic intermediates, hormones, and other signaling molecules and secondary metabolites) (<1.5 KDa) that are presented in a biological pattern such as a single organism. A single analytical platform cannot sample the whole metabolome/lipidome due to the chemical variety of the said metabolites. Mass spectrometry approaches are among the most trustworthy analytical platforms that ensure precise and structural quantitative data for complicated biological samples (Koal and Deigner, 2010; Dudley et al., 2010).

In addition to the ongoing development of new techniques for assessing the metabolome, the current clinically applicable approaches can be divided into two broad categories as nuclear magnetic resonance (NMR)-based and chromatography/mass spectrometry (MS)-based approaches. Both approaches have advantages and disadvantages (Mishur and Rea, 2012).

MS-based metabolomics has been utilized in various areas of disease research. Nevertheless, it is a difficult and long process to investigate metabolites in-depth. For multi-omic studies in neurology, mass spectrometry imaging (IMS) seems a strong instrument. IMS combines the multichannel (m/z) measurement capacity of mass spectrometers and a surface sampling process allowing for the quick investigation and mapping of intact proteins, released glycans, proteolytic digested peptides, glycolipids, small metabolites and phospholipids in brain tissues (Xu and Li, 2019). MS is regarded as a multipurpose instrument with high sensitivity and specificity and is frequently used worldwide. MS technology has been implemented in different main disciplines that ensure technical support for identifying and exploring endogenous substances in living beings (Yang et al., 2019). It is possible to combine all chemical isolation techniques, such as capillary electrophoresis (CE) or gas-liquid chromatography (GC) and liquid-chromatography (LC) with MS detection (König, 2011). Some sources of ionization in MS have the ability to ionize molecules. Matrix-assisted laser desorption/ionization (MALDI), desorption electrospray ionization (DESI), and secondary ion mass spectrometry (SIMS) are now included as ionization sources in the most important IMSI studies (Buchberger et al., 2018; Chandra et al., 2000; Cooks et al., 2006).

Mass Spectrometry Approach in Neurology

Neurological diseases are important health problems, and there is a need for research to improve early diagnosis and/or develop more efficient treatment approaches. Despite the presence of numerous imaging methods and techniques to investigate the mentioned diseases, the available approaches are usually costly and time-consuming. MALDI-IMS represents a label-free, creative, and ever-developing technique for tissue histopathology generating 2D ion density maps that represent the dispersion of an analyte across a tissue section. The ability to identify the spatial dispersion of hundreds of analytes in one imaging study without needing any preliminary information is one of the primary advantages of MALDI-IMS over other imaging modalities (Schnackenberg et al., 2022). Despite the fact that MALDI-IMS was basically developed for the spatial profiling of peptides and proteins, it can detect N-linked glycans, lipids, neurotransmitters, metabolites, and small molecule drugs (Ryan, 2019). Moreover, MALDI-IMS has the ability to detect hundreds of analytes at the same time in one imaging study. The increased productivity has led IMS to become effective in numerous disciplines, such as psychiatry and neurology (Chen et al., 2019). MALDI-IMS is quite appropriate for detecting lipid types long associated with neurological diseases, such as Parkinson's, Huntington's, Alzheimer's, and multiple sclerosis. Many lipids are ionized because a phosphate group or nitrogen center is present, resulting in the abundant detection of negative or positive ions by MALDI. The majority of lipids have molecular weights below 1000 DA, the mass range ensuring the ultimate sensitivity in MS. Therefore, incorporating IMS platforms into neurological research has provided a comprehensive assessment of diseases by brain regions and the matching of specific classes of lipids to disease-relevant brain regions (Zemski, 2011; Shariatgorji et al., 2014).

Alternative ionization approaches are available in IMS, which have demonstrated that different applications, e.g., desorption electrospray ionization (DESI) and secondary ion mass spectrometry (SIMS), are also useful. DESI imaging has been employed for assessing lipid dynamics in vascular dementia rat models, metabolite and lipid profiles in human brain tumors, and chemical dynamics in fetal pig brain development (Severiano et al., 2020; Jarmusch et al., 2016). SIMS imaging has been used in clinical samples taken from Alzheimer's patients, in addition to many studies on protein and lipid localization in the brains of Alzheimer's disease animal models. Unlike other ionization approaches, an energy-absorbing matrix is needed in MALDI. Nevertheless, MALDI is the most commonly used method, although a matrix material is needed for ionization (Carlred et al., 2014; Lazar et al., 2012).

Stroke

Cell death occurs immediately because of the interrupted blood flow to the brain. The researchers focused on imaging gangliosides, involved in the formation of brain disease following a stroke. MALDI-IMS was implemented as a novel instrument for better investigation of gangliosides in stroke. In the early assessment of gangliosides using MALDI-IMS, it was found that stroke is caused by middle cerebral artery occlusion (MCAO) in mice. After injury and reperfusion, mice were sacrificed at different time points from MCAO to day 28. Unique profiles of various ganglioside types, including disialotetrahexosylganglioside (GD), trisialotetrahexosyl ganglioside (GT1b), mono-sialotetrahexosylganglioside (GM1), mono sialotrihexosylganglioside (GM2), and monosialodihexosylgaglycoside (GM3), the highest expression of the brain regions and the changes occurring 3-7 days after reperfusion related to secondary neuron death and neuroinflammation, respectively, were evaluated. The research results verified previous studies describing GM1 in white matter tracts and GD1a in the gray matter after stroke and detected GM2 and GM3 in the gray matter at the border of the infarcted region for the first time (Whitehead et al., 2011). It has been reported that post-stroke, GM1 and GD1 decrease in brain tissue, ganglioside disorder occurs, and GM2 and GM3 accumulate specifically in brain tissue (Caughlin et al., 2019).

The MALDI-IMS platforms were also used to investigate the effect of stroke on other types of lipids. In a study in which MALDI-IMS was used with in vivo PET imaging to evaluate lipids after stroke recovery, stroke-induced lipid changes were detected (Henderson et al., 2018). Especially 1-palitoyl-2-hydroxy-sn-glycero-3-phosphocol (LPC 16:0) and sphingomyelin (SM) N-palmitoyl D-erythro-sphingosylphosphorylcholine (SM d18:1/16:0) indicated up-regulation at the injury site three months after stroke. 1-palmitoyl-2-oleoyl-glycero-3-phosphocholine (16:0/18:1 PC, POPC), phosphatidylcholines (PCs), and 1,2-dipalmitoyl sn-glycero-3-phosphocholine (16: 0/16:0 PC, DPPC found in healthy tissue) indicated down-regulation at the scar site. It is impossible to determine lipids using other imaging methods such as MRI and PET; therefore, in lipidomic brain studies, this work emphasizes an important advantage of using MALDI-IMS (Henderson et al., 2018). Mulder et al. (Mulder et al., 2019) used the mentioned approach to assess lipids in healthy tissue within, adjacent to, and surrounding the infarct core of mouse brains collected following transient MCAO (tMCAO)-induced stroke. The findings revealed an increase in sodium species of LPCs and PCs according to potassium species in the infarct core in the first 24 hours after a stroke. Another study used MALDI-IMS to assess alterations in the brains of wild-type mice after N-methyl-D-aspartate receptor (NMDA) subunit GluN2D knockdown (GluN2D-/-) and MCAO-induced stroke. The NMDA receptor-mediated neuronal death was determined after ischemic stroke (Andrews et al., 2020). The changes in endogenous analytes in brain tissue after stroke and the impacts of the suggested stroke treatments were evaluated by MALDI-IMS studies. A neuroprotective agent should cross the blood-brain barrier (BBB) to be able to protect against ischemic conditions, e.g., stroke. In their study, Wang et al. (Wang et al., 2018) showed the potential of IMS to assess the uptake and effects of drugs in brain tissue. The therapeutic effect of chloroquine after stroke was researched. Chloroquine accumulation in lysosomes disrupts the normal function of enzymes that catabolize complex gangliosides. Therefore, chloroquine can prevent ganglioside dysregulation and inhibit the catabolism of gangliosides after stroke. In the current research, chloroquine pretreatment was shown to prevent GM2 and GM3 upgradings and consumption of GD1 and GM1 after a stroke (Caughlin et al., 2019). Recently, MALDI-IMS has also been used to assess alterations in brain metabolites and the impacts of cell therapies after neonatal stroke. Either mesenchymal stem/stromal cells (MSCs) or CD43+ cells were administered intravenously forty-eight hours after stroke induction by MCAO, and all metabolites except glucose decreased significantly in the infarct core after MCAO. Glucose, carnitine, and glutamate increased significantly in the peri-infarct regions (0.4 mm border of infarct) (Tanaka et al., 2020).

Multiple Sclerosis

Multiple sclerosis represents a debilitating disease when the central nervous system (CNS) is attacked by the immune system of the body. The formation of demyelinating lesions in the brain is one of the characteristics of multiple sclerosis. Nevertheless, the occurrence and repair mechanisms of the lesions have not been well understood. Axons are protected by the remyelination of lesions, and the hypothesis that the degree of remyelination can affect the severity of the disease in subjects has been established. For the purpose of better understanding the roles of certain proteins in multiple sclerosis, IMS was used to evaluate peptides in brain tissues after death, taken from diagnosed patients (Maccarrone et al., 2017). The research aimed to detect dissimilarly expressed proteins and peptides in normal white matter, gray matter, and lesions associated with multiple sclerosis. Depending on the degree of myelination, different patterns of proteins and peptides were demonstrated. Plaques with low remyelination levels were related to 7 low molecular weight compounds that could be protein degradation products. From the MALDI-IMS dataset, the patterns of protein/peptide changes also showed the existence of cortical lesions, but the normal histological analysis could not detect lesions; however, their existence was confirmed by immunostaining. Furthermore, while the peptide, thymosin beta-4, was found in partially remyelinated lesions in white matter, it was not identified in completely remyelinated lesions. It has been demonstrated that thymosin beta-4 plays a role in cell migration and can be involved in the differentiation of oligodendrocyte progenitor cells to induce lesion remyelination (Maccarrone et al., 2017). IMS was used to research the impacts on demyelination/remyelination and especially lipid composition in a multiple sclerosis mouse model. Myelin is rich in lipids, and it has been indicated that changes in lipid profiles are involved in multiple sclerosis (Sekera et al., 2020; Grajchen et al., 2018). Bowman et al. (Bowman et al., 2020) assessed the distribution of lipids in brain tissue taken from post-mortem patients with active multiple sclerosis lesions. By conducting histological analysis, they revealed that lipid signals were associated with cellular-level characteristics, such as cell nuclei, neutral lipids, CD68, monocyte lineage protein cluster, and myelinated areas.

Teriflunomide, an immunomodulatory agent, has been approved in the United States and Europe for the treatment of recurrent forms of multiple sclerosis. It has been argued by the studies that the drug may have a direct impact on the CNS compartment due to the ability of the drug to cross the BBB. The impacts of the drug on brain metabolites were evaluated after a four-day treatment to assess the ability of the teriflunomide to cross the BBB, and imaging findings revealed that the drug could not reach the CNS compartment. Nevertheless, endogenous metabolites in the brain were affected by drug administration. Among the twenty-four metabolites assessed, considerable alterations were observed in mice administered teriflunomide for the adenine and uracil nucleotides, uridine diphosphate (UDP)-glucose, glucose-6-phosphate, and glutathione. Because the imaging findings show that the drug did not cross the BBB, it is likely that the changed metabolites are due to drug administration, which is due to an indirect mechanism of action that remains uncertain. Furthermore, it was assumed that an indirect mechanism might probably involve drug interaction with cells that line the BBB and therefore activate CNS cells (Rzagalinski et al., 2019).

Parkinson's Disease

Parkinson's disease (PD) represents a neurodegenerative disease, which impacts movement and is usually described as a dopamine deficiency disorder. Moreover, different non-dopamine neurotransmitter systems are impacted at motor onset and become more apparent with the disease progression (Perry et al., 1991). In 2012, a MALDI-IMS study was carried out to clarify the site-specific distribution profiles of neuropeptides in the rat brain of a PD animal model (Hanrieder et al., 2012). Concerning neuropeptide characterization, MALDI-IMS reveals novel molecular mechanisms of neuropeptide modulation of neuronal transmission and has advantages, especially in determining unknown peptide processing products. On the other hand, conventionally utilized antibody-based approaches aimed at previously observed post-translational changes and known peptide sequences. In the present research, MALDI IMS investigated a relationship between des-tyrosine alpha-neoendorphine levels and the severity of dyskinesia. It has been reported that removing N-terminal tyrosine may represent a previously unknown mechanism of functional inactivation of dynorphins in the striatum since it reduces the opioid-receptor binding of dynorphin (Hanrieder et al., 2012). PD represents a degenerative brain disease that impacts nerve cells in the substantia nigra and basal ganglia. Because the neurotransmitter dopamine is generated by nerve cells in the substantia nigra, there is great interest in monitoring neurotransmitter distribution in the brain concerning disease development. It has historically been challenging to reach this by means of MALDI-IMS. Nevertheless, a MALDI-IMS method has recently been developed to obtain a comprehensive map of neurotransmitter networks using Parkinson's brain samples from postmortem human tissues and animal models (Shariatgorji et al., 2019).

Alzheimer's Disease

Alzheimer's disease (AD) represents a lethal neurodegenerative disease, which demolishes important mental functions, especially memory. The high levels of amyloid-β (Aβ, beta-amyloid) peptides forming Aβ plaques and accumulated hyperphosphorylated tau protein inducing neurofibrillary tangles (NFTs) in the brain are the main neuropathological characteristics of AD. Moreover, in recent years, studies have strongly indicated that lipids play a very important role in AD pathology (Chew et al., 2020). There have been quite a low number of tools to evaluate lipids in tissues until recent times. MALDI-IMS was applied for the investigation of both AD-related peptides and lipids and is an advantageous tool for increasing knowledge about the disease in question, considering that it is capable of visualizing the spatial dispersion of analytes. MALDI-IMS was used to show the spatial dispersion of a wide variety of Aβ species in the autopsied brains of humans. It was found that the accumulation profile of Aβ1-41 was largely different in its accumulation capacity from Aβ1-42, which was demonstrated to determine the location of accumulation of the C-terminus of the Aβ structure in AD brains. The distribution of various types of Aβ was also revealed in the same parts of autopsied human brains without particular probes (Kakuda et al., 2017). A new three-mode, high-resolution (10 μm) MALDI-IMS method was developed by another group for the analysis of both lipids and proteins in the identical tissue section. When the above-mentioned method was performed on a transgenic AD mouse model, the co-localization of plaque-associated Aβ isoforms and different lipid species was revealed (Kaya et al., 2017a; Kaya et al., 2017b). With increasing evidence, since lipids have been shown to be involved in the pathology of AD, the usage of MALDI-IMS to detect AD-associated lipids has appeared. A protocol using MALDI-IMS was published for spatial mapping of lipids in brain tissues from the brains of patients with Alzheimer's disease and normal human brains (O'Rourke et al., 2019). The expression of two different types of lipids was shown in the gray and white matter of the inferior temporal gyrus (ITG) of a patient with AD compared to a neurologically normal individual. Human hippocampus samples were analyzed with the objective of identifying 43 lipids that differed considerably between AD and normal tissue. It was concluded in further imaging research that the majority of the alterations noticed in AD brains were specific to the dentate gyrus (DG) and cornu ammonis (CA1) regions, and it was hypothesized that each hippocampal subarea had its own function (Mendis et al., 2016). Lipid changes are likely to be specific to every region of the brain. MALDI-IMS will continue to participate in attempts to support identifying AD-related peptides and enhancing new therapies for the treatment of AD.

Epilepsy

Childhood absence epilepsy (CAE) has a genetic source known to be associated with mutations in genes involved in the calcium, sodium, and potassium channels and in GABAA receptor subunit genes. In children, CAE may lead to behavioral, cognitive, and emotional disorders. Few studies assessed protein alterations in CAE models. An IMS approach was used with the objective of visualizing the potential protein markers of CAE along the intact brain section using mouse BS/Orl and BR/Orl strains. Two strains revealed contrasting epileptic characteristics with BS/Orl (Lagarrigue et al., 2012).

Amyotrophic Lateral Sclerosis (ALS)

Few metabolomic studies have been conducted on ALS. In an untargeted metabolomic assessment of ALS plasma, reductions in 4-vinylphenol sulfate and catechol sulfate were measured. They are microbial host metabolites in that vinyl phenol and catechol represent microbial metabolites of the gastrointestinal flora. However, these metabolites are sulfated in the human liver (Lawton et al., 2012).

Genetic Diseases

Most studies have focused on changes in lipid profiles. A recent study used LC/MS and IMS to assess glycosphingolipids (GSL) in the brains of mice with Gaucher disease. Gaucher disease increases the risk of developing Lewy body disease and Parkinson's disease. The accumulation of GSL species (possibly associated with a mutation in GBA1) has been correlated with Gaucher disease. Nevertheless, the relationship between GSL accumulation and disease pathology is not clearly understood. Jones et al., used a Farber's disease murine model and introduced an IMS method to detect ceramides in kidney tissue. Ceramides were not previously determined in the tissue by employing other imaging methods (Jones et al., 2017).

Mass Spectrometry Approach in Psychiatry

Recently, there has been an increase in attempts to discuss psychiatric disorders at the molecular level to understand the relevant molecular and pathophysiological mechanisms. An attempt to explore presumed biomarkers specific to psychiatric disorders was an important step (Alawieh et al., 2012). Biomarker investigation mainly uses "omic" technologies (genomic, transcriptomic and proteomic), as demonstrated, for example, in the transcriptomic profiling of mood disorders or psychosis and the proteomic profiling of bipolar disorder (Herberth, 2011; Kurian et al., 2011). Proteomics began to be increasingly studied, although transcriptomics and genomics were among the first tools used. Nevertheless, there are individual and common advantages and difficulties in all approaches. Confirming or validating the identified proteins is a common difficulty for both proteomics and genomics (Schmidt et al., 2011).

Psychiatric disorders may inherently have an adaptive pathway that regulates down-regulation of multiple genes through epigenetic mechanisms. For example, it is argued that DNA methylations or histone modifications combined with glutamatergic and GABAergic gene promoters are crucial in the pathogenesis of bipolar disorder and schizophrenia, as indicated by reduced protein levels of GABAergic neuronal markers (RELN, glutamic acid decarboxylase, and reelin). In psychiatric disorders, there are numerous possible genetic sources from which biomarkers can be obtained. Nevertheless, non-genomic biomarkers, including peptide/protein biomarkers, are also promising. Differential gel-based quantitative proteomics is an available common approach in the mass spectrometric characterization of proteins (Unlu et al., 1997). It is composed of separating samples (from controls with defects and influenced) by gel electrophoresis (usually 2D-gel electrophoresis). Then, the gel bands are analyzed by MS/LC-MS and tryptic digestion for protein quantification and identification. Ditzen et al. (Ditzen et al., 2006) identified enolase phosphatase (EP) and glyoxalase I (GLX1) as protein markers that might be risk markers for anxiety in a trait anxiety mouse model. In a different study, the said technique was employed for the identification of 59 potential biomarkers in the cerebral cortex and 11 in the amygdala in the postmortem brain tissue of suicide victims (Kékesi et al., 2012). Most of the said proteins have already been suggested as psychiatric protein biomarkers. In another research concentrating on major depressive disorder (MDD) in a rat model, MALDI-TOF-MS and 2D-gel were used to identify 27 potential protein markers with roles in oxidative metabolism, transcription, neurogenesis, and signal transduction (Mu et al., 2007). The exact molecular etiology and a different definition of many psychiatric disorders have not yet been well identified. Thus, there is a great requirement to discover new proteins and molecular biomarkers for monitoring, forecasting, categorizing, or treating psychiatric disorders (Roy et al., 2012).

The presence of sufficient model systems that fully mimic pathophysiological conditions in the brain is another difficulty. Neuropsychiatric and cognitive symptoms, e.g., hallucinations or suicidal thoughts, are difficult to evaluate in any model organism. With regard to human research, the problem is the presence of well-characterized human material obtained following international standard protocols. Furthermore, there is a need for large sample pools for highly efficient analyses and data, as well as because of individual variability. Concerning databases, programs, or software utilized in proteomics and genomics, well-characterized and identified genes and proteins have a higher risk of detection compared to those having unknown functions (Ngounou Wetie et al., 2013).

MS may and will take an essential part in detecting psychiatric biomarkers. There have been some innovations and developments in the area of MS, particularly, and proteomics, in general. Elevated machine sensitivity that allows detecting proteins present at low concentrations and advanced software that allows not only protein detection but also the analysis of the whole protein pathway are among them. The above-mentioned developments turn the discipline in question into a discipline with an increasing potential of benefit in order to improve the comprehensibility of the molecular mechanisms that underlie the pathophysiology of psychiatric disorders. MS has some potential advantages with regard to potential diagnostic use. Firstly, MS is capable of identifying all proteins in a sample, while targeting the protein of interest is required in other techniques. Secondly, the analysis of biomaterials, e.g., urine, saliva, or blood, is appropriate and does not require intervention (in the case of saliva and urine). Thirdly, newly developed machines are extremely sensitive, which increases the potential of peripheral body fluids to reflect the protein content of the central nervous system in an actual way. Ultimately, protein marker alterations can possibly precede behavioral changes by indicating in advance whether a treatment is effective. This can be beneficial, especially in psychiatry, because the impacts of treatment in people with psychiatric problems are usually not immediately measured (Ngounou Wetie et al., 2013).

Conclusion

MALDI-IMS represents a promising novel technology, which can be used for assessing the spatial dispersions of analyte(s) concerning tissue histology. The well-defined brain structure causes MALDI-IMS to be an especially beneficial tool in neurological studies for the purpose of identifying the target regions for therapy and focus areas for a better understanding of the mechanisms of disease or injury. Despite the confirmed success of MALDI-IMS in various neurological and psychiatric studies, there are areas that should be addressed in: the existing databases and commercially available software for multimodal analysis are needed to identify compounds of higher molecular weight, develop more broadly, and load and standardize imaging experiments.

References

Abu-Asab, M. S., Chaouchi, M., Alesci, S., Galli, S., Laassri, M., Cheema, A. K., Atouf, F., VanMeter, J., Amri, H.(2011). Biomarkers in the age of omics: time for a systems biology approach. *OMICS*, 15, 105–112. https://doi.org/10.1089/omi.2010.0023.

Alawieh, A., Zaraket, F. A., Li, J. L., Mondello, S., Nokkari, A., Razafsha, M., Fadlallah, B., Boustany, R. M., Kobeissy, F. H. (2012). Systems biology, bioinformatics, and biomarkers in neuropsychiatry. *Front Neurosci*, 6, 187. https://doi.org/10.3389/fnins.2012.00187.

Andrews, W.T., Donahu, D., Holmes, A., Balsara, R., Castellino, F. J., Hum- mon, A. B. (2020). In situ metabolite and lipid analysis of GluN2D-/- and wild-type mice after ischemic stroke using MALDI MSI. *Anal Bioanal Chem*, 412, 6275–6285. https://doi.org/10.1007/s00216-020-02477-z.

Bowman, A. P., Bogie, J. F. J., Hendriks, J. J. A., Haidar, M., Belov, M., Heeren, R. M. A, Ellis, S. R. (2020). Evaluation of lipid coverage and high spatial resolution MALDI-imaging capabilities of oversampling combined with laser post-ionization. *Anal Bioanal Chem*, 412, 2277–2289. https://doi.org/10.1007/s00216-019-02290-3.

Buchberger, A. R., DeLaney, K., Johnson, J., & Li, L. (2018). Mass spectrometry imaging: A review of emerging advancements and future insights. *Analytical Chemistry,* 90, 240–265. https://doi.org/10.1021/acs.analchem.

Carlred, L., Gunnarsson, A., Solé-Domènech, S., Johansson, B., Vukojević, V., Terenius, L., Codita, A., Winblad, B., Schalling, M., Höök, F., Sjövall, P. (2014). Simultaneous imaging of amyloid-β and lipids in brain tissue using antibody-coupled liposomes and time-of-fight secondary ion mass spectrometry. *J Am Chem Soc*, 136, 9973–9981. https://doi.org/10.1021/ja5019145.

Caughlin, S., Hepburn, J., Liu, Q., Wang, L., Yeung, K. K., Cechetto, D. F., Whitehead, S. N. (2019) Chloroquine restores ganglioside homeostasis and improves pathological and behavioral outcomes post-stroke in the rat. *Mol Neurobiol*, 56, 3552–3562. https://doi.org/10.1007/s12035-018-1317-0.

Chandra, S., Smith, D. R., & Morrison, G. H. (2000). Subcellular imaging by dynamic SIMS ion microscopy. *Analytical Chemistry*, 72, 104A–114A. https://doi.org/10.1021/ac002716i.

Chen, K., Baluya, D., Tosun, M., Li, F., Maletic-Savatic, M. (2019). Imaging mass spectrometry: a new tool to assess molecular underpinnings of neurodegeneration. *Metabolites*, 9, 135. https://doi.org/10.3390/metabo9070135.

Chew, H., Solomon, V. A., Fonteh, A. N. (2020). Involvement of lipids in Alzheimer's disease pathology and potential therapies. *Front Physiol*, 11, 598. https://doi.org/10.3389/fphys.2020.00598.

Cooks, R. G., Ouyang, Z., Takats, Z., & Wiseman, J. M. (2006). Detection technologies ambient mass spectrometry. *Science*, 311, 1566–1570. https://doi.org/10.1126/science.1119426

Ditzen, C., Jastorff, A. M., Kessler, M. S., Bunck, M., Teplytska, L., Erhardt, A., Krömer, S. A., Varadarajulu, J., Targosz, B. S., Sayan-Ayata, E. F., Holsboer, F., Landgraf, R., Turck, C. W. (2006). Protein biomarkers in a mouse model of extremes in trait anxiety. Mol Cell *Proteomics,* 5, 1914-1920. . https://doi.org/10.1074/mcp.M600088-MCP200.

Dudley, E., Yousef, M., Wang, Y., Griffiths, W. J. (2010). Targeted metabolomics and mass spectrometry. *Adv Protein Chem Struct Biol*, 80, 45–83. https://doi.org/10.1016/B978-0-12-381264-3.00002-3.

Fiehn, O. (2001). Combining genomics, metabolome analysis, and biochemical modelling to understand metabolic networks. *Comparative and Functional Genomics,* 2, 155-168. https://doi.org/10.1002/cfg.82.

Grajchen, E., Hendriks, J. J. A., Bogie, J. F. J. (2018). The physiology of foamy phagocytes in multiple sclerosis. *Acta Neuropathol Commun,* 6, 124. https://doi.org/10.1186/s40478-018-0628-8.

Hanrieder, J., Ljungdahl, A., Andersson, M. (2012). MALDI imaging mass spectrometry of neuropeptides in Parkinson's disease. *J Vis Exp,* 60, 3445. https://doi.org/10.3791/3445.

Henderson, F., Hart, P. J., Pradillo, J. M., Kassiou, M., Christie, L., Williams, K. J., Boutin, H., McMahon, A. (2018). Multi-modal imaging of long-term recovery post-stroke by positron emission tomography andmatrix-assisted laser desorption/ionization mass spectrometry. *Rapid Commun Mass Spectrom,* 32, 721–729. https://doi.org/10.1002/rcm.8090.

Herberth, M., Koethe, D., Levin, Y., Schwarz, E., Krzyszton, N. D., Schoeffmann, S., Ruh, H., Rahmoune, H., Kranaster, L., Schoenborn, T., Leweke, M. F., Guest, P. C., Bahn, S. (2011). Peripheral profiling analysis for bipolar disorder reveals markers associated with reduced cell survival. *Proteomics,* 11, 94-105. https://doi.org/10.1002/pmic.201000291.

Ibanez, C., Valdes, A., Garcia-Canas, V., Simo, C., Celebier, M., Rocamora-Reverte, L., Gomez-Martinez, A., Herrero, M., Castro-Puyana, M., Segura-Carretero, A., Ibanez, E., Cifuentes, A. (2012). Global Foodomics strategy to investigate the health benefits of dietary constituents. *J Chromatogr A*, 1248, 139-153. https://doi.org/10.1016/j.chroma.2012.06.008.

Jarmusch, A., Pirro, V., Baird, Z., Hattab, E., Cohen-Gadol, A., Cooks, R. (2016). Lipid and metabolite profiles of human brain tumors by desorption electrospray ionization-MS. *PNAS,* 113, 1486–1491. https://doi.org/10.1073/pnas.15233061

Jones, E., Zhang, W., Zhao, X., Quiason, C., Dale, S., Shahidi-Latham, S., Grabowski, G., Setchell, K., Drake, R., Sun, Y. (2017). Tissue localization of glycosphingolipid accumulation in a Gaucher disease mouse brain by LC-ESI-MS/MS and high-resolution MALDI imaging mass spectrometry. *SLAS Discov,* 22, 1218–1228. https://doi.org/10.1177/2472555217719372.

Kakuda, N., Miyasaka, T., Iwasaki, N., Nirasawa, T., Wada-Kakuda, S., Takahashi-Fujigasaki, J., Murayama, S., Ihara Y., Ikegawa, M. (2017). Distinct deposition of amyloid-β species in brains with Alzheimer's disease pathology visualized with MALDI imaging mass spectrometry. *Acta Neuropathol Commun*, 5, 73. https://doi.org/10.1186/s40478-017-0477-x.

Kaya, I., Brinet, D., Michno, W., Baskurt, M., Zetterberg, H., Blenow, K., Hanrieder, J.(2017a). Novel trimodal MALDI imaging mass spectrometry (IMS3) at 10 μm reveals spatial lipid and peptide correlates implicated in Aβ plaque pathology in Alzheimer's disease. *ACS Chem Neurosci*, 8, 2778–2790. https://doi.org/10.1021/acschemneuro.7b00314.

Kaya, I., Michno, W., Brinet, D., Iacone, Y., Zanni, G., Blennow, K., Zetterberg, H., Hanrieder, J. (2017b). Histology-compatible MALDI mass spectrometry based imaging of neuronal lipids for subsequent immunofuorescent staining. *Anal Chem*, 89, 4685–4694. https://doi.org/10.1021/acs.analchem.7b00313.

Kékesi, K. A., Juhász, G., Simor, A., Gulyássy, P., Szegő, E. M., Hunyadi-Gulyás, E., Darula, Z., Medzihradszky, K. F., Palkovits, M., Penke, B., Czurkó, A. (2012). Altered functional protein networks in the prefrontal cortex and amygdala of victims of suicide. *PLoS One*, 7, e50532. https://doi.org/10.1371/journal.pone.0050532.

Koal, T., Deigner, H. P. (2010). Challenges in mass spectrometry based targeted metabolomics. *Curr Mol Med*, 10, 216–226. https://doi.org/10.2174/156652410790963312.

König, S. (2011). Urine molecular profiling distinguishes health and disease: new methods in diagnostics? Focus on UPLC-MS. *Expert Reviews in Molecular Diagnosis*, 11, 383–39. https://doi.org/10.1586/erm.11.13.

Kurian, S. M., Le-Niculescu, H., Patel, S. D., Bertram, D., Davis, J., Dike, C., Yehyawi, N., Lysaker, P., Dustin, J., Caligiuri, M., Lohr, J., Lahiri, D. K., Nurnberger, JI. Jr., Faraone, S. V., Geyer, M. A., Tsuang, M. T., Schork, N. J., Salomon, D. R., Niculescu, A. B. (2011). Identification of blood biomarkers for psychosis using convergent functional genomics. *Mol Psychiatry*, 16, 37-58. https://doi.org/10.1038/mp.2009.117.

Lagarrigue, M., Alexandrov, T., Dieuset, G., Perrin, A., Lavigne, R., Baulac, S., Thiele, H., Martin, B., Pineau, C. (2012). New analysis workflow for MALDI imaging mass spectrometry: application to the discovery and identification of potential markers of childhood absence epilepsy. *J Proteome Res,* 11, 5453-63. https://doi.org/10.1021/pr3006974.

Lawton, K. A., Cudkowicz, M. E., Brown, M. V., Alexander, D., Caffrey, R., Wulff, J. E. (2012). Biochemical alterations associated with ALS. *Amyotroph Lateral Scler,* 13, 110–118. https://doi.org/10.3109/17482968.2011.619197.

Lazar, A., Bich, C., Panchal, M., Desbenoit, N., Petit, V., Touboul, D., Dau- phinot, L., Marquer, C., Laprévote, O., Brunelle, A., Duyckaerts, C. (2012). Ti me-of-fight secondary ion mass spectrometry (TOF-SIMS) imaging reveals cholesterol overload in the cerebral cortex of Alzheimer disease patients. *Acta Neuropathol,* 125, 133–144. https://doi.org/10.1007/s00401-012-1041-1.

Maccarrone, G., Nischwitz, S., Deininger, S. O., Hornung, J., König, F. B., Stadelmann, C., Turck, C. W., Weber, F. (2017). MALDI imaging mass spectrometry analysis-A new approach for protein mapping in multiple sclerosis brain lesions. *J Chromatogr B Analy Technol Biomed Life Sci*, 1047, 131–140. https://doi.org/10.1016/j.jchromb.2016.07.001.

Mendis, L. H., Grey, A. C., Faull, R. L. M., Curtis, M. A. (2016). Hippocampal lipid differences in Alzheimer's disease: a human brain study using matrix-assisted laser desorption/imaging mass spectrometry. *Brain Behav*,6, e00517. https://doi.org/10.1002/brb3.517.

Mishur, R. J., Rea, S. L. (2012). Applications of mass spectrometry to metabolomics and metabonomics: detection of biomarkers of aging and of age-related diseases. *Mass Spectrom Rev,* 31, 70–95. https://doi.org/10.1002/mas.20338.

Mu, J., Xie, P., Yang, Z. S., Yang, D. L., Lv, F. J., Luo, T. Y., Li, Y. (2007). Neurogenesis and major depression: implications from proteomic analyses of hippocampal proteins in a rat depression model. *Neurosci Lett*, 416, 252-256. https://doi.org/10.1016/j.neulet.2007.01.067.

Mulder, I. A., Ogrinc, Potočnik, N., Broos, L. A. M., Prop, A., Wermer, M. J. H., Heeren, R. M. A., van den Maagdenberg, A. M. J. M. (2019.) Distinguishing core from penumbra by lipid profiles using mass spectrometry imaging in a transgenic mouse model of ischemic stroke. *Sci Rep,* 9, 1090. https://doi.org/10.1038/s41598-018-37612-5.

Ngounou Wetie, A. G., Sokolowska, I., Wormwood, K., Beglinger, K., Michel, T.M., Thome, J., Darie, C. C., Woods, A. G. (2013) Mass spectrometry for the detection of potential psychiatric biomarkers. *J Mol Psychiatry*, 1, 8. https://doi.org/10.1186/2049-9256-1-8.

Nordström, A., Lewensohn, R. (2010). Metabolomics: moving to the clinic. *J Neuroimmune Pharmacol*, 5, 4–17. https://doi.org/10.1155/2015/354671

O'Rourke, M. B., Smith, C. C., De La Monte, S. M., Sutherland, G. T., Padula, M. P. (2019). Higher mass accuracy MALDI-TOF/TOF lipid imaging of human brain tissue in Alzheimer's disease. *Curr Protoc MolBiol*., 126, e86. https://doi.org/10.1002/cpmb.86.

Perry, E. K., McKeith, I., Thompson, P., Marshall, E., Kerwin, J., Jabeen, S., Edwardson, J. A., Ince, P., Blessed, G., Irving, D., Perry, R. H. (1991). Topography, extent, and clinical relevance of neurochemical deficits in dementia of Lewy body type, Parkinson's disease, and Alzheimer's disease. *Ann NY Acad Sci*, 640, 197–202. https://doi.org/10.1111/j.1749-6632.1991.tb00217.x.

Roy, U., Woods, A. G., Sokolowska, I., Darie, C. C. (2014). Utility of computational structural biology in mass spectrometry. *Adv Exp Med Biol*, 806, 107-128. https://doi.org/10.1007/978-3-319-06068-2_6.

Ryan, D. J., Spraggins, J. M., Caprioli, R. M. (2019). Protein identification strategies in MALDI imaging mass spectrometry: a brief review. *Curr Opin Chem Biol*, 48, 64–72. https://doi.org/10.1016/j.cbpa.2018.10.023.

Rzagalinski, I., Hainz, N., Meier, C., Tschernig, T., Volmer, D. A. (2019). Spatial and molecular changes of mouse brain metabolism in response to immunomodulatory treatment with terifunomide as visualized by MALDI-MSI. *Anal Bioanal Chem*, 411, 353–365. https://doi.org/10.1007/s00216-018-1444-5.

Schmidt, H. D., Shelton, R. C., Duman, R. S. (2011). Functional biomarkers of depression: diagnosis, treatment, and pathophysiology. *Neuropsychopharmacology*, 36, 2375-94. https://doi.org/10.1038/npp.2011.151.

Schnackenberg, L. K., Thorn, D. A., Barnette, D., Jones, E. E. (2022). MALDI imaging mass spectrometry: an emerging tool in neurology. *Metab Brain Dis*, 37, 105-121. https://doi.org/10.1007/s11011-021-00797-2.

Sekera, E. R., Saraswat, D., Zemaitis, K. J., Sim, F. J., Wood, T. D. (2020). MALDI mass spectrometry imaging in a primary demyelination model of murine spinal cord. *J Am Soc Mass Spectrom*, 31, 2462-2468. https://doi.org/10.1021/jasms.0c00187.

Severiano, D., Oliveira-Lima, O., Vasconcelos, G., Marques, B., Carvalho, G., Freitas, E., Xavier, C., Gomez, M., Pinheiro, A., Gomez, R., Boniek, V., Pinto, M. (2020). Cerebral lipid dynamics in chronic cerebral hypoperfusion model by DESI-MS imaging. *Neuroscience*, 426, 1–12 https://doi.org/10.1016/j.neuroscience.2019.11.014.

Shariatgorji, M., Svenningsson, P., Andrén, P. E. (2014). Mass spectrometry imaging, an emerging technology in neuropsychopharmacology. *Neuropsychopharmacology*, 39, 34–49 https://doi.org/10.1038/npp.2013.215.

Shariatgorji, M., Nilsson, A., Fridjonsdottir, E., Vallianatou, T., Käll-back, P., Katan, L., Sävmarker, J., Mantas, I., Zhang, X., Bezard, E., Svenningsson, P., Odell, L. R., Andrén, P. E. (2019). Comprehensive mapping of neurotransmitter networks by MALDI-MS imaging. *Nat Methods,* 16, 1021–1028. https://doi.org/10.1038/s41592-019-0551-3.

Tanaka, E., Ogawa, Y., Fuji, R., Shimonaka, T., Sato, Y., Hamazaki, T., Nagamura-Inoue, T., Shintaku, H., Tsuji, M. (2020). Metabolomic analysis and mass spectrometry imaging after neonatal stroke and cell therapies in mouse brains. *Sci Rep*, 10, 21881. https://doi.org/10.1038/s41598-020-78930-x.

Unlu, M., Morgan, M. E. and Minden, J. S. (1997) Difference gel electrophoresis: A single gel method for detecting changes in protein extracts. *Electrophoresis*, 18, 2071-2077 https://doi.org/10.1002/elps.1150181133.

Wang, J. S. H., Freitas-Andrade, M., Bechberger, J. F., Naus, C. C., Yeung, K. K., Whitehead, S.N. (2018). Matrix-assisted laser desorption/ionization imaging mass spectrometry of intraperitoneally injecteddanegaptide (ZP1609) for treatment of stroke-reperfusion injury in mice. *Rapid Commun Mass Spectrom,* 32, 951–958. https://doi.org/10.1002/rcm.8115.

Whitehead, S. N., Chan, K. H., Gangaraju, S., Slinn, J., Li, J., Hou, S. T. (2011). Imaging mass spectrometry detection of gangliosides species in the mouse brain following transient focal cerebral ischemia and long-term recovery. *PLoS One*, 6, e20808 https://doi.org/10.1371/journal.pone.0020808.

Xu, G., Li, J (2019). Recent advances in mass spectrometry imaging for multiomics application in neurology. *J Comp Neurol*, 527, 2158-2169. https://doi.org/10.1002/cne.24571.

Yang, Q., Zhang, A. H., Miao, J. H., Sun, H., Han, Y., Yan, G. L., Wu, F. F., Wang, X. J. (2019) Metabolomics biotechnology, applications, and future trends: a systematic review. *RSC Adv*, 9, 37245-37257. https://doi.org/10.1039/c9ra06697g.

Zemski, Berry, K. A., Hankin, J. A., Barkley, R. M., Spraggins, J. M., Caprioli, R. M., Murphy, R. C. (2011) MALDI imaging of lipid biochemistry in tissues by mass spectrometry. *Chem Rev, 111*, 6491–6512. https://doi.org/10.1021/cr200280p

Chapter 18

Nutritional Metabolomics and Their Implications in Clinical Studies

Semra Türkoğlu*, PhD
Department of Nutrition and Dietetics, Health Sciences Faculty,
Firat University, Elazığ, Turkey

Abstract

Metabolomics deals with small molecule metabolites, and one of their main purposes is to identify those small molecules that make differences in the metabolic effects of different diets. Thus, deepening our knowledge of the interactive and regulatory roles of human health and nutrition. Metabolomics, pharmacology, and toxicology have also been widely adopted, but they are relatively new to human nutrition. Today, scientists play an important role in the health status of people by finding new bioactive food components that prevent cancer, obesity, diabetes, cardiovascular and chronic diseases, as well as prolong life and improve physical and mental health. In this context, the use of high-throughput metabolomics techniques contributes to the development of nutritional models, the benefits of a diet to metabolism, and the improvement of physiological responses to this diet. That is, it provides a better understanding of the effects of genes, enzymes, proteins, metabolites, and microenvironments at the cellular level. Metabolomics can assist in the design of nutritional programs and improve our understanding of nutrition and the role of nutrients in promoting and maintaining cellular functions and overall health. The purpose of this section is to make a general assessment of nutritional metabolomics, to emphasize the effects of nutritional metabolomics on clinical studies, and to contribute to the scientific literature on these issues.

* Corresponding Author's E-mail: smrturkoglu@hotmail.com.

In: Metabolomics and Clinical Approach
Editors: Sevgi Durna Daştan and Taner Daştan
ISBN: 979-8-89113-095-1

Keywords: nutritional metabolomics, metabolites, clinical studies

Introduction

Nutritional metabolomics is a highly efficient and sensitive approach that has emerged to determine the effects of different nutritional approaches on chronic diseases with varying metabolic phenotypes and to describe and characterize the biochemical reactions underlying the effects (Mihalik et al., 2012; Purushotham et al., 2012). Challenges have arisen due to the associations of the consumption of certain foods with the disease, the ability to identify new correlations, complex metabolic pathways, and individual variability in digestion, as well as newly discovered metabolites (Kim & Milner, 2011; Lodge, 2010). This section discusses progress toward making these approaches manageable for nutritional research. The aim of metabolomics is to identify metabolites used in the diagnosis of disease or providing treatment control. In this way; It allows dietary recommendations to be made according to the patient's metabolic profile and genetic structure. One of the main goals of metabolomics is to identify these small molecules that differentiate between the effects of different diets while deepening our knowledge of the interactive and regulatory roles of human health and nutrition (Gibney et al., 2005).

Metabolomics analyzes the compounds in food components, determines their metabolites in body fluids and biological tissues, and investigates the physiological responses of the nutrition program (Llorach et al., 2012). All natural and unnatural food components are often referred to as the "food metabolome." The food metabolome provides important insights into the complex interactions between nutrition and health (Rubio et al., 2012).

The number of different non-nutrient molecules in the food source is greater than the number of nutrients. For instance, plants produce and accumulate secondary metabolites for defense, growth, reproduction, and similar mechanisms that are not essential nutrients. Until recently, the potential metabolic effects of these secondary metabolites, phytochemicals, were mostly ignored in conventional nutrition (Cassidy & Dalais, 2003). In fact, all of these non-nutritive metabolites, along with the potential metabolic effects of food components, must be accounted for in the metabolome. At the same time the thousands of compounds in foods such as coffee, red wine, fruit, vegetables, and fish, there are also non-nutrients, some of which are man-made or randomly generated, that occur in foods (Gibney et al., 2005).

Clinical Studies

Many reviews and comments have revealed the difficulties and limitations of the application of metabolism to nutrition, diet, and health (German et al., 2004; Scalbert et al., 2009; Wishart, 2008; Zeisel et al., 2005). Most of these studies have focused on the determination of nutritional metabolomics to determine nutritional states and their effects on disease (Rezzi et al., 2007).

Scientists can obtain more nutritious foods with changes that will occur as a result of food processing according to the metabolomic information and molecular content of the food (Heuberger et al., 2010; Beleggia, 2011). In recent studies, it has been found that products obtained from organic agriculture contain much more antioxidants and phenolic compounds than products obtained from conventional agriculture (Novotna et al., 2012). In similar applications, metabolomics is beginning to show an effect on the study of food conversion (Heuberger et al., 2010). Food-derived metabolites affect cell metabolism by three main mechanisms: proteins, enzymes, and micro-interactions. The composition with respect to a variety of metabolites directly determines the chemical-physical properties of large macromolecules. For instance, trials to change the composition of the nerve membranes of animals have shown a change, especially in those fed a diet containing fatty acids (Beleggia et al., 2011). The altered composition affects the shape and flexibility of membranes, as well as the functions of ion channels and intramembrane proteins (Rapoport et al., 2011). Nutritional metabolites regulate pathways for energy supply and energy metabolism. For example, sugars can enter the tricarboxylic acid (TCA) cycle and electron transport system via glycolysis to produce energy-rich metabolites such as adenosine triphosphate. In metabolism, when adenosine triphosphate is in excess, sugar metabolism is involved in fatty acid synthesis (Bocarsly et al., 2010). There is evidence from recent research that high fructose corn syrup-rich foods and beverages lead to fatty liver and diabetes, and subsequently chronic inflammatory diseases. Alternatively, some metabolites, such as B-complex vitamins, modify or aid the catalytic activity of cofactors. For example, thiamine pyrophosphate (vitamin B1), a thiamine derivative, catalyzes many biochemical pathways as a cofactor in glycolysis and the TCA, including the complex of the pyruvate dehydrogenase enzyme. Nutritional metabolites can act as messenger signals. Likewise, Nicotinamide adenine dinucleotide (NAD) is an important coenzyme involved in various energy metabolism pathways, including glycolysis, oxidative phosphorylation, and fatty acids oxidation. For example, it has been shown that fasting, calorie limitation, and low-carbohydrate diets may ultimately be responsible for increased lifespan, modulation of enzyme activities and gene expression in animal models (Sassone-Corsi, 2013). Some nutritional metabolites can modulate cell metabolism by acting as antioxidants to reduce cell pollutants that cause oxidation-induced damage. Antioxidants can interact with unstable compounds such as free radicals, metals, and oxygen. In this way, it prevents the propagation of the formation of reactive oxygen species (ROS) or oxidative stress, which can damage all components of the cell, including protein, lipid, and DNA (Sassone-Corsi, 2013). In summary, a better understanding of the micro-level effects of genes, proteins, enzymes, and metabolites at the cellular level and their effect on cell functions can help the design of nutrition programs with a metabolomic approach in order to increase general health (Sassone-Corsi, 2013). Epidemiological studies for some diseases such as cancer, cardiovascular diseases, and Alzheimer's suggest that dietary habits can significantly reduce the risk of diseases (Snigdha et al., 2012). Today, studies on nutrition programs enriched with natural antioxidants, vitamins and phytochemicals, and regular food supplements are continuing (Manach et al., 2009). For example, a certain genetic polymorphism may occur, that is, the risk of catching the disease, the response to treatment, and the different side effects of the drugs taken (Cornelis & El-Sohemy 2007). With this evidence, a combination of genomics and metabolomics suggests that the most appropriate nutritional recommendations for individuals can be created. Like protein and carbohydrates, fats are among the largest classes of foods. The metabolomic analysis is called lipidomics because the solubility of lipids is different from carbohydrates and proteins (Wenk, 2005). Lipomic approaches can be applied to develop appropriate diagnostic methods to monitor nutritional imbalances or deficiencies in lipids as the ratio of omega-3 fatty acids to omega-6 fatty acids (Moco et al., 2006).

Food frauds are common occurrences in foodstuffs such as fruit juice and oils (Ogrinc et al., 2003). In this context, the metabolite profile of the fraudulent product can be easily detected by using it to extract the product-specific characteristics (such as aroma, color, amino acid profile, and vitamin content) that cannot be made by other methods. In recent years, important steps have been taken to determine the essential food components necessary for the development and continuity of human health, with studies conducted by food scientists and biochemists. Mandatory food supplements, such as minerals and vitamins, are frequently used in the treatment of nutritional deficiencies with nutritional programs (Lindon et al., 2013). Today, nutrition scientists are looking for new methods to be used in the prevention and treatment of obesity, diabetes, cardiovascular, and chronic diseases (Gibney et al., 2005). At the same time, studies are conducted to identify new bioactive food components that delay aging, provide weight loss, improve mental and physical health, and prevent diseases such as cancer and heart diseases. The use of metabolomic techniques in this context provides benefits such as improving food consumption patterns, improving physiological responses to any diet and drug use, and new components can be discovered (Clarke & Haselssen, 2008; Sébédio, 2017). In the evaluation of the vitamin D level, 25-hydroxyvitamin D[25(OH)D] is preferred because it has a long half-life. However, to evaluate the pathophysiological role of vitamin D metabolites in various diseases, it is necessary to examine the whole metabolome. For this, some metabolomic studies are thought to be necessary to know the total 2 (OH) D levels as well as various metabolites such as free/bioavailable forms, vitamin D binding protein (DBP), parathormone, and 1alpha,25-dihydroxyvitamin D3, 3-epi-25-Hydroxyvitamin D3, 24,25-dihydroxy vitamin D3 in order to make an accurate clinical interpretation of vitamin D. In metabolomic studies to determine the effects and functions of vitamin D metabolites in diseases and nutritional status, it becomes easier to evaluate the efficacy of treatment with cholecalciferol or ergocalciferol. Metabolomics has been evaluated as a universal and standard analytical method that covers all vitamin D metabolites (Erdem & Akbas, 2018). The use of slimming tablets is very popular today, as it causes rapid weight loss. However, aristolochic acid, which is used in herbal slimming tablets of Chinese origin, has been shown to have damage at the gene level in the bone marrow of rats and to be associated with gene mutations by metabolomic methods in another study (Yaman, 2015).

Some metabolomic studies in the World conducted on rats, diets containing whole grain (n=10) or refined wheat flour (n=10) were applied to two groups for two weeks. The whole grain consuming group was given 60 g/100 g of whole grain flour, while the other group was given the same amount of refined wheat flour. Among the markers of oxidative stress, isoprostanes and malondialdehydes, vitamin E and C, and lipid levels (liver and plasma triglyceride and cholesterol) were measured by metabolomic techniques. It has been shown that some TCA intermediates, aromatic amino acids, and hippuric acid were significantly higher in the urine of rats fed whole grain flour, thus causing a change in the basal metabolic rate. In addition, increased levels of reduced glutathione and betaine have been reported. This is considered a sign of reduced oxidative stress and good redox status (Fardet et al., 2007). In a comprehensive study that grouped dietary patterns and examined the effects on the serum levels of 1003 women, 163 metabolites were examined. In this study, seven different parameters were selected by taking food consumption records. These are coffee, garlic, vegetables and fruits, alcohol, consumption of red meat, low-energy diet, and traditional British diet (consumption of fried fish and potatoes, meat, savory pies, and vegetables). A correlation was found between garlic, coffee, vegetable intake, low energy diets, and metabolite profile. As a result of these dietary patterns, plasma carnitines, glycerophospholipids, and sphingolipids were found to be reduced. No association was found between meat consumption, high alcohol intake, and the traditional British diet and these metabolites (Menni et al., 2013). In another study, 77 mildly obese individuals were fed a low-energy diet for 8 weeks. These individuals were then randomly divided into two groups, one high glycemic index group and the other low glycemic index diet group, followed by urine samples collected for 6 weeks. The metabolite profiles of both groups were examined using the NMR technique. As a result, it has been shown that there is no relationship between the glycemic index and Cpeptide levels (Rasmussen et al., 2012). Obesity has become an important public health problem in recent years with the increase in prevalence and incidence. However, the underlying biochemical and metabolic pathways are not fully understood. The metabolic approach, identifying biomarkers related to obesity, helps clarify these mechanisms. In one study, branched chain amino acids (BCAA), organic acids, non-esterified fatty acids, phospholipids, and acylcarnitines were identified as potential biological products for obesity. This suggests an association between high BCAA and other amino acids with obesity. In addition, it has been reported that β-oxidation deregulation is associated with the development of obesity (Rauschert et al., 2014; Yılmaz & Özpınar, 2019). Krishnan et al., used metabolomics in different groups to classify the glycemic indices response to different diets. Twenty-four healthy premenopausal women aged 20-50 years were included in the study. The researchers identified blood sugar, leptin, and insulin as covariates. The study revealed three different biologically significant subgroups, one with higher leptin levels and the other with higher insulin resistance. Wang et al., evaluated the response of 23 healthy individuals to dietary carotenoids in watermelon and tomato juice. The study revealed five metabolic subsets of carotenoids in juices. These different metabolic consequences appear to be induced by genetic variants of the carotenoid-metabolizing enzyme β-carotene 15, 15'-monooxygenase 1. The study by Li et al., included 1500 participants, 760 women, and 740 men aged 18 to 90 years. In this study, the researchers evaluated twenty-six fatty acids. Identified four subgroups of participants with different fatty acid patterns related to their dietary habits, demographics, and metabotype. Another study evaluated the metabolic phenotypes of 19 women (postmenopausal) with a mean age of 61 years. 189 metabolites were evaluated. Two different metabolic subgroups were identified in relation to fasting and satiety metabolic profiles (Moazzami et al., 2014).

Conclusion

The metabolomics approach is a new and promising technology for use in nutritional research and in determining the relationship between nutrition and health. At the same time as metabolomics, a step towards personalization in nutrition can be taken (Wishart et al., 2007). Prevention and treatment of diseases through nutrition can be treated by classifying individuals into certain groups based on the metabolome. It can be transformed into a routine analysis and foresight method in the future by defining the nutritional needs of individuals and their individual differences, and by developing personalized nutrition programs suitable for individual nutritional needs with such a strategy, giving importance to preventive medicine practices that should be included in diet specialists. Thanks to the rapid development of technologies used in metabolomics profiling, there is a need for a database that collects nutritional metabolomics in order to evaluate the relationship of metabolomics with health, which can be analyzed today.

References

Beleggia, R., Platani C., Papa R., Chio, A., Barros, E., Mashaba, C., Wirth, J., Fammartino, A., Sautter, C., Conner, S., Rauscher, J., Stewart, D., Cattivelli L. (2011). Metabolomics and food processing: from semolina to pasta. *J Agric Food Chem.*, 59, 9366-9377. https://doi.org/10.1021/jf2022836.

Bocarsly, M. E., Powell, E. S., Avena, N. M., Hoebel, B. G. (2010). High-fructose corn syrup causes characteristics of obesity in rats: increased body weight, body fat and triglyceride levels. *Pharmacol Biochem Behav.*, 97, 101-106. https://doi.org/10.1016/j.pbb.2010.02.012.

Cassidy, A., Dalais, F. S. (2003). Phytochemicals. In: Gibney MJ, Macdonald I, Roche H, eds. *Nutrition & Metabolism* (pp. 307-317). Oxford, United Kingdom: Blackwell Science.

Clarke, C. J., Haselssen, J. N. (2008). Metabolic profiling as a tool for understanding mechanisms of toxicity. *Toxicol Pathol.*, 36(1), 140-147. https://doi.org/10.1177/0192623307310.

Cornelis, M. C., El-Sohemy, A. (2007). Coffee, caffeine, and coronary heart disease. *Curr Opin Clin Nutr Metab Care.*, 10, 745-751. https://doi.org/10.1097/MOL.0b013e3280127b04.

Dettmer, K., Hammock, B. D. (2004). Metabolomics – a new exciting field within the "omics" sciences. *Environ Health Persp.*, 112, 396-7. https://doi.org/10.1289/ehp.112-1241997.

Erdem, K.B., Akbas, H. (2018). Vitamin D and Metabolomics. *Turkish Journal of Clinical Biochemistry*, 16(2), 127-194.

Fardet, A., Canlet, C., Gottardi, G., Lyan, B., Llorach, R., Rémésy, C., Mazur, A., Paris, A., Scalbert, A. (2007). Whole-Grain and Refined Wheat Flours Show Distinct Metabolic Profiles in Rats as Assessed by a 1H NMR-Based Metabonomic Approach. *J Nutr.*, 137(4), 923-929. https://doi.org/10.1093/jn/137.4.923.

German, J. B., Bauman, D. E., Burrin, D. G., Failla, M. L., Freake, H. C., King, J. C., Klein, S., Milner, J. A., Pelto, G. H., Rasmussen, K. M., Zeisel, S. H. (2004). Metabolomics in the opening decade of the 21st century: building the roads to individualized health. *J Nutr.,* 134, 2729–32. https://doi.org/10.1093/jn/134.10.2729.

Gibney, M. J., Walsh, M., Brennan, L., Roche, H. M., German, B., Ommen, B. (2005). Metabolomics in human nutrition: opportunities and challenges. *Am J Clin Nutr.*, 82, 497-503. https://doi.org/10.1093/ajcn.82.3.497.

Heuberger, A. L., Lewis, M. R., Chen, M. H., Brick, M. A., Leach, J. E., Ryan, E. P. (2010). Metabolomic and functional genomic analyses reveal varietal differences in bioactive compounds of cooked rice. *Plos One*, 5, 2915. https://doi.org/10.1371/journal.pone.0012915.

Kim, Y. S., Milner, J. A. (2011). Bioactive food components and cancer-specific metabonomic profiles. *J Biomed Biotechnol.*, 2011, 721213. https://doi.org/10.1155/2011/721213.

Krishnan, S., Newman, J. W., Hembrooke, T. A., Keim, N. L. (2012). Variation in metabolic responses to meal challenges differing in glycemic index in healthy women: is it meaningful? *Nutr Metabol.* 9, 26. https://doi.org/10.1186/1743-7075-9-26.

Li, K., Brennan, L., McNulty, B. A., Bloomfield, J. F., Duff, D. J., Devlin, N. F., Gibney, M. J., Flynn, A., Walton. J., Nugent, A. P. (2016). Plasma fatty acid patterns reflect dietary habits and metabolic health: a cross-sectional study. *Mol Nutr Food Res.,* 60, 2043–52. https://doi.org/10.1002/mnfr.201500711.

Lindon, J. C., Holmes, E., Bollard, M. E., Stanley, E. G., Nicholson, J. K. (2013). Metabonomics technologies and their applications in physiological monitoring, drug safety assessment and disease diagnosis. *Biomarkers*, 9, 1-31. https://doi.org/10.1080/13547500410001668379.

Llorach, R., Garcia-Aloy, M., Tulipani, S., Vazquez-Fresno, R., Andres-Lacueva, C. (2012). Nutrimetabolomic strategies to develop new biomarkers of intake and health effects. *J Agric Food Chem.*, 60, 8797-8808. https://doi.org/10.1021/jf301142b.

Lodge, J. K. (2010). Symposium 2: Modern approaches to nutritional research challenges: Targeted and non-targeted approaches for metabolite profiling in nutritional research. *Proc Nutr Soc.*, 69, 95–102. https://doi.org/10.1017/S0029665109991704.

Manach, C., Hubert, J., Llorach, R., Scalbert, A. (2009). The complex links between dietary phytochemicals and human health deciphered by metabolomics. *Mol Nutr Food.*, 53, 1303-1315. https://doi.org/10.1002/mnfr.200800516.

Menni, C., Zhai, G., Macgregor, A., Prehn, C., Römisch-Margl, W., Suhre, K., Adamski, J., Cassidy, A., Illig, T., Spector, T. D., Valdes, A. M. (2013). Targeted metabolomics profiles are strongly correlated with nutritional patterns in women. *Metabolomics*, 9(2), 506- 514. https://doi.org/10.1007/s11306-012-0469-6.

Mihalik, S. J., Michaliszyn, S. F., de las Heras, J., Bacha, F., Lee, S., Chace, D. H., DeJesus, V. R., Vockley, J., Arslanian, S. A. (2012). Metabolomic profiling of fatty acid and amino acid metabolism in youth with obesity and type 2 diabetes: evidence for enhanced mitochondrial oxidation. *Diabetes Care*, 35, 605–611. https://doi.org/10.2337/DC11-1577.

Moazzami, A. A., Shrestha, A., Morrison, D. A., Poutanen, K., Mykkänen, H. (2014). Metabolomics reveals differences in postprandial responses to breads and fasting metabolic characteristics associated with postprandial insulin demand in postmenopausal women. *J. Nutr.,* 144, 807–14. https://doi.org/10.3945/jn.113.188912.

Moco, S., Bino, R. J., Vorst, O., Verhoeven, H. A., Groot, J., Beek, T. A. (2006). A liquid chromatography-mas spectrometry-based metabolome database for tomato. *Plant Physiol.,* 141, 1205-1218. https://doi.org/10.1104/pp.106.078428.

Novotna, H., Kmiecik, O., Galazka, M., Krtková, V., Hurajová, A., Schulzová, V., Hallmann, E., Rembiałkowska, E., Hajšlová, J. (2012). Metabolomic fingerprinting employing DART-TOFMS for authentication of tomatoes and peppers from organic and conventional farming. *Food Addit Contam Part A Chem Anal Control Expo Risk Assess.*, 29, 1335-1346. https://doi.org/10.1080/19440049.2012.690348.

Ogrinc, N., Kosir, I. J., Spangenberg, J. E., Kidric, J. (2003). The application of NMR and MS methods for detection of adulteration of wine, fruit juices and olive oil. *Anal Bioanal Chem.*, 376, 424-430. https://doi.org/10.1007/s00216-003-1804-6.

Purushotham, A., Xu, Q., Li, X. (2012). Systemic SIRT1 insufficiency results in disruption of energy homeostasis and steroid hormone metabolism upon high-fat-diet feeding. *FASEB J.*, 26, 656-667. https://doi.org/10.1096/fj.11-195172.

Rapoport, S. I., Ramadan, E., Basselin, M. (2011). Docosahexaenoic acid (DHA) incorporation into the brain from plasma, as an in vivo biomarker of brain DHA metabolism and neurotransmission. *Prostaglandins Other Lipid Mediat.* 96, 109-113. https://doi.org/10.1016/j.prostaglandins.2011.06.003.

Rasmussen, L. G., Winning, H., Savorani, F., Ritz, C., Engelsen, S. B., Astrup, A., Larsen, T. M., Dragsted, L. O. (2012). Assessment of dietary exposure related to dietary GI and fibre intake in a nutritional metabolomic study of human urine. *Genes Nutr.*, 7(2), 281-293. https://doi.org/10.1007/s12263-011-0250-x.

Rauschert, S., Uhl, O., Koletzko, B., Hellmuth, C. (2014). Metabolomic biomarkers for obesity in humans: a short review. *Ann. Nutr. Metab.*, 64, 314-324. https://doi.org/10.1159/000365040.

Rezzi, S., Ramadan, Z., Fay, L. B., Kochhar, S. (2007). Nutritional metabonomics: applications and perspectives. *Journal of proteome research,* 6, 513–25. https://doi.org/10.1021/pr060522z.

Rubio-Aliaga, I., Kochhar, S., Silva-Zolezzi, I. (2012). Biomarkers of nutrient bioactivity and efficacy: a route toward personalized nutrition. *J Clin Gastroenterol.*, 46, 545-554. https://doi.org/10.1097/MCG.0b013e3182548df2.

Sassone-Corsi, P. (2013). Physiology. When metabolism and epigenetics converge. *Science,* 339, 148-150. https://doi.org/10.1126/science.1233.

Scalbert, A., Brennan, L., Fiehn, O., Hankemeier, T., Kristal, B. S., van Ommen, B., Pujos-Guillot, E., Verheij, E., Wishart, D., Wopereis, S. (2009). Mass-spectrometry-based metabolomics: limitations and recommendations for future progress with particular focus on nutrition research. Metabolomics. 5, 435–58. https://doi.org/10.1007/s11306-009-0168-0.

Sébédio, J. L. (2017). Metabolomics, nutrition, and potential biomarkers of food quality, intake, and health status. *Adv Food Nutr Res.* 82, 83-116. https://doi.org/10.1016/bs.afnr.2017.01.001.

Snigdha, S., Astarita, G., Piomelli, D., Cotman, C. W. (2012). Effects of diet and behavioral enrichment on free fatty acids in the aged canine brain. *Neuroscience*, 202, 326-333. https://doi.org/10.1016/j.neuroscience.2011.12.002.

Wang, T. T., Edwards, A. J., Clevidence, B. A. (2013). Strong and weak plasma response to dietary carotenoids identified by cluster analysis and linked to beta-carotene 15, 15'-monooxygenase 1 single nucleotide polymorphisms. *J Nutr Biochem*, 24, 1538–46. https://doi.org/10.1016/j.jnutbio.2013.01.001.

Wenk, M. R. (2005). The emerging field of lipidomics. *Nat Rev Drug Discov*, 4, 594-610. https://doi.org/10.1038/nrd1776.

Wishart DS. (2008). Metabolomics: applications to food science and nutrition research. *Trends Food Sci Technol.,* 19, 482–93. https://doi.org/10.1016/j.tifs.2008.03.003.

Wishart, D. S., Tzur, D., Knox, C., Eisner, R., Guo, A. C., Young, N., Cheng, D., Jewell, K., Arndt, D., Sawhney, S., Fung, C., Nikolai, L., Lewis, M., Coutouly, M. A., Forsythe, I., Tang, P., Shrivastava, S., Jeroncic, K., Stothard, P., Amegbey, G., Block, D., Hau, D. D., Wagner, J., Miniaci, J., Clements, M., Gebremedhin, M., Guo, N., Zhang, Y., Duggan, G. E., Macinnis, G. D., Weljie, A. M., Dowlatabadi, R., Bamforth, F., Clive, D., Greiner, R., Li, L., Marrie, T., Sykes, B. D., Vogel, H. J., Querengesser, L. (2007). HMDB: the human metabolome database. *Nucleic Acids Res.*, 35, 521-526. https://doi.org/10.1093/nar/gkl923.

Yaman, Ö. (2015). An overview of metabolomic studies in medicine. *Journal of Bahri Dagdas Animal Research*. 3(1), 33-46.

Yılmaz, I., Özpınar, H. (2019). Metabolomic Applications in Nutrition and Food: An Overview, *IGUSABDER*, 8, 827-839.

Zeisel, S. H., Freake, H. C., Bauman, D. E., Bier, D. M., Burrin, D. G., German, J. B., Klein, S., Marquis, G. S., Milner, J. A. Pelto, G. H., Rasmussen, K. M. (2005). The nutritional phenotype in the age of metabolomics. *J Nutr.* 135, 1613–6. https://doi.org/10.1093/jn/135.7.1613.

Chapter 19

Metabolome in Urology Practices: Signatures in Plasma and Urine

Aydemir Asdemir*, **MD**
Department of Urology, Faculty of Medicine, Sivas Cumhuriyet University, Sivas, Turkey

Abstract

Comparing the vast variation in biochemical processes seen in tumor cells with normal cells can be considered the initiation of metabolomics research, which is now used in different medical fields. Currently, there is an undisputed need for clinically relevant biomarkers that can be used for the diagnosis and prognosis of urologic cancer types, e.g., prostate, bladder, and metabolomics can be considered promising at this stage. Novel and relevant biomarkers are required for specialized diagnosis, monitoring, and treatment of a particular disease, which would also contribute to the improvement, enhancement, and personalization of a designed therapy. While considerable progress has been made in determining important biomarkers, more challenges remain to be solved for the further integration of metabolomics into clinical practices. This chapter reviews relevant metabolomics research conducted in the field urology.

Keywords: urine, plasma, metabolome, signature, urology

---

* Corresponding Author's Email: aydemirasdemir@hotmail.com.

In: Metabolomics and Clinical Approach
Editors: Sevgi Durna Daştan and Taner Daştan
ISBN: 979-8-89113-095-1

Introduction

Metabolomics is a primer for integrative evaluation of all metabolism processes, i.e., metabolites, of a given biological specimen. Since metabolites of a given system, i.e., metabolome, are the final results from all interactions of genome-to-proteome, metabolomics can be considered as the highly specific indicator of a particular phenotype. Therefore, metabolomics is particularly useful in the study of the discovery of drugs (Wishart, 2008), the identification of disease biomarkers (Brindle et al., 2003; Dunne et al., 2005; Kaddurah-Daouk et al., 2004; Mendrick & Schnackenberg, 2009; Ng et al., 2011) and environment-gene interactions (Bundy et al., 2009; Montoliu et al., 2012; Nicholson et al., 2012; Viant, 2008). Biological fluids, in other words, bio-fluids have the potential of representing the integrative nature of a biological system through the complexity of its metabolome, they would be used for revealing interorganal connections, and the role of the host–microbiota interaction. Also, collecting them is simple and less invasive. Hematologic samples of blood serum- plasma, and urinary samples are the generally used fluid specimens for metabolomics methodology (Zhang, 2012).

The results of analyses come from Omics Sciences have been very useful and helpful in characterizing metabolic conditions such as metabolic syndrome and diabetes and also in identifying congenital metabolism disorders (Garcia-Cazorla et al., 2015; Lamari et al., 2015). Such disorders are related to metabolites and/or lipids that are easily identified as abnormal. They are significant outliers.

Proteomics, genomics, metabolomics, and transcriptomics are parts of the whole. Each of the omics can analyze their respective coverage as a whole in a system-wide manner, and cancer research in systems biology utilizes the omics processes (Trock, 2011; He et al., 2012).

For the physiological status of a biological system, metabolomics can provide an idea. For instance, a particular difference in the normal metabolic pattern might be an indicator of a particular disease; therefore, the normal metabolic profile has the prospect of a place for biomarker identifications for clinical practice (Ramautar et al., 2013). The prospect of metabolites unravelling and distinguishing the reasons behind the phenotypic variation in a given state is clearly promising (Monteiro et al., 2014a).

Metabolomics is the integrative study in which the metabolites come from endogenous and exogenous sources in a given system, which includes all metabolism products to foreign substances such as drugs and nutrients. Metabolites can offer some clues about some disorders and illnesses such as different cancers (Trock, 2011; Aboud & Weiss, 2013; Monteiro et al., 2013; Weiss and Kim, 2012; Monteiro et al., 2014b).

The metabolic phenotypes presented by neoplasms are rather peculiar. This may be because of cancer development and progression. Metabolomics can be used as a plausible approach to expose metabolic aberrations, relevant biomarkers, and uncovering pharmaceutical target sites (Monteiro et al., 2014a; Aboud & Weiss, 2013; Monteiro et al., 2015).

Important Metabolomics Studies in the Urology Field

The metabolite patterns of plasma or serum samples from patients having low- and high-grade bladder cancer were investigated by Cao et al. (2012), which applied the human nuclear magnetic resolution (H-NMR) technique to serum samples to determine cancerous stages in patients and contrast patients to control. In their study, they used individuals who show urinary calculi along with hematuria, which is the case for bladder cancer, as control, and they managed to distinguish bladder cancer patients from both normal control patients and others who show only calculi by contrasting metabolite profiles. Alterations in serum metabolite profiles in patients were observed as increases in lipids, some aminoacids, glucose, lactate, and citrate having bladder cancer in contrast to the healthy and calculi groups. Between grades, the low-grade bladder cancer patients showed an increase in glucose, but showed decreases for tyrosine, glycine, phenylalanine, and lactate (Cao et al., 2012). In another study, Bansal et al. (2013) utilized the H-NMR method on serum samples to achieve differentiation between patients with low- or high-grade bladder cancer and healthy individuals. In conclusion, they achieved a distinction between healthy and patients with cancer. They have determined striking differences in serum levels of glutamine, dimethylamine (DMA), histidine, malonate, valine, and lactate between healthy and cancer patients. The validity of these approaches was further supported by a further double-blind study that used 106 bladder cancer suspects and provided feasibility for early diagnosis (Bansal et al., 2013). To research metabolic pathways disturbed in non-muscle invasive bladder cancer, a metabolomics approach using H-NMR was conducted in urinary samples (Srivastava et al., 2010). The decreased urinary amounts of phenylalanine, citrate and hippuric acid were determined compared to controls. Gamagedara et al. (2012) designed a creatinine-normalized liquid chromatography mass spectrometry (LC-MS) methodology to calculate levels of urinary taurine, phenylalanine, and hippuric acid.

Because Taurine's increase in bladder cancer, urine is correlated with its increases in bladder cancer, and taurine has the prospect of the relevant diagnostic biomarker for bladder cancer (Tripathi et al., 2013).

Pasikanti et al. (2010) achieved a 100% sensitive GC-TOF-MS application for the discrimination of patients having bladder cancer from healthy individuals, therefore, researchers managed to provide a solid foundation for metabolomics in different stages of cancer, even though further studies with larger datasets are required. As ribitol, valine, uridine, citrate, gluconic acid, glycerol, and melibiose, 15 of the 32 products of significantly altered metabolites were detected. Kynurenine's potential role in the grow of bladder cancer due to altered tryptophan process was determined by Pasikanti et al. (Pasikanti et al., 2013). Metabolic upregulation of tryptophan results in higher concentrations of *N*-acetyltryptophan (Alberice et al., 2013; Pasikanti et al., 2013), tryptophan (Putluri et al., 2011; Alberice et al., 2013), kynurenine (Dettmer et al., 2013; Putluri et al., 2011). As well as acetylcarnitine, isovalerylcarnitine, carnitine, and octenoylcarnitine were observed to increase in bladder cancer urines. Another bladder cancer urine study (Alberice et al., 2013; Putluri et al., 2011) results are consistent with this. In the cancer group, they found that 2,6-dimethylhptanoyl carnitine, decanoylcarnitine and glutarylcarnitine levels decreased. In non-muscle invasive bladder cancer the levels of carnitines were lower than muscle invasive bladder cancer (Jin et al., 2014). To distinguish grades of cancer, they can be useful. Acetyl-CoA's urinary levels in bladder cancer patients were found elevated (Jin et al., 2014). Citrate levels decreased in bladder cancer (Cao et al., 2012; Srivastava et al., 2010; Pasikanti et al., 2010; Pasikanti et al., 2013; Dettmer et al., 2013).

The excessive activities of cancer cells alter the normal metabolism of purines and pyrimidines. Also, pyrimidine metabolism was found to be upregulated in bladder cancer, which are related metabolites for transcription and indicate highly active states of neoplasms (Pasikanti et al., 2010; Pasikanti et al., 2013). As for the pyrimidine synthesis, ureidosuccinic acid's decreased levels may reflect its higher consumption (Shen et al., 2019). Enhancements in the purine metabolism can be attributed to an increase in hypoxanthine and a decrease in uric acid, inosinic acid, and adenosine (Alberice et al., 2013). In the process of purine catabolism, hypoxanthine formed first and became uric acid. Adenosine and inosinic acid deteriorations in bladder cancer cases are explained by this bioprocess.

Various research was conducted to investigate proteins having higher mass and associated modifications (Kreunin et al., 2007), which focused on glycoproteins in urinary metabolisms. As alpha-1B-glycoprotein important biomarkers were described by them. Further glycoprotein biomarkers associated with bladder cancer were also emphasized (Yang et al., 2011). Linden et al. also highlighted alpha-1-antitrypsin (A1AT) in their study (Linden et al., 2012; Lei et al., 2013). Some higher levels of mass urinary proteins were found to be consistent with bladder cancer (Li et al., 2011; Li et al., 2012). Sensitivity (89-92%) and specificity (85-86% for healthy individuals) of the Apo-A1-biomarker were proposed and supported (Lei et al., 2013; Li et al., 2014). Chen et al. also observed differentiated urinary status of ApoA1 (Chen et al., 2010). In the same research, a six-peptide panel was presented as carrying diagnostic ratio, which was further supported in the following studies using NMR on different samples (Chen et al., 2010, 2012).

Sarcosine, which is a glycine derivative that has N-methyl group, can be determined in urine, that is strikingly increased in prostate cancer in stages of metastasis. It was determined as an alternative metabolite, which is known to be overexpressed in invasive prostate cancer cell lines but is relatively benign. The GNMT (glycine-N-methyl transferase), which is a sarcosine generating enzyme from glycine precursors, knockdown was used to hinder cancerous invasion from prostate cancer. Similarly, SARDH (sarcosine dehydrogenase) knockdown was used to inhibit the cancerous phenotype in benign prostate epithelia by degradation of sarcosine. The sarcosine pathway's components are coordinately regulated by the ERG gene and the androgenic receptor fusion product. Taken together, the obtained results eagerly indicate sarcosine as a relevant metabolite for the deduction of cancerous invasion and metastasis profiles. The promising aspect of sarcosine as a clinically relevant biomarker is further maintained by the fact that benign samples did not provide noticeable sarcosine levels. Further supporting this fact is the detection of pronounced levels of sarcosine in more than 79% of all metastatic examples analysed (Sreekumar et al., 2009).

For the prostate cancer, as a metabolic intermediary of glycine biosynthesis, sarcosine was proposed as a urinary biomarker by Seekumar et al. (2009) since it is almost indiscernible in healthy individuals, yet highly pronounced in metastatic PCa (Sreekumar et al., 2009). Although the importance of sarcosine in carcinogenesis is unknown. But carcinogenesis makes alterations to the biosynthesis pathway of sarcosine. In the metabolism of PCa tissues, GNMT is in the critical position. It catalyzes the transformation from glycine to sarcosine (Cernei et al., 2013). Using urine as the matrix, other studies also achieved similar results (Jiang et al., 2010; Stabler et al., 2011; Bianchi et al., 2011; Cao et al., 2011; Khan et al., 2013). The clinical relevance of sarcosine as a biomarker was examined using different cell lines (primary and immortal benign prostate epithelial cells and immortal PC cells), and sarcosine levels were determined to be pronounced in immortal PCa lines (Sreekumar et al., 2009; Putluri et al., 2011). Gene expression modifications for the biosynthesis of enzymes contributing to sarcosine metabolism impact normal stages of the cell cycle, which is also noticeable in cellular metabolism of PCa (Sreekumar et al., 2009; Khan et al., 2013). Nevertheless, some studies reported insignificant results for urinary sarcosine differences for prostate cancer compared to control groups (Wu et al., 2011; Jentzmik et al., 2010), and these contrasting results could be the results of individual variations or variations in experimental methodology (Issaq & Veenstra, 2011).

In the urine of PCa patients, common metabolic patterns were observed in amino and organic acids, fatty acids, sphingolipids, and carbohydrates. The use of carbohydrates for energy production by cancer cells causes dysregulation of carbohydrate degradation. Alterations in carnitine patterns were also determined. The results showed disturbances in Krebs cycle energy metabolism that can be explained by the Warburg effect and changes in m-aconitase activity (Wu et al., 2011; Struck-Lewicka et al., 2015).

For the discrimination of low and high grades of PCa, the prospect of sarcosine as a clinical biomarker was reinforced by different studies that employed various methods, namely fluorometrics, LC-MS, and H-NMR, which were pointed to the increased plasma levels of sarcosine in PCa patients (Lucarelli et al., 2012; Koutros et al., 2013; Kumar et al., 2015).

Differences in certain biosynthesis pathways and associated metabolites were found in the serum/plasma samples from the patients with PCa. For cell proliferation abnormalities, the alteration in fatty acids is needed to provide energy (Zang et al., 2014; Crowe et al., 2008; Johansson et al., 2009; Zhou et al., 2012; Miyagi et al., 2011; Giskeodegard et al., 2015; Osl et al., 2008). The high levels serum glucose samples were related to increases in cancer recurrence even after rigorous treatment approaches such as radical prostatectomy and radiotherapy at the time of PCa diagnosis (Wright et al., 2013; Kumar et al., 2015; Pandeya et al., 2014).

Metabolomics results obtained from plasma and serum samples can be used to distinguish profile changes in cases of medications. Research investigated fasting plasma samples for metabolite profiling of patients with prostate cancer before and three months after androgen deprivation therapy, which was provided results for increases in majority of bile acids and decreases in steroid levels that were apparent during the course of treatment (Saylor et al., 2012). After 3 months of treatment, very low-level metabolites related to fatty acid metabolism were also observed, which was coupled with decreases in catabolism of carnitines, ketones, and other compound structures of keto-acids (Saylor et al., 2012).

To discover new biomarkers for cancer metabolomics can be successfully used due to the particular property of metabolite profiles as being the final phenotype in the cases of disease states.

Metabolic profiles are affected by different factors with diverse effects, e.g., age, diet, drugs, and others, which is the prime reason behind the interpretive challenges. The statistical platforms used, the analytical procedures and sample preparation are additional problems. While metabolomics is undisputedly a powerful field of research for the discoveries of significant biomarkers to provide clinical applications in numerous disease conditions, the vast amounts of data and inherent variations in such datasets are the most obvious technical and analytical setbacks in the field. However, the promising features are still bright.

Increases in amino acids, lactate, and choline were reported in nearly all research conducted on prostate cancer that used different samples of prostate fluids, urine, blood, tissues, and cell lines.

Using GC- and LC-MS, uniform metabolomics analysis of urinary, blood, and tissue levels had been accomplished, which otherwise requires both cell line and in vivo studies. Among all metabolites analyzed, three metabolites (cinnamoylglycine, nicotinamide, and cysteine-glutathione disulfide) provided highly critical changes from serum and tissue samples, which also supported the validity of serum samples in metabolite changes in contrast to tissue samples for developing pharmaceutical targets as evident in tryptophan degradation and PPAR-alpha antagonism (Sheila et al., 2012).

In all three matrices (plasma, urine, tissue) of the suite of identified metabolites, an apparent correlation between metabolic profiles was evident for tissue and serum samples, which in turn supports the notion of metabolic variation seen in different compartments (Sheila et al., 2012).

Research by Ganti et al. (2011) presented the feasibility of urinary acylcarnitines in humans for metabolic alterations in tissue samples, as was shown in patients with RCC, which was also supported by xenograft models.

Tissue cysteine-glutathione disulfide (CSSG) had the most increased magnitude of alterations among all measured metabolites (Sheila et al., 2012). This compound was below the detectable range in urine and changed in that matrix insignificantly. For kidney cancer, the clinical relevance of oxidative stress was emphasized from the striking differentiations in GSSG, GSH and CSSG levels in the samples (Kim et al., 2011).

The metabolic products in the nicotinamide and tryptophan pathways intersect in the metabolite quinolinate and were represented very well. The tryptophan metabolism pathway has been regularly observed in (Sheila et al., 2012) RCC metabolomics and proteomics studies (Kim et al., 2011, Perroud et al. 2008), and in other research a low amount of tryptophan in serum has been observed in all grades of RCCs (Lin et al., 2011). Among the analyzed metabolites, quinolinate was found to be proliferative for certain ccRCC cell lines (Kim et al., 2011).

In general, human steroid hormone precursors were observed to be the most down-regulated in urogenital schistosomiasis cases. To produce testosterone, estrogens, and estradiol, these steroid precursors are required. The host steroids are much reduced after urogenital schistosomiasis. Santos et al. (2014) demonstrated that a high amount of infertility occurs along with urogenital schistosomiasis. Botelho et al. suggested that this form of infertility may be due to hormonal imbalances (Botelho et al., 2017). Adewale et al. (2018) presented the notable reduction of precursor compounds for sex hormones in cases of urogenital schistosomiasis in humans.

Gouveia *et al.* (2015) detected four molecules called m/z 269, 228, 204 and 369 which were estrogen-related parasite molecules (Gouveia et al., 2015). These were significant enough to be considered as biomarkers on *S. haematobium, nevertheless, further validations of the proposed biomarkers are needed to establish standards and reveal structures.*

In urogenital schistosomiasis associated-bladder pathology cases, correlations were observed for phosphatidylcholine (PC) and phosphatidylethanolamine (PE). Bagnoli et al., 2016 suggested that increased PCs may have a role in induction of cancer (Bagnoli et al., 2016). Also, Zinrajh et al. (2014) suggested this in their study about colorectal and non-small-cell lung cancers (Zinrajh et al., 2014).

Azordegan et al. (2013) found GGM in pathologies of bladder without tumours. Baez et al. (1997) suggested increases for benzenamines of adrenochrome and 3-Succinoylpyridine, in cases of urogenital schistosomiasis infection.

Mostafa et al. detected 3-Succinoylpyridine, a nicotine metabolite, in the urine of schistosomiasis patients (Mostafa et al., 1999). It is suggested that they have a role in carcinogenesis. Also, Felicia et al. (Felicia et al., 2000) found 3SP in the urine of tobacco smokers in abundance in infection-only cases. Thus, Mostafa et al. have suggested that in urogenital schistosomiasis infection quinones could be formed (Mostafa et al., 1999).

Conclusion

Since metabolic profiles are the final phenotypes of a given disease condition, metabolomics has the convincing prospect of being a useful diagnostic method in the urology field. Metabolomics is a powerful tool for this aim. For example, prostate cancer, bladder cancer and kidney cancer. For detection, for disease progression, and for the therapeutic response, they could be used. But there are some challenges and limitations, such as insufficient samples in research for clinical validation even though quantitative methods are increasingly employed. The standardized qualification and quantification tests and methods are lack, and because of this, understanding the diagnosis and therapy can be challenging and takes too long. Even when the same samples were analyzed, there is some weak relationship and small overlap between biomarkers. The storage of samples, different handling, and work environmental conditions may support the dynamic, reliable, and sensitive metabolic profile. Different analytical techniques covering different metabolites had been used. These are some of the factors affecting results along with other diverse factors, e.g., genetics, lifestyle, environment, and medical history. Urine is especially prone to changes from such factors. Therefore, it may lead to errors in analysis. In the case of urinary metabolomics, this is more important. Despite the related difficulties, they can be used to detect therapeutic targets and to indicate of cancer prognosis. Therefore, further studies are still needed to establish truly sensitive, specific, and affordable non-invasive methods to use in clinical practice for the urology field.

References

Aboud, O. A., Weiss, R. H. (2013). New opportunities from the cancer metabolome. *Clin Chem,* 59: 138–146. https://doi.org/10.1373/clinchem.2012.184598.

Adewale, S. A., Mundhe, S. D., Awobode, H. O., Onile, O. S., Agunloye, A. M., Isokpehi, R. D., Shouche, Y. S., Santhakumari, B., Anumudu, C. I. (2018). Metabolite profiling for biomarkers in Schistosoma haematobium infection and associated bladder pathologies. *PLoS neglected tropical diseases*, 12(4): e0006452. https://doi.org/10.1371/journal.pntd.0006452.

Alberice, J. V., Amaral, A. F. S., Armitage, E. G., Lorente, J. A., Algaba, F., Carrilho, E., Marquez, M., Garcia, A., Malats, N., Barbas, C. (2013). Searching for urine biomarkers of bladder cancer recurrence using a liquid chromatography-mass spectrometry and capillary electrophoresis-mass spectrometry metabolomics approach. *J Chromatogr,* 1318: 163– 70. https://doi.org/10.1016/j.chroma.2013.10.002.

Azordegan, N., Fraser, V., Le, K., Hillyer, L. M., Ma, D. W., Fischer, G. (2013). Carcinogenesis alters fatty acid profile in breast tissue. *Mol Cell Biochem*, 374: 223–232. https://doi.org/10.1007/s11010-012-1523-4.

Bundy, J. G., Davey, M. P., Viant, M. R. (2009). Environmental metabolomics: a critical review and future perspectives. Metabolomics, 5: 3–21. https://doi.org/0.1007/s11306-008-0152-0.

Brindle, J. T., Antti, H., Holmes, E., Tranter, G., Nicholson, J. K., Bethell, H. W. L., Clarke, S., Schofield, P. M., McKilligin, E., Mosedale, D. E., Grainger, D. J. (2003). Rapid and noninvasive diagnosis of the presence and severity of coronary heart disease using 1H-NMR-based metabonomics. *Nat Med,* 9: 477–477. https://doi.org/10.1038/nm1202-802.

Bansal, N., Gupta, A., Mitash, N., Shakya, P. S., Mandhani, A., Mahdi, A. A., Sankhwar, S. N., Mandal, S. K. (2013). Low- and high-grade bladder cancer determination via human serum-based metabolomics approach. *J Proteome Res*, 12: 5839– 50. https://doi.org/10.1021/pr400859w.

Bianchi, F., Dugheri, S., Musci, M., Bonacchi, A., Salvadori, E., Arcangeli, G., Cupelli, V., Lanciotti, M., Masieri, L., Serni, S. (2011). Fully automated solid-phase microextraction-fast gas chromatography–mass spectrometry method using a new ionic liquid column for high-throughput analysis of sarcosine and *N*-ethylglycine in human urine and urinary sediments. *Anal Chim Acta.*, 707:197–203.

Botelho, M. C., Alves, H., Richter, J. (2017). Estrogen catechols detection as biomarkers in schistosomiasis induced cancer and infertility. *Lett Drug Des Discov*, 14(2): 135–138. https://doi.org/10.2174/1570180813666160720165057.

Bagnoli, M., Granata, A., Nicoletti, R., Krishnamachary, B., Bhujwalla, Z. M., Canese, R., Podo, F., Canevari, S., Iorio, E., Mezzanzanica, D. (2016). Choline metabolism alteration: a focus on ovarian cancer. *Front Oncol*, 6:153. https://doi.org/10.3389/fonc.2016.00153.

Baez, S., Segura-Aguilar, J., Widersten, M., Johansson, A., Mannervik, B. (1997). Glutathione transferases catalyse the detoxication of oxidized metabolites (o-quinones) of catecholamines and may serve as an antioxidant system preventing degenerative cellular processes. *Biochem J*, 324: 25–28. https://doi.org/10.1042/bj3240025.

Cao, M., Zhao, L., Chen, H., Xue, W., Lin D. (2012). NMR-based metabolomic analysis of human bladder cancer. *Anal Sci*, 28: 451– 6. https://doi.org/10.2116/analsci.28.451.

Chen, Y. T., Chen, C. L., Chen, H. W., Chung, T., Wu, C. C., Chen, C. D., Hsu, C. W., Chen, M. C., Tsui, K. H., Chang, P. L., Chang, Y. S., Yu, J. S. (2010). Discovery of novel bladder cancer biomarkers by comparative urine proteomics using iTRAQ technology. *Journal of Proteome Research*, 9(11):5803–15. https://doi.org/10.1021/pr100576x.

Chen, Y. T., Chen, H. W., Domanski, D., Smith, D. S., Liang, K. H., Wu, C. C., Chen, C. L., Chung, T., Chen, M. C., Chang, Y. S., Parker, C. E., Borchers, C. H., Yu, J. S. (2012). Multiplexed quantification of 63 proteins in human urine by multiple reaction monitoring-based mass spectrometry for discovery of potential bladder cancer biomarkers. *Journal of Proteomics*, 75(12):3529–45. https://doi.org/10.1016/j.jprot.2011.12.031.

Cernei, N., Heger, Z., Gumulec, J., Zitka, O., Masarik, M., Babula, P., Eckschlager, T., Stiborova, M., Kizek, R., Adam, V. (2013). Sarcosine as a potential prostate cancer biomarker - a review. *Int J Mol Sci.* 14:13893–13908. https://doi.org/10.3390/ijms140713893.

Cao, D. L., Ye, D. W., Zhang, H. L., Zhu, Y., Wang, Y. X., Yao, X. D. (2011). A multiplex model of combining gene-based, protein-based, and metabolite-based with positive and negative markers in urine for the early diagnosis of prostate cancer. *Prostate*, 71:700–710. https://doi.org/10.1002/pros.21286.

Crowe, F. L., Allen, N. E., Appleby, P. N. (2008). Fatty acid composition of plasma phospholipids and risk of prostate cancer in a case–control analysis nested within the European Prospective Investigation into Cancer and Nutrition. *Am J Clin Nutr*, 88:1353–1363. https://doi.org/10.3945/ajcn.2008.26369.

Dunne, V. G., Bhattachayya, S., Besser, M., Rae, C., Griffin, J. L. (2005). Metabolites from cerebrospinal fluid in aneurysmal subarachnoid haemorrhage correlate with vasospasm and clinical outcome: a pattern-recognition H-1 NMR study. *NMR Biomed*, 18: 24–33. https://doi.org/10.1002/nbm.918.

Dettmer, K., Vogl, F. C., Ritter, A. P., Zhu, W., Nürnberger, N., Kreutz, M., Oefner, P. J., Gronwald, W., Gottfried, E. (2013). Distinct metabolic differences between various human cancer and primary cells. *Electrophoresis*, 34: 2836– 47. https://doi.org/10.1002/elps.201300228.

Felicia, N. D., Rekha, G. K., Murphy, S. E. (2000). Characterization of cytochrome P450 2A4 and 2A5 catalysed 4-(methylnitrosamino)-1-(3-pyridyl)-1-butanone (NNK) metabolism. *Arch. Biochem Biophys*, 384: 418–424. https://doi.org/10.1006/abbi.2000.2128.

Gamagedara, S., Shi, H., Ma, Y. (2012). Quantitative determination of taurine and related biomarkers in urine by liquid chromatography–tandem mass spectrometry. *Analytical and bioanalytical chemistry*, 402: 763-770. https://doi.org/10.1007/s00216-011-5491-4.

Garcia-Cazorla, A., Mochel, F., Lamari, F., Saudubray, J. M. (2015). The clinical spectrum of inherited diseases involved in the synthesis and remodeling of complex lipids, A tentative overview. *Journal of inherited metabolic disease,* 38:19–40. https://doi.org/10.1007/s10545-014-9776-6.

Giskeodegard, G. F., Hansen, A. F., Bertilsson, H., Gonzalez, S. V., Kristiansen, K. A., Bruheim, P., Mjos, S. A., Angelsen, A., Bathen, T. F., Tessem, M. B. (2015). Metabolic markers in blood can separate prostate cancer from benign prostatic hyperplasia. *Br J Cancer*, 113:1712–1719. https://doi.org/10.1038/bjc.2015.411.

Ganti, S., Taylor, S., Kim, K., Hoppel, C. L., Guo, L., Yang, J., Evans, C, Weiss, R. H. (2011). Urinary acylcarnitines are altered in kidney cancer. *Int J Cancer*, 130(12): 2791-2800. https://doi.org/10.1002/ijc.26274.

Gouveia, M. J., Santos, J., Brindley, P. J., Rinaldi, G., Lopes, C., Santos, L. L., da Costa, J. M., Vale, N. (2015). Estrogen-like metabolites and DNA-adducts in urogenital schistosomiasis-associated bladder cancer. *Cancer Letters*, 359: 226–232. https://doi.org/10.1016/j.canlet.2015.01.018.

He, J. C., Chuang, P. Y., Ma'ayan, A., Iyengar, R. (2012). Systems biology of kidney diseases. *Kidney Int*. 81:22–39. https://doi.org/10.1038/ki.2011.314.

Issaq, H. J., Veenstra, T. D. (2011). Is sarcosine a biomarker for prostate cancer? *J Sep Sci*, 34:3619–3621. https://doi.org/10.1002/jssc.201100572.

Jiang, Y., Cheng, X., Wang, C., Ma, Y. (2010;). Quantitative determination of sarcosine and related compounds in urinary samples by liquid chromatography with tandem mass spectrometry. *Anal Chem*, 82:9022–9027. https://doi.org/10.1021/ac1019914.

Jentzmik, F., Stephan, C., Miller, K., Schrader, M., Erbersdobler, A., Kristiansen, G., Lein, M., Jung, K. (2010). Sarcosine in urine after digital rectal examination fails as a marker in prostate cancer detection and identification of aggressive tumours. *Eur Urol*, 58:12–18. https://doi.org/10.1016/j.eururo.2010.01.035.

Jin, X., Yun, S. J., Jeong, P. Kim, I. Y., Kim, W. J., Park, S. (2014). Diagnosis of bladder cancer and prediction of survival by urinary metabolomics. *Oncotarget* 5: 1635– 45. https://doi.org/10.18632/oncotarget.1744.

Johansson, M., Van Guelpen, B., Vollset, S. E., Hultdin, J., Bergh, A., Key, T., Midttun, O., Hallmans, G., Ueland, P. M., Stattin, P. (2009). One-carbon metabolism and prostate cancer risk: prospective investigation of seven circulating B vitamins and metabolites. *Cancer Epidemiol Biomarkers Prev*, 18:1538–1543. https://doi.org/10.1158/1055-9965.EPI-08-1193.

Kaddurah-Daouk, R., Beecher, C., Kristal, B., Maston, W., Bogdanov, M. (2004). Bioanalytical advances for metabolomics and metabolic profiling. *Pharmagenomics*, 4: 46–52.

Kreunin, P., Zhao, J., Rosser, C., Urquidi, V., Lubman, D. M., Goodison, S. (2007). Bladder cancer associated glycoprotein signatures revealed by urinary proteomic profiling. *Journal of Proteome Research*, 6(7):2631–9. https://doi.org/10.1021/pr0700807.

Khan, A. P., Rajendiran, T. M., Ateeq, B., Asangani, I. A., Athanikar, J. N., Yocum, A. K., Mehra, R., Siddiqui, J., Palapattu, G., Wei, J. T. (2013). The role of sarcosine metabolism in prostate cancer progression. *Neoplasia*, 15:491–501. https://doi.org/10.1593/neo.13314.

Koutros, S., Meyer, T. E., Fox, S. D., Issaq, H. J., Veenstra, T. D., Huang, W. Y., Yu, K., Albanes, D., Chu, L. W., Andriole, G. (2013). Prospective evaluation of serum sarcosine and risk of prostate cancer in the Prostate, Lung, Colorectal and Ovarian Cancer Screening Trial. *Carcinogenesis*, 34:2281–2285. https://doi.org/10.1093/carcin/bgt176.

Kumar, D., Gupta, A., Mandhani, A., Sankhwar, S. N. (2015). Metabolomics-derived prostate cancer biomarkers: fact or fiction? *J Proteome Res*, 14:1455–1464. https://doi.org/10.1021/pr5011108.

Kim, K., Taylor, S. L., Ganti, S., Guo, L., Osier, M. V., Weiss, R. H. (2011). Urine Metabolomic Analysis Identifies Potential Biomarkers and Pathogenic Pathways in Kidney Cancer. *OMICS*, 15:293–303. https://doi.org/10.1089/omi.2010.0094.

Lamari, F., Mochel, F., Saudubray, J. M. (2015). An overview of inborn errors of complex lipid biosynthesis and remodelling. *Journal of inherited metabolic disease,* 38:3–18. https://doi.org/10.1007/s10545-014-9764-x.

Linden, M., Lind, S. B., Mayrhofer, C., Segersten, U., Wester, K., Lyutvinskiy, Y., Zubarev, R., Malmström, P. U., Pettersson, U. (2012). Proteomic analysis of urinary biomarker candidates for nonmuscle invasive bladder cancer. *Proteomics*, 12(1):135–44. https://doi.org/10.1002/pmic.201000810.

Lei, T., Zhao, X., Jin, S., Meng, Q., Zhou, H., Zhang, M. (2013). Discovery of potential bladder cancer biomarkers by comparative urine proteomics and analysis. *Clinical Genitourinary Cancer*, 11(1):56–62. https://doi.org/10.1016/j.clgc.2012.06.003.

Li, H., Li, C., Wu, H., Zhang, T., Wang, J., Wang, S., Chang, J. (2011). Identification of Apo-A1 as a biomarker for early diagnosis of bladder transitional cell carcinoma. *Proteome science,* 9(1):21. https://doi.org/10.1186/1477-5956-9-21.

Li, F., Chen, D. N., He, C. W., Zhou, Y., Olkkonen, V. M., He, N., Chen, W., Wan, P., Chen, S. S., Zhu, Y. T., Lan, K. J., Tan, W. L. (2012). Identification of urinary Gc-globulin as a novel biomarker for bladder cancer by two-dimensional fluorescent differential gel electrophoresis (2D-DIGE). *Journal of Proteomics*, 77:225–36. https://doi.org/10.1016/j.jprot.2012.09.002.

Li, C., Li, H., Zhang, T., Li, J., Liu, L., Chang, J. (2014). Discovery of Apo-A1 as a potential bladder cancer biomarker by urine proteomics and analysis. *Biochemical and Biophysical Research Communications*, 446(4):1047–52. https://doi.org/10.1016/j.bbrc.2014.03.053.

Lucarelli, G., Fanelli, M., Larocca, A. M., Germinario, C. A., Rutigliano, M., Vavallo, A., Selvaggi, F. P., Bettocchi, C., Battaglia, M., Ditonno, P. (2012). Serum sarcosine increases the accuracy of prostate cancer detection in patients with total serum PSA less than 4.0 ng/ml. *Prostate*, 72:1611–1621. https://doi.org/10.1002/pros.22514.

Lin, L., Huang, Z., Gao, Y., Yan, X., Xing, J., Hang, W. (2011). LC-MS based serum metabonomic analysis for renal cell carcinoma diagnosis, staging, and biomarker discovery. *J Proteome Res*, 10:1396–405. https://doi.org/10.1021/pr101161u.

Montoliu, I., Genick, U., Ledda, M., Collino, S., Martin, F. P., le Coutre, J., Rezzi, S. (2013). Current status on genome-metabolome-wide associations: an opportunity in nutrition research. *Genes Nutr*, 8: 19–27. https://doi.org/10.1007/s12263-012-0313-7.

Mendrick, D. L., Schnackenberg, L. (2009). Genomic and metabolomic advances in the identification of disease and adverse event biomarkers. *Biomark Med,* 3: 605–615. https://doi.org/10.2217/bmm.09.43.

Monteiro, M., Carvalho, M., de Lourdes Bastos, M., de Pinho, P. (2014a). Biomarkers in renal cell carcinoma: a metabolomics approach. *Metabolomics,* 10:1210–1222. https://doi.org/10.1007/s11306-014-0659-5.

Monteiro, M. S., Carvalho M, Bastos, M. L., de Pinho, P., G. (2013). Metabolomics analysis for biomarker discovery: advances and challenges. *Curr Med Chem,* 20:257–271. https://doi.org/10.2174/092986713804806621.

Monteiro, M., Carvalho, M., Henrique, R., Jeronimo, C., Moreira, N., de Lourdes Bastos, M., de Pinho, P. G. (2014b). Analysis of volatile human urinary metabolome by solid-phase microextraction in combination with gas chromatography–mass spectrometry for biomarker discovery: application in a pilot study to discriminate patients with renal

cell carcinoma. *Eur J Cancer,* 50:1993–2002. https://doi.org/10.1016/j.ejca.2014.04.011.
Monteiro, M. S., Carvalho, M., Bastos, M. dL., Pinho, P. G. (2015). Identification and data processing methods in metabolomics: Potentiality of volatile organic compounds to discriminate patients with cancer by using chemometric tools. *Future Science Ltd.,* pp. 166–184. https://doi.org/10.4155/fseb2013.14.178.
Miyagi, Y., Higashiyama, M., Gochi, A., Akaike, M., Ishikawa, T., Miura, T., Saruki, N., Bando, E., Kimura, H., Imamur, F. (2011). Plasma free amino acid profiling of five types of cancer patients and its application for early detection. *PLoS One*, 6: e24143. https://doi.org/10.1371/journal.pone.0024143.
Mostafa M. H., Sheweita S. A., O'Connor P. J. (1999). Relationship between schistosomiasis and bladder cancer, Clin Microbiol Rev. 12: 97–111. https://doi.org/10.1128/CMR.12.1.97.
Nicholson, J. K., Holmes, E., Kinross, J. M., Darzi, A. W., Takats, Z., Lindon, J. C. (2012). Metabolic phenotyping in clinical and surgical environments. *Nature,* 491: 384–392. https://doi.org/10.1038/nature11708.
Ng, D. J. Y., Pasikanti, K. K., Chan, E. C. Y. (2011). Trend analysis of metabonomics and systematic review of metabonomics-derived cancer marker metabolites. *Metabolomics*, 7: 155–178. https://doi.org/10.1007/s11306-010-0250-7.
Osl, M., Dreiseitl, S., Pfeifer, B., Weinberger, K., Klocker, H., Bartsch, G., Schafer, G., Tilg, B., Graber, A., Baumgartner, C. (2008). A new rule-based algorithm for identifying metabolic markers in prostate cancer using tandem mass spectrometry. *Bioinformatics*, 24:2908–2914. https://doi.org/10.1093/bioinformatics/btn506.
Pasikanti, K. K., Esuvaranathan, K., Ho, P. C., Mahendran, R., Kamaraj, R., Wu, Q. H., Chiong, E., Chan, E. C. (2010). Noninvasive urinary metabolomic diagnosis of human bladder cancer. *J Proteome Res*, 9: 2988– 95.
Pasikanti, K. K., Esuvaranathan, K., Hong, Y., Mahendran, R., Raman Nee Mani, L., Chiong, E., Chan, E. C. (2013). Urinary metabotyping of bladder cancer using two-dimensional gas chromatography time-of-flight mass spectrometry. *J Proteome Res*, 12: 3865– 73. https://doi.org/10.1021/pr4000448.
Putluri, N., Shojaie, A., Vasu, V. T., Vareed, S. K., Nalluri, S., Putluri, V., Thangjam, G. S., Panzitt, K., Tallman, C. T., Butler, C., Sana, T. R., Fischer, S. M., Sica, G., Brat, D. J., Shi, H., Palapattu, G. S., Lotan, Y., Weizer, A. Z., Terris, M. K., Shariat, S. F., Michailidis, G., Sreekumar, A. (2011). Metabolomic profiling reveals potential markers and bioprocesses altered in bladder cancer progression. *Cancer Res*, 71: 7376– 86. https://doi.org/10.1158/0008-5472.CAN-11-1154.
Putluri, N., Shojaie, A., Vasu, V. T., Nalluri, S., Vareed, S. K., Putluri, V., Vivekanandan-Giri, A., Byun, J., Pennathur, S., Sana, T. R. (2011). Metabolomic profiling reveals a role for androgen in activating amino acid metabolism and methylation in prostate cancer cells. *PLoS One*, 6:e21417. https://doi.org/ 10.1371/journal.pone.0021417.
Pandeya, D. R., Mittal, A., Sathian, B., Bhatta, B. (2014). Role of hyperinsulinemia in increased risk of prostate cancer: a case control study from Kathmandu Valley. *Asian Pac J Cancer Prev*, 15:1031–1033. https://doi.org/10.7314/apjcp.2014.15.2.1031.

Perroud, B., Ishimaru, T., Borowsky, A. D., Weiss, R. H. (2008). Grade-dependent proteomics characterization of kidney cancer. *Mol Cell Proteomics*, 8:971–85. https://doi.org/10.1074/mcp.M800252-MCP200.

Ramautar, R. Berger, R., van der Greef, J., Hankemeier, T. (2013). Human metabolomics: strategies to understand biology. *Curr Opin Chem Biol*, 17:841–846. https://doi.org/10.1016/j.cbpa.2013.06.015.

Srivastava, S., Roy, R., Singh, S. Kumar, P., Dalela, D., Sankhwar, S. N., Goel, A., Sonkar, A. A. (2010). Taurine - a possible fingerprint biomarker in non-muscle invasive bladder cancer: a pilot study by 1H NMR spectroscopy. *Cancer Biomarker*, 6: 11– 20. https://doi.org/10.3233/CBM-2009-0115.

Shen, C., Sun, Z., Chen, D., Su, X., Jiang, J., Li, G., Lin, B., Yan, J. (2019). Developing urinary metabolomic signatures as early bladder cancer diagnostic markers. *Omics* 19: 1– 11. https://doi.org/10.1089/omi.2014.0116.

Sreekumar, A., Poisson, L. M., Rajendiran, T. M., Khan, A. P., Cao, Q., Yu, J., Laxman, B., Mehra, R., Lonigro, R. J., Li, Y. (2009). Metabolomic profiles delineate potential role for sarcosine in prostate cancer progression. *Nature*, 457:910–914. https://doi.org/10.1038/nature07762.

Stabler, S., Koyama, T., Zhao, Z., Martinez-Ferrer, M., Allen, R. H., Luka, Z., Loukachevitch, L. V., Clark, P. E., Wagner, C., Bhowmick, N. A. (2011). Serum methionine metabolites are risk factors for metastatic prostate cancer progression. *PLoS One*, 6:e22486. https://doi.org/10.1371/journal.pone.0022486.

Struck-Lewicka, W. Kordalewska, M., Bujak, R., Yumba Mpanga, A., Markuszewski, M., Jacyna, J., Matuszewski, M., Kaliszan, R., Markuszewski, M. J. (2015). Urine metabolic fingerprinting using LC-MS and GC-MS reveals metabolite changes in prostate cancer: A pilot study. *J Pharm Biomed Anal,* 111:351–361. https://doi.org/10.1016/j.jpba.2014.12.026.

Saylor, P. J., Karoly, E. D., Smith, M. R. (2012). Prospective study of changes in the metabolomic profiles of men during their first three months of androgen deprivation therapy for prostate cancer. *Clin Cancer Res*, 18:3677–3685. https://doi.org/10.1158/1078-0432.CCR-11-3209.

Sheila, G., Sandra, L., Taylor S., Omran Abu, A., Joy, Y., Christopher E., Michael, V. O., Danny, C. A., Kyoungmi, K., Weiss R. H. (2012 Jul 15). Kidney tumor biomarkers revealed by simultaneous multiple matrix metabolomics analysis. *Cancer Res*, 72(14): 3471–3479. https://doi.org/10.1158/0008-5472.CAN-11-3105.

Santos, J., Gouveia, M. J., Vale, N., Delgado, M. L., Goncalves, A., da Silva, J .M., Oliveira, C., Xavier, P., Gomes, P., Santos, L. L., Lopes, C., Barros, A., Rinaldi, G., Brindley, P. J., da Costa, J. M., Sousa, M., Botelho, M. C. (2014). Urinary estrogen metabolites and self-reported infertility in women infected with Schistosoma haematobium. *PLoS ONE*, 9(5): e96774. https://doi.org/10.1371/journal.pone.0096774.

Trock, B. J. (2011). Application of metabolomics to prostate cancer. *Urol Oncol,* 29:572–581. https://doi.org/10.1016/j.urolonc.2011.08.002.

Tripathi, P., Somashekar, B. S., Ponnusamy, M., Gursky, A., Dailey, S., Kunju, P., Lee, C. T., Chinnaiyan, A. M., Rajendiran, T. M., Ramamoorthy, A. (2013). HR-MAS NMR tissue metabolomic signatures cross-validated by mass spectrometry distinguish bladder cancer from benign disease. *J Proteome Res*, 12: 3519– 28. https://doi.org/10.1021/pr4004135.

Viant, M. R. (2008). Recent developments in environmental metabolomics. *Mol Biosyst,* 4: 980–986. https://doi.org/10.1039/b805354e.

Wishart, D. S. (2008). Applications of metabolomics in drug discovery and development. *Drugs R D*, 9: 307–322. https://doi.org/10.2165/00126839-200809050-00002.

Weiss, R. H., Kim, K. (2012). Metabolomics in the study of kidney diseases. *Nat Rev Nephrol,* 8:22–33. https://doi.org/10.1038/nrneph.2011.152.

Wu, H., Liu, T., Ma, C., Xue, R., Deng, C., Zeng, H., Shen, X. (2011). GC/MS-based metabolomic approach to validate the role of urinary sarcosine and target biomarkers for human prostate cancer by microwave-assisted derivatization. *Anal Bioanal Chem*, 401:635–646. https://doi.org/10.1007/s00216-011-5098-9.

Wright, J. L., Plymate, S. R., Porter, M. P., Gore, J. L., Lin, D. W., Hu, E., Zeliadt, S. B. (2013). Hyperglycemia and prostate cancer recurrence in men treated for localized prostate cancer. *Prostate Cancer Prostatic Dis*, 16:204–208. https://doi.org/ 10.1038/pcan.2013.5.

Yang, N., Feng, S., Shedden, K., Xie, X., Liu, Y., Rosser, C. J., Lubman, D. M., Goodison, S. (2011). Urinary glycoprotein biomarker discovery for bladder cancer detection using LC/MS-MS and label-free quantification. *Clinical Cancer Research* 17(10):3349–59. https://doi.org/10.1158/1078-0432.CCR-10-3121.

Zhang, A., Sun, H., Wang, P., Han, Y., Wang, X. (2012). Recent and potential developments of biofluid analyses in metabolomics. *J. Proteom*, 75:1079–1088. https://doi.org/10.1016/j.jprot.2011.10.027.

Zang, X., Jones, C. M., Long, T. Q., Monge, M. E., Zhou, M., Walker, L. D., Mezencev, R., Gray, A., McDonald, J. F., Fernandez, F. M. (2014). Feasibility of detecting prostate cancer by ultraperformance liquid chromatography–mass spectrometry serum metabolomics. *J Proteome Res*, 13:3444–3454. https://doi.org/10.1021/ pr500409q.

Zhou, X., Mao, J., Ai, J., Deng, Y., Roth, M. R., Pound, C., Henegar, J., Welti, R., Bigler, S. A. (2012). Identification of plasma lipid biomarkers for prostate cancer by lipidomics and bioinformatics. *PLoS One*, 7:e48889. https://doi.org/10.1371/journal. pone.0048889.

Zinrajh, D., Hörl, G., Jürgens, G., Marc, J., Sok, M., Cerne, D. (2014). Increased phosphatidylethanolamine N-methyltransferase gene expression in non-small-cell lung cancer tissue predicts shorter patient survival. *Oncology Letters*, 7: 2175–2179. https://doi.org/10.3892/ol.2014.2035.

Chapter 20

Metabolomic Applications in Food Science and Nutrition

Ayse Burcu Aktas*, PhD
Department of Biochemistry, Faculty of Science,
Sivas Cumhuriyet University, Sivas, Turkey

Abstract

The definition of metabolomics encloses an efficient description of small molecule metabolites present in different biological matrices. Metabolomics has shown up as a prominent tool for various areas including health diseases, drug research, plant science, food science, and nutrition. The metabolomics has recently been used to investigate some parameters in particular for food quality, processing, and the safety of both raw materials and final products. Food metabolomics has also a position in human nutrition research. This book chapter focuses on the novel and potential applications of metabolomics in food science and nutrition by summarizing some metabolomic analysis of food components, metabolomics from the preferential, presumable, and informative approaches in food processing, food microbiology, food safety, food quality, and benefits of foodomics in human nutrition and related health diseases.

Keywords: metabolomics, foodomics, food science, food processing, food analyses, nutrition

* Corresponding Author's Email: burcuaktas@cumhuriyet.edu.tr.

In: Metabolomics and Clinical Approach
Editors: Sevgi Durna Daştan and Taner Daştan
ISBN: 979-8-89113-095-1

Introduction

Metabolomics is a discipline to explain the performances of metabolites by identifying, quantifying, and detailing their mechanisms of action. There are several advanced instruments and techniques to investigate the metabolomes of various samples, including fundamentally nuclear magnetic resonance (NMR), mass spectrometry (MS), and vibrational spectrometry (VS) or combinations of other techniques. Generally, all these instrumental techniques are aimed to isolate, determine, quantify, characterize structures, and explain their functions on the metabolic pathways. Since metabolomes are complex molecules, it is highly needed to conduct many of these techniques together to better understand the whole mechanism (Fraga-Corral et al., 2022; Zhang et al., 2012).

Metabolomics has great potential to figure out the major problems of food science. Moreover, metabolomics is considered as an effective technique for further agricultural needs (Green et al., 2007; Hall et al., 2008). The engagements of informative, discriminative, and predictive metabolomics have been used for food quality, process, nutrition, and food component analysis (Cevallos-Cevallos et al., 2009). This book chapter covers a review of current metabolomics applications in food quality, safety, microbiology, processing, and nutrition.

Metabolomics in Food Science

Analysis of Food Metabolomics

The analysis of food metabolomics has been used in food safety control, including foodborne pathogens, toxins, some allergens, pesticides, antibiotics, food quality (in terms of organoleptic properties and nutritional value), food authenticity, and food traceability (Cook and Nightingale, 2018).

There are six main steps for metabolomics analysis including sample preparation, metabolite extraction, derivatization, metabolite separation, detection, and data treatment. In general, the essential steps for metabolomics analysis are detection and data analysis. The steps could be selected according to the purpose of the study, sample type, instrument type, and detection method (Pinu, 2015). Some of the metabolomics studies related to different food samples are summarized in Table 1. Since the metabolomic analyses of foods are quite varied, most studies could be classified as discriminative. The informative metabolomic analyses are mostly interested in the recognition and quantification of certain metabolites to obtain detailed information about the food sample. The untargeted metabolomics solely focuses on the identification of some groups of metabolites to obtain patterns or fingerprints, whereas targeted metabolomics demands higher purification and selective extraction stages (Alonso et al., 2015). Some metabolomics studies are predictive means that statistical models are constructed to estimate a variable that is difficult to quantify based on the metabolite profile and abundance (Table 1).

Table 1. The metabolomics studies of different food samples

Sample and purpose	Analysis Type	Instrumentation	Data Analysis	Reference
Blueberries: polyphenol composition	Untargeted/ informative	UHPLC-MS	Principal Component Analysis (PCA)	Zhao et al., 2017
Cheese: Production control	Untargeted/ informative	IMS	Compound identification	Vautz et al., 2006
Honey: determinations of residues	Untargeted/ discriminative/ predictive	NMR	Partial Least Square (PLS)	Li et al., 2016
Meat: quality/safety	Targeted/ discriminative	HILIC-MS/MS	MRL Validation	Dasenaki et al., 2016
Olive oil: classification	Untargeted/ predictive	GC-HRMS	Orthogonal partial least squares discriminant analysis (OPLS-DA)	Sales et al., 2017
Maize: GMO identification	Untargeted/ discriminative	CE-TOF-MS	PCA	Levandi et al., 2008
Vinegar: Metabolic profile	Untargeted/ discriminative	GC-MS	Hierarchical cluster analysis (HCA)	Pinu et al., 2016
Fermented vegetable juice: monitoring metabolites	Untargerted/ discriminative/ predictive	NMR	PCA OPLS-DA	Tomita et al., 2017
Coffee: determination of product origin	Untargeted/ predictive/ discriminative	UHPLC-(Q)ToF MS	PCA PLS-DA	Ossa et al., 2018
Almonds: discrimination	Untargerted/ discriminative/ predictive	UHPLC-(Q)ToF	PCA PLS-DA	Solsona et al., 2018
Tea	Targeted	GC-MS	MRL Validation	Saito-Shida et al., 2015
Shellfish: drug residue	Targeted	LC/GC-MS-MS	Compound identification	Chang et al., 2016
Wheat	Untargeted	UHPLC-(Q)ToF	PCA OPLS-DA	Rubert et al., 2017a

Metabolomics in Food Quality

The main target of food quality states is to ensure the appropriate organoleptic and desired characteristics of the product. The research related to food quality aims to evaluate the impacts of food processes on food compounds. The improvement in metabolomic techniques has allowed the monitoring of some quality parameters of foods during processing. The metabolomics methods have been commonly employed to identify the chemical composition of food products (Cossignani et al., 2014). The taste quality of white tea was evaluated by non-targeted metabolomics in combination with multivariate analysis (Yue et al., 2019). A metabolomic data-based prediction model was constructed which could separate green, yellow, and white teas according to unique tea metabolites (Zhang et al., 2019). The two-dimensional liquid chromatography was utilized in the determination of anthocyanins of different aged red wines and also to make the comparison of metabolites of aged red wines (Willemse et al., 2015). An untargeted metabolomics technique was used to distinguish the volatile compounds of grape juices according to various fungal infections performed by *Botrytis cinerea, Penicillium expansum, Aspergillus niger,* or *A. carbonarius* (Schueuermann et al., 2019).

Food authenticity and quality are closely related to each other. Food adulteration exposes defects in quality by incorporating prohibited ingredients or poor products, causing a health threat to customers. Therefore, food authenticity has great importance in the food industry for maintaining nutritional benefits, origin, and production standards. The metabolomics-based methods effectively specify the discrimination potential between adulterated and authentic foods. Moreover, metabolomics has been used to define the protected designation of origin (PDO) of food products. A prediction model was performed to discriminate adulterated Bordeaux wine in terms of geographical origin with LC-QTOF-MS (Lin et al., 2014). The different ingredients of the milk powders were analyzed by metabolomics coupled with 2DLC and monosaccharides were found in various trademarks and types of milk powder (Ma et al., 2014).

Metabolomics-based methods have been extensively used in examining the ingredients stated on the label of fruits, rice, and different vegetables (potatoes, peppers, white cabbage), clarifying differences in established production systems of wheat and maize, detecting the origin of olive oil, vinegar, wine, almonds, cocoa beans, honey, coffee species, saffron, and citrus fruit juices (Li et al., 2021).

Metabolomics in Food Microbiology

The foodborne pathogens, particularly *Salmonella spp.*, *Listeria monocytogenes*, *Campylobacter jejuni*, and *Shigella spp.*, spoilage microorganisms (such as Pseudomonas spp., *Acinetobacter spp.*, and *Botrytis spp.*), and currently emerging pathogens have appeared as a result of the internationalization of the food supply chain and food consumption trends (Li and Zhu, 2017). Traditional laboratory techniques are primarily time-consuming and labor-intensive. A large number of microbial biomarkers with varying levels of microbial contamination have been identified using metabolomics-based methods. These methods have demonstrated significant promise in the early detection of microbial contamination. The GC-MS has been used to characterize three prominent foodborne pathogens, *E. coli O157:H7*, *L. monocytogenes*, and *S. enterica*. Several potential pathogen-specific biomarkers were discovered, allowing the rapid differentiation of food samples containing pathogens (Jadhav et al., 2019). Furthermore, metabolomics has the ability to determine some antimicrobial compounds responsible for the antimicrobial characteristics of foods (Cevallos-Cevallos et al., 2009).

Despite the fact that this technique is promising in identifying metabolic shifts in different stages of microorganisms and providing important information on pathogen microorganisms, it is challenging to develop a universal method for removing bacterial cultures during metabolomics research. The extracellular and intracellular metabolites of microorganisms are typically difficult to distinguish from each other and also to identify. Moreover, metabolites are relatively unstable and could be quickly degraded during the handling and processing of samples. The current improvements in microbial metabolomics are not optimal. Therefore, more sensitive and reproducible analytical tools, as well as appropriate sample treatment techniques, are required to successfully determine the complexity of metabolites for metabolomics analysis (Li et al., 2021).Metabolomics in Food Safety

The foods could be contaminated with foodborne causative agents (pathogens and biotoxins), and some physical and chemical materials (pesticides and metals) which cause to foodborne illnesses throughout the critical steps of food processes. Metabolomics is able to evaluate the safety conditions of foods during processing and pre- and post-harvest periods and storage. Generally, untargeted discriminative analysis has been used for food safety. The MS/NMR-based metabolomics analysis is superior for the detection and quantification of pathogens, chemical contaminants, prohibition compounds, and natural toxins (Rešetar et al., 2015).

Foodborne pathogens and their toxins do not remarkably the change characteristic properties (flavor, texture, or appearance) of foods. As a result, microbial contaminants are the most frequently reported foodborne causative agents. Microbial metabolomics may also be used to explain how environmental factors affect complex biological systems (Anderson et al., 2014). The metabolomic applications for food microbiology are discussed in the previous section.

Foodborne biotoxins are classified into two groups: intrinsic foodborne biotoxins and extrinsic foodborne biotoxins. These toxins are synthesized and released into the environment during pathogen growth and cause common foodborne outbreaks. Metabolomics is able to detect toxins in the early stages to ensure food safety. Mass spectroscopy, in particular, could profile metabolites associated with microbial contamination, and NMR could also directly define microbial toxins (Kleigrewe et al., 2012). Some natural toxins are known to be lethal since they are extremely toxic at lower concentrations. As a result, preparation methods should be improved to provide sensitive and high-throughput detection. For example, the addition of multiple antibody immunoaffinity columns prior to HPLC-MS/MS was selectively determined different toxins with a reduction in the detection limit (Zhang et al., 2016).

Fungicides, pesticides, antibiotics, and nanomaterials are examples of xenobiotics that can contaminate food via the atmosphere, soil, and water. These xenobiotics negatively affect whole living organisms even at low levels. Metabolomics can detect various groups of xenobiotics in various food matrices (Li et al., 2021).

The metabolomics methods have been developed to control veterinary drug residues and antibiotics in animals following alterations in metabolites in biological tissues (Kaufmann et al., 2015). Liquid chromatography combined with electrospray ionization and tandem mass spectrometry (LC-ESI-MS/MS) has been utilized in the quantification and identification of 115 different veterinary drug and pharmaceutical residues in milk powder, egg, and fish tissue (Dasenaki and Thomaidis, 2015). A targeted analysis has been performed by investigating 20 different antibiotic residues in dairy products including powdered milk, commercial milk, and raw milk (Wang et al., 2017).

The pesticides are widely used in agricultural productions. Pesticides are receiving much more attention since the presence of residues in foods involves health risks. For multi-residue pesticide analyses in various foods, the combination of QuEChERS (Quick, Easy, Cheap, Effective, Rugged, and

Safe) with solid-phase extraction (SPE) or solid-phase micro-extraction (SPME) has been achieved. The QuEChERS approach was optimized for the determination of mycotoxins and pesticides in coffee. It was observed that 117 pesticides and 30 mycotoxins were present in raw coffee (González-Curbelo et al., 2015; Reichert et al., 2018).

The new genetic engineering developments and genetically engineered (GE) crops with genomic modifications have been produced and allowed for the cultivation of genetically modified (GM) crops. The unknown health threat of GM foods is a source of health concerns among consumers, and they have been restricted in many countries. It is critical to estimate the addition of genetically modified foods and/or food ingredients to the food supply and to evaluate risk parameters using metabolomics techniques. Untargeted metabolomics is routinely involved in the differentiation of conventional foods, transgenic foods, and genetically modified foods (Cevallos-Cevallos et al., 2009; Li et al., 2021). There have been comprehensive researches related to wheat (Shewry et al., 2007), soybean (García-Villalba et al., 2008), barley (Kogel, 2010) and potato (Shepherd et al., 2015) differentiate genetic modification for food safety.

Metabolomics in Food Processing

Food processing comprises the all over changes in physical and chemical structure that are created by components of foods that could be detected by metabolomics. Informative metabolomics is able to determine undesired effects pre-processing and during processing including degradation of compounds and nutrients, and synthesis of new compounds like toxins (Cevallos-Cevallos et al., 2009). The fermentation process of cheonggukjang has been monitored by informative and discriminative untargeted analysis by using nuclear magnetic resonance, and the final products were separated according to the fermentation time (Choi et al., 2007). Metabolomics could also be used to decide the suitability of raw materials for a certain process. While some potato varieties are favored for frying, others are used in the baking industry. The flow infusion electrospray-ionization mass spectrometry (FI-ESI-MS) and compound identification were aided by GC-MS to determine the differences between potato varieties (Beckmann et al., 2007).

Targeted and untargeted metabolomics have been widely used to measure the effects of process parameters on the metabolite composition of foods. There are several metabolomics studies related to different food processes; the effects of storage conditions on red wine (Arapitsas et al., 2016), the influences of blending and heating on Tiger nut milk (Rubert et al., 2017b), carrot, tomato, broccoli (Lopez-Sanchez et al., 2015), and banana (Chen et al., 2020), the impacts of energy stages on mung beans sprout (Chen et al., 2019), and the consequences of heat processing on Brassica vegetables (Hennig et al., 2014).

Metabolomics for Nutrition

Foodomics is a discipline that focuses on food and nutrition to explain the relationship between ingredients of food with quality and safety, daily diet, health, and diseases via developed omics technologies and chemometrics, bioinformatics, and biostatistics to enhance consumer's beneficence, health, and knowledge. The main subjects of foodomics could be summarized into three groups;

1. Human health (food consumption related to human health)
2. Food resources (plant and animal origin of food)
3. Food Processing (Picone et al., 2019; Zotti et al., 2016).

Nowadays, foodomics is used to better understand the molecular connections between human health, nutrition, and food. In particular, foodomics has been used for developing novel nutraceutical and functional foods. The effects of bee pollen (BP) on inflammatory bowel disease were investigated utilizing metabolomics analysis by using ultra-performance liquid chromatography in tandem with quadrupole time of flight-mass spectrometry (UPLC-Q-TOF/MS). It was discovered that the BP extract's regulatory mechanism protects cellular metabolic pathways from DSS-induced Caco-2 cell metabolism disorders (Li et al., 2019). The metabolomic methods were used to assess the anti-proliferative potential of Passiflora mollissima seeds on HT-29 human colon cancer cells. The results confirm that foodomics enabled the identification of genes, comprising polyamine and glutathione metabolism, or the inactivation of NUPR1 transcription could be involved in fluctuations in intracellular ceramide concentrations (Ballesteros-Vivas et al., 2020).

One of the most important and challenging aspects of nutrition is the monitoring food consumption of consumers. It is a simple way to precisely control the health of consumers by monitoring the food that a person has consumed. The food frequency questionnaires (FFQs) fill out by consumers revealed some findings on the positive or negative effects of certain foods or diets. It has also been observed that FFQ recall for retrospective diet studies is not good enough. Moreover, FFQ does not provide direct information about plasma levels of circulating nutrients or micronutrients (Wishart, 2008). Food consumption monitoring combined with metabolomics provides detailed knowledge of blood, urine, or saliva from volunteers in diet intervention studies. Foods are complex molecules and have many more components and metabolites. Food-specific biomarkers could be found in either blood or urine. The presence of these biomarkers proves the consumption of a certain food or the amount of the compound increases significantly over a period of time. It is known that the substantial difference between urine and blood is the percentages of metabolites to non-metabolites. Generally, urine has a significantly higher proportion of non-metabolites than blood. In a study on biomarkers of onion consumption, 11 relatively high abundance quercitin metabolites were discovered in urine, whereas only 5 lower abundance quercitin metabolites were found in the blood (Mullen et al., 2004). Therefore, metabolomic studies could be a solution to the problems of food consumption questionnaires used in probable diet objection or food interference studies.

Conclusion

Metabolomics has achieved great progress, with exciting findings associated with food analysis through the development of analytical techniques. The application of metabolomics in food processing, food quality control, and food safety is satisfactory with appropriate statistical analyses. Furthermore, targeted metabolomics should be improved with the automation, fast, and precision of entire metabolite quantitation. The untargeted metabolomics should be refined to control analytical data quality and develop a more reliable standardization of protocols. Comprehensive attention should be paid to food microbiology and nutrition for future aspects.

References

Alonso, A., Marsal, S., & Julià, A. (2015). Analytical methods in untargeted metabolomics: state of the art in 2015. *Frontiers in bioengineering and biotechnology*, *3*, 23. https://doi.org/10.3389/fbioe.2015.00023.

Anderson, J., Bogart, N., Clarke, A., Nelson, L., Warren, B., & Jespersen, L. (2014). Food safety management in the global food supply chain. *Perspectives in Public Health*, *134*(4), 181-181. https://doi.org/10.1177/1757913914538139.

Arapitsas, P., Della Corte, A., Gika, H., Narduzzi, L., Mattivi, F., & Theodoridis, G. (2016). Studying the effect of storage conditions on the metabolite content of red wine using HILIC LC–MS based metabolomics. *Food chemistry*, *197*, 1331-1340. https://doi.org/10.1016/j.foodchem.2015.09.084.

Ballesteros-Vivas, D., Alvarez-Rivera, G., León, C., Morantes, S. J., Ibánez, E., Parada-Alfonso, F., Cifuentes, A., & Valdés, A. (2020). Foodomics evaluation of the anti-proliferative potential of Passiflora mollissima seeds. *Food Research International*, *130*, 108938. https://doi.org/10.1016/j.foodres.2019.108938.

Beckmann, M., Enot, D. P., Overy, D. P., & Draper, J. (2007). Representation, comparison, and interpretation of metabolome fingerprint data for total composition analysis and quality trait investigation in potato cultivars. *Journal of Agricultural and Food Chemistry*, *55*(9), 3444-3451. https://doi.org/10.1021/jf0701842.

Bedair, M., & Sumner, L. W. (2008). Current and emerging mass-spectrometry technologies for metabolomics. *TrAC Trends in Analytical Chemistry*, *27*(3), 238-250. https://doi.org/10.1016/j.trac.2008.01.006.

Cevallos-Cevallos, J. M., Reyes-De-Corcuera, J. I., Etxeberria, E., Danyluk, M. D., & Rodrick, G. E. (2009). Metabolomic analysis in food science: a review. *Trends in Food Science & Technology*, *20*(11-12), 557-566. https://doi.org/10.1016/j.tifs.2009.07.002.

Chaleckis, R., Meister, I., Zhang, P., & Wheelock, C. E. (2019). Challenges, progress and promises of metabolite annotation for LC–MS-based metabolomics. *Current opinion in biotechnology*, *55*, 44-50. https://doi.org/10.1016/j.copbio.2018.07.010.

Chang, G. R., Chen, H. S., & Lin, F. Y. (2016). Analysis of banned veterinary drugs and herbicide residues in shellfish by liquid chromatography-tandem mass spectrometry (LC/MS/MS) and gas chromatography-tandem mass spectrometry (GC/MS/MS). *Marine Pollution Bulletin*, *113*(1-2), 579-584. https://doi.org/10.1016/j.marpolbul.2016.08.080.

Chen, L., Wu, J. E., Li, Z., Liu, Q., Zhao, X., & Yang, H. (2019). Metabolomic analysis of energy regulated germination and sprouting of organic mung bean (Vigna radiata) using NMR spectroscopy. *Food Chemistry*, *286*, 87-97. https://doi.org/10.1016/j.foodchem.2019.01.183.

Chen, L., Zhao, X., Wu, J. E., He, Y., & Yang, H. (2020). Metabolic analysis of salicylic acid-induced chilling tolerance of banana using NMR. *Food Research International*, 128, 108796. https://doi.org/10.1016/j.foodres.2019.108796.

Choi, H. K., Yoon, J. H., Kim, Y. S., & Kwon, D. Y. (2007). Metabolomic profiling of Cheonggukjang during fermentation by 1H NMR spectrometry and principal components analysis. *Process Biochemistry*, *42*(2), 263-266. https://doi.org/10.1016/j.procbio.2006.07.014.

Cook, P. W., & Nightingale, K. K. (2018). Use of omics methods for the advancement of food quality and food safety. *Animal Frontiers*, *8*(4), 33-41. https://doi.org/10.1093/af/vfy024.

Cossignani, L., Urbani, E., Simonetti, M. S., Maurizi, A., Chiesi, C., & Blasi, F. (2014). Characterisation of secondary metabolites in saffron from central Italy (Cascia, Umbria). *Food chemistry*, *143*, 446-451. https://doi.org/10.1016/j.foodchem.2013.08.020.

Cozzolino, D., Flood, L., Bellon, J., Gishen, M., & De Barros Lopes, M. (2006). Combining near infrared spectroscopy and multivariate analysis as a tool to differentiate different strains of *Saccharomyces cerevisiae*: a metabolomic study. *Yeast*, *23*(14-15), 1089-1096. https://doi.org/10.1002/yea.1418.

Dasenaki, M. E., & Thomaidis, N. S. (2015). Multi-residue determination of 115 veterinary drugs and pharmaceutical residues in milk powder, butter, fish tissue and eggs using liquid chromatography–tandem mass spectrometry. *Analytica Chimica Acta*, *880*, 103-121. https://doi.org/10.1016/j.aca.2015.04.013.

Dasenaki, M. E., Michali, C. S., & Thomaidis, N. S. (2016). Analysis of 76 veterinary pharmaceuticals from 13 classes including aminoglycosides in bovine muscle by hydrophilic interaction liquid chromatography–tandem mass spectrometry. *Journal of Chromatography A*, *1452*, 67-80. https://doi.org/10.1016/j.chroma.2016.05.031.

Fraga-Corral, M., Carpena, M., Garcia-Oliveira, P., Pereira, A. G., Prieto, M. A., & Simal-Gandara, J. (2022). Analytical metabolomics and applications in health, environmental and food science. *Critical Reviews in Analytical Chemistry*, *52*(4), 712-734. https://doi.org/10.1080/10408347.2020.1823811.

Gallo, M., & Ferranti, P. (2016). The evolution of analytical chemistry methods in foodomics. *Journal of Chromatography A*, *1428*, 3-15. https://doi.org/10.1016/j.chroma.2015.09.007.

García-Villalba, R., León, C., Dinelli, G., Segura-Carretero, A., Fernández-Gutiérrez, A., Garcia-Cañas, V., & Cifuentes, A. (2008). Comparative metabolomic study of transgenic versus conventional soybean using capillary electrophoresis–time-of-flight mass spectrometry. *Journal of Chromatography A*, *1195*(1-2), 164-173. https://doi.org/10.1016/j.chroma.2008.05.018.

González-Curbelo, M. Á., Socas-Rodríguez, B., Herrera-Herrera, A. V., González-Sálamo, J., Hernández-Borges, J., & Rodríguez-Delgado, M. Á. (2015). Evolution and applications of the QuEChERS method. *TrAC Trends in Analytical Chemistry*, *71*, 169-185. https://doi.org/10.1016/j.trac.2015.04.012.

Green, R. D., Qureshi, M. A., Long, J. A., Burfening, P. J., & Hamernik, D. L. (2007). Identifying the future needs for long-term USDA efforts in agricultural animal genomics. *International journal of biological sciences*, *3*(3), 185. https://doi.org/10.7150/ijbs.3.185.

Hall, R. D., Brouwer, I. D., & Fitzgerald, M. A. (2008). Plant metabolomics and its potential application for human nutrition. *Physiologia plantarum*, *132*(2), 162-175. https://doi.org/10.1111/j.1399-3054.2007.00989.x.

Hennig, K., De Vos, R. C. H., Maliepaard, C., Dekker, M., Verkerk, R., & Bonnema, G. (2014). A metabolomics approach to identify factors influencing glucosinolate thermal degradation rates in Brassica vegetables. *Food chemistry*, *155*, 287-297. https://doi.org/10.1016/j.foodchem.2014.01.062.

Jadhav, S. R., Shah, R. M., Karpe, A. V., Beale, D. J., Kouremenos, K. A., & Palombo, E. A. (2019). Identification of putative biomarkers specific to foodborne pathogens using metabolomics. In *Foodborne bacterial pathogens* (pp. 149-164). Humana, New York, NY.

Kaufmann, A., Butcher, P., Maden, K., Walker, S., & Widmer, M. (2015). Reliability of veterinary drug residue confirmation: high resolution mass spectrometry versus tandem mass spectrometry. *Analytica Chimica Acta*, *856*, 54-67. https://doi.org/10.1016/j.aca.2014.11.034.

Kleigrewe, K., Aydin, F., Hogrefe, K., Piecuch, P., Bergander, K., Würthwein, E. U., & Humpf, H. U. (2012). Structure elucidation of new fusarins revealing insights in the rearrangement mechanisms of the Fusarium mycotoxin fusarin C. *Journal of agricultural and food chemistry*, *60*(21), 5497-5505. https://doi.org/10.1021/jf3009469.

Kogel, K. H. (2010). Transcriptome and metabolome profiling of field-grown transgenic barley lack induced differences but show cultivar-specific variances. *Proceedings of the National Academy of Sciences*, *107*(14), 6198-6203. https://doi.org/10.1073/pnas.1001945107.

Levandi, T., Leon, C., Kaljurand, M., Garcia-Canas, V., & Cifuentes, A. (2008). Capillary electrophoresis time-of-flight mass spectrometry for comparative metabolomics of transgenic versus conventional maize. *Analytical chemistry*, *80*(16), 6329-6335. https://doi.org/10.1021/ac8006329.

Li, H., & Zhu, J. (2017). Targeted metabolic profiling rapidly differentiates Escherichia coli and Staphylococcus aureus at species and strain level. *Rapid Communications in Mass Spectrometry*, *31*(19), 1669-1676. https://doi.org/10.1002/rcm.7949.

Li, Q., Liang, X., Guo, N., Hu, L., Prasad, M. P., Wu, Y., Xue, X., Wu, L., & Wang, K. (2019). Protective effects of Bee pollen extract on the Caco-2 intestinal barrier dysfunctions induced by dextran sulfate sodium. *Biomedicine & Pharmacotherapy*, *117*, 109200. https://doi.org/10.1016/j.biopha.2019.109200.

Li, S., Tian, Y., Jiang, P., Lin, Y., Liu, X., & Yang, H. (2021). Recent advances in the application of metabolomics for food safety control and food quality analyses. *Critical Reviews in Food Science and Nutrition*, *61*(9), 1448-1469. https://doi.org/10.1080/10408398.2020.1761287.

Li, Y., Zhang, J., Jin, Y., Wang, L., Zhao, W., Zhang, W., Zhai, L., Zhang, Y., Zhang, Y., & Zhou, J. (2016). Hybrid quadrupole-orbitrap mass spectrometry analysis with accurate-mass database and parallel reaction monitoring for high-throughput screening and quantification of multi-xenobiotics in honey. *Journal of Chromatography A*, *1429*, 119-126. https://doi.org/10.1016/j.chroma.2015.11.075.

Lin, L., Xu, D., Shen, X., Zhang, Z., Chen, L., & Wang, C. (2014). Traceability of the wine in Bordeaux region from France based on liquid chromatography-quadrupole-time of flight tandem mass spectrometry. *Journal of Food Safety and Quality*, *5*(9), 2649-2656.

Lopez-Sanchez, P., De Vos, R. C. H., Jonker, H. H., Mumm, R., Hall, R. D., Bialek, L., Leenman, R., Strassburg, K., Vreeken, R., Hankemeier, T., Schumm, S., & Van Duynhoven, J. (2015). Comprehensive metabolomics to evaluate the impact of industrial processing on the phytochemical composition of vegetable purees. *Food Chemistry*, *168*, 348-355. https://doi.org/10.1016/j.foodchem.2014.07.076.

Ma, J., Hou, X., Zhang, B., Wang, Y., & He, L. (2014). The analysis of carbohydrates in milk powder by a new "heart-cutting" two-dimensional liquid chromatography method. *Journal of Pharmaceutical and Biomedical Analysis*, *91*, 24-31. https://doi.org/10.1016/j.jpba.2013.11.006.

Mullen, W., Boitier, A., Stewart, A. J., & Crozier, A. (2004). Flavonoid metabolites in human plasma and urine after the consumption of red onions: analysis by liquid chromatography with photodiode array and full scan tandem mass spectrometric detection. *Journal of Chromatography A*, *1058*(1-2), 163-168. https://doi.org/10.1016/j.chroma.2004.08.117.

Ossa, D. E. H., Gil-Solsona, R., Peñuela, G. A., Sancho, J. V., & Hernández, F. J. (2018). Assessment of protected designation of origin for Colombian coffees based on HRMS-based metabolomics. *Food chemistry*, *250*, 89-97. https://doi.org/10.1016/j.foodchem.2018.01.038.

Picone, G., De Noni, I., Ferranti, P., Nicolai, M. A., Alamprese, C., Trimigno, A., Brodkorb, A., Portmann, R., El, S. H., & Capozzi, F. (2019). Monitoring molecular composition and digestibility of ripened bresaola through a combined foodomics approach. *Food Research International*, *115*, 360-368. https://doi.org/10.1016/j.foodres.2018.11.021.

Pinu, F. R. (2015). Metabolomics - The new frontier in food safety and quality research. *Food Research International*, *72*, 80-81. https://doi.org/10.1016/j.foodres.2015.03.028.

Pinu, F. R., de Carvalho-Silva, S., Trovatti Uetanabaro, A. P., & Villas-Boas, S. G. (2016). Vinegar metabolomics: An explorative study of commercial balsamic vinegars using gas chromatography-mass spectrometry. *Metabolites*, *6*(3), 22. https://doi.org/10.3390/metabo6030022.

Reichert, B., de Kok, A., Pizzutti, I. R., Scholten, J., Cardoso, C. D., & Spanjer, M. (2018). Simultaneous determination of 117 pesticides and 30 mycotoxins in raw coffee, without clean-up, by LC-ESI-MS/MS analysis. *Analytica Chimica Acta*, *1004*, 40-50. https://doi.org/10.1016/j.aca.2017.11.077.

Rešetar, D., Pavelić, S. K., & Josić, D. (2015). Foodomics for investigations of food toxins. *Current Opinion in Food Science*, *4*, 86-91. https://doi.org/10.1016/j.cofs.2015.05.004.

Rubert, J., Monforte, A., Hurkova, K., Pérez-Martínez, G., Blesa, J., Navarro, J. L., Stranka, M., Soriano, J. M., & Hajslova, J. (2017b). Untargeted metabolomics of fresh and heat treatment Tiger nut (Cyperus esculentus L.) milks reveals further insight into food quality and nutrition. *Journal of chromatography A*, *1514*, 80-87. https://doi.org/10.1016/j.chroma.2017.07.071.

Rubert, J., Righetti, L., Stranska-Zachariasova, M., Dzuman, Z., Chrpova, J., Dall'Asta, C., & Hajslova, J. (2017a). Untargeted metabolomics based on ultra-high-performance liquid chromatography–high-resolution mass spectrometry merged with chemometrics: A new predictable tool for an early detection of mycotoxins. *Food chemistry*, *224*, 423-431. https://doi.org/10.1016/j.foodchem.2016.11.132.

Saito-Shida, S., Nemoto, S., & Teshima, R. (2015). Multiresidue determination of pesticides in tea by gas chromatography-tandem mass spectrometry. *Journal of*

Environmental Science and Health, Part B, *50*(11), 760-776. https://doi.org/10.1080/03601234.2015.1058092.

Sales, C., Cervera, M. I., Gil, R., Portolés, T., Pitarch, E., & Beltran, J. (2017). Quality classification of Spanish olive oils by untargeted gas chromatography coupled to hybrid quadrupole-time of flight mass spectrometry with atmospheric pressure chemical ionization and metabolomics-based statistical approach. *Food chemistry*, *216*, 365-373. https://doi.org/10.1016/j.foodchem.2016.08.033.

Schueuermann, C., Steel, C. C., Blackman, J. W., Clark, A. C., Schwarz, L. J., Moraga, J., Collado, I. G., & Schmidtke, L. M. (2019). A GC–MS untargeted metabolomics approach for the classification of chemical differences in grape juices based on fungal pathogen. *Food chemistry*, *270*, 375-384. https://doi.org/10.1016/j.foodchem.2018.07.057.

Shepherd, L. V. T., Hackett, C. A., Alexander, C. J., McNicol, J. W., Sungurtas, J. A., Stewart, D., McCue, K. F., Belknap, W. R., & Davies, H. V. (2015). Modifying glycoalkaloid content in transgenic potato–Metabolome impacts. *Food chemistry*, *187*, 437-443. https://doi.org/10.1016/j.foodchem.2015.04.111.

Shewry, P. R., Baudo, M., Lovegrove, A., Powers, S., Napier, J. A., Ward, J. L., Baker, J. M., & Beale, M. H. (2007). Are GM and conventionally bred cereals really different? *Trends in Food Science & Technology*, *18*(4), 201-209. https://doi.org/10.1016/j.tifs.2006.12.010.

Solsona, R., Boix, C., Ibáñez, M., & Sancho, J. V. (2018). The classification of almonds (Prunus dulcis) by country and variety using UHPLC-HRMS-based untargeted metabolomics. *Food Additives & Contaminants: Part A*, *35*(3), 395-403. https://doi.org/10.1080/19440049.2017.1416679.

Tomita, S., Saito, K., Nakamura, T., Sekiyama, Y., & Kikuchi, J. (2017). Rapid discrimination of strain-dependent fermentation characteristics among Lactobacillus strains by NMR-based metabolomics of fermented vegetable juice. *PLoS One*, *12*(7), e0182229. https://doi.org/10.1371/journal.pone.0182229.

Vautz, W., Zimmermann, D., Hartmann, M., Baumbach, J. I., Nolte, J., & Jung, J. (2006). Ion mobility spectrometry for food quality and safety. *Food additives and contaminants*, *23*(11), 1064-1073. https://doi.org/10.1080/02652030600889590.

Wang, L., Yang, B., Zhang, X., & Zheng, H. (2017). Novel two-dimensional liquid chromatography–tandem mass spectrometry for the analysis of twenty antibiotics residues in dairy products. *Food Analytical Methods*, *10*(6), 2001-2010. 1–2010 https://doi.org/10.1007/s12161-016-0763-4.

Willemse, C. M., Stander, M. A., Vestner, J., Tredoux, A. G., & De Villiers, A. (2015). Comprehensive two-dimensional hydrophilic interaction chromatography (HILIC)× reversed-phase liquid chromatography coupled to high-resolution mass spectrometry (RP-LC-UV-MS) analysis of anthocyanins and derived pigments in red wine. *Analytical chemistry*, *87*(24), 12006-12015. https://doi.org/10.1021/acs.analchem.5b03615.

Wishart, D. S. (2008). Metabolomics: applications to food science and nutrition research. *Trends in food science & technology*, *19*(9), 482-493. https://doi.org/10.1016/j.tifs.2008.03.003.

Yue, W., Sun, W., Rao, R. S. P., Ye, N., Yang, Z., & Chen, M. (2019). Non-targeted metabolomics reveals distinct chemical compositions among different grades of Bai Mudan white tea. *Food chemistry*, *277*, 289-297. https://doi.org/10.1016/j.foodchem.2018.10.113.

Zhang, A., Sun, H., Wang, P., Han, Y., & Wang, X. (2012). Modern analytical techniques in metabolomics analysis. *Analyst*, *137*(2), 293-300. https://doi.org/10.1039/C1AN15605E.

Zhang, Q., Wu, S., Li, Y., Liu, M., Ni, K., Yi, X., Shi, Y., Ma, L., Willmitzer, L., & Ruan, J. (2019). Characterization of three different classes of non-fermented teas using untargeted metabolomics. *Food Research International*, *121*, 697-704. https://doi.org/10.1016/j.foodres.2018.12.042.

Zhang, Z., Hu, X., Zhang, Q., & Li, P. (2016). Determination for multiple mycotoxins in agricultural products using HPLC–MS/MS via a multiple antibody immunoaffinity column. *Journal of Chromatography B*, *1021*, 145-152. https://doi.org/10.1016/j.jchromb.2016.02.035.

Zhao, Y., Wu, X., Yu, L., & Chen, P. (2017). Retention of polyphenols in blueberries (Vaccinium corymbosum) after different cooking methods, using UHPLC–DAD–MS based metabolomics. *Journal of Food Composition and Analysis*, *56*, 55-66. https://doi.org/10.1016/j.jfca.2016.12.003.

Zotti, M., Del Coco, L., De Pascali, S. A., Migoni, D., Vizzini, S., Mancinelli, G., & Fanizzi, F. P. (2016). Comparative analysis of the proximate and elemental composition of the blue crab Callinectes sapidus, the warty crab Eriphia verrucosa, and the edible crab Cancer pagurus. *Heliyon*, *2*(2), e00075. https://doi.org/10.1016/j.heliyon.2016.e00075.

Chapter 21

The Use of Metabolomics in Neonatology

Murat Doğan*, MD

Department of Pediatric Emergency, Kayseri City Hospital, Kayseri, Turkey

Abstract

Recently, many articles and reviews on metabolomics have been published in the fields of perinatology, obstetrics, and pediatrics. Metabolomics, which lies at the end point of the "omics cascade," allows for the detection of alterations in systems-level metabolites within biological pathways, thus providing insights into the mechanisms that underlie various physiological conditions and pathologies. Metabolomics, along with transcriptomics, has an essential role in discovering connections between genetic regulation, metabolite phenotyping, and biomarker identification. Biomarkers discovered through metabolomics may shed some light on the etiology of certain newborn pathological conditions (such as preterm birth, intrauterine growth retardation, asphyxia, metabolic diseases, neurological disorders, organ pathologies, sepsis, nutritional problems) and their adverse effects on infant development and improve current clinical conditions.

Keywords: metabolomics, metabolic diseases, neonatology

Introduction

Metabolites are the substrates and products of metabolic reactions, which require enzymes, minerals, lipids, peptides, amino acids, vitamins, and other

* Corresponding Author's E-mail: doktormurat033@hotmail.com.

In: Metabolomics and Clinical Approach
Editors: Sevgi Durna Daştan and Taner Daştan
ISBN: 979-8-89113-095-1

cofactors. Metabolomics refers to the "systematic identification and quantification of the small molecule metabolic products of a biological system at a specific point in time." In recent years, the new field of metabolomics, which is included in the "omics" subclass of scientific studies, has received a great deal of attention in both clinical and academic health. This collection of small, low-weight molecules is called the metabolome, which is the fingerprint of metabolism at a given time (Dettmer et al., 2007; Wishart et al., 2012).

Metabolomics measurement is evaluated by Mass Spectrometry (MS) or Nuclear Magnetic Resonance Spectroscopy (NMR) of all metabolites in a biological sample. By using high throughput technologies, metabolomics allows the identification and measurement of recognizable metabolites in a given biological sample. The available biological sample tissues can come from the mother (plasma, urine, vaginal fluids, milk, and hair), the fetus/newborn (amniotic fluid, umbilical cord blood, plasma, urine, meconium, saliva, and other fluids from the infant), or the placenta. The most commonly used biological sample is plasma, which is easy to obtain and rich in proteins and metabolites. According to the results of human and animal studies, metabolomics has a very important place in revealing the difference between physiological and pathological conditions together with the detection of specific biomarkers. Any abnormal metabolite concentration may be a sign of a dysfunctional or impaired metabolic pathway, indicating the presence of a disease (Horgan et al., 2009).

In conclusion, the outcomes of metabolomics analyses could be useful in the diagnosis of a disease, the identification of therapeutic targets, the detection of disease-specific markers, and offer solutions for prevention, monitoring of drug efficacy, and safety, identifying neonatal and pediatric disease onset, early diagnosis, and prognosis (Ismail et al., 2019; Mazzone et al., 2015).

The Potential of Metabolomics in Pediatrics

Fetal life and the perinatal period are crucial phases for the neonatal. The triggers and the conditions to which the fetus is exposed represent essential factors influencing the development of the newborn. Intrauterine factors in perinatal life can lead to negative consequences that will affect fetal development. Metabolomics application can provide great advantages in understanding, diagnosis and treatment of conditions such as preterm birth,

IUGR, asphyxia, metabolic diseases, neuropsychiatric disorders, sepsis, and nutritional problems (Ismail et al., 2019; Mussap et al., 2013).

Metabolomics and Asphyxia

The potential role of metabolomics in perinatal asphyxia is an interesting topic. Asphyxia is one of the most important causes of neonatal death or cerebral palsy, which leads to disability and poor neurodevelopment (Mussap et al., 2013; Locci et al., 2018). During asphyxia, disrupted cellular homeostasis causes significant metabolic changes, and studies of the metabolome may provide a pathophysiological 'snapshot' of these conditions. Krebs cycle intermediates (hypoxanthine, acylcarnitine, succinate) play an important role in perinatal asphyxia. Hypoxanthine, a purine metabolite, is elevated under hypoxic conditions. Hypoxanthine is oxidized to uric acid by xanthine oxidase when reoxygenated (Saugstad, 1988). The overproduction of reactive oxygen products, including hydrogen peroxide, free radicals, proteases, caspases, superoxide anion radicals, and reactive nitrogen species, causes mitochondrial dysfunction and cell death (Liu et al., 2011). As a result of asphyxia, fatty acid oxidation is incomplete, and fatty acid coenzyme A esters increase, resulting in the production of acylcarnitines (Rebouche, 2004). Debuf et al., found that acylcarnitines were promising in their study of perinatal asphyxia biomarkers. Some studies detected the occurrence of specific metabolic perturbations in the urine of asphyxiated newborns. One of them analyzed that mediators such as maleic acid, glycine, and sorbitol varied in relation to asphyxia, while aspartic acid, glucose, ornithine, asparagine, gluconic acid and L-lysine were mostly affected by kidney damage (Fanos et al., 2014). In another study, they found that acidosis and hypoxaemia determined variations in metabolites involved in energy demand, oxidative stress (lactate, threonine, hydroxysovalerate, glucose), and kidney damage (Longini et al., 2015). As a result, it was determined that citrate, α-ketoglutarate, dimethylamine, acetone, acetate, glutamine, pyruvate, succinate, and arginine were decreased in urine profiles of asphyxia babies (Locci et al., 2018). These data highlight that metabolomics can be used in the diagnosis of asphyxia patients.

Metabolomics in Intrauterine Growth Retardation (IUGR) and Preterm Birth

Intrauterine growth retardation (IUGR) is a fetal growth retardation disorder in which the expected fetal weight for gestational age is below the 10% percentile. IUGR causes a significantly increased risk of stillbirth, neonatal death, and perinatal morbidity. IUGR is in most cases caused by uteroplacental insufficiency, but it can also be caused by many different factors such as congenital anomalies, infections, and drug and substance use (Ergaz et al., 2005). Studies have shown that low maternal manganese and selenium levels are associated with IUGR and low birth weight. It has been determined that iron deficiency is associated with growth retardation, preterm birth, and deterioration of cognitive functions and neurological development (Hofstee et al., 2018). It has been shown that the incidence of preterm birth is reduced in women who are supplemented with calcium (Villar et al., 2006). Studies have found that low levels of selenium in maternal and cord blood are associated with preterm birth, suggesting that adequate maternal selenium may protect against preterm births (Dobrzynski et al., 1998).

Metabolomics and Neonatal Nutrition

Breastfeeding is the most important step in newborn nutrition. Breast milk (BM) contains water, vitamins, minerals, lipids, carbohydrates, proteins, growth-factors (GFs), chemokines, immunoglobulins (Ig), cytokines, hormones, specific microbiome, immune cells, and multipotent stem cells. BM is the most suitable food for newborns and especially for premature babies (Dessì et al., 2016; Kaingade et al., 2017). BM oligosaccharides (HMOs) regulate the neonatal gut microbiome, provide immune system development, protect against infections, and may reduce the rate of development of necrotizing enterocolitis (NEC) (Fanos et al., 2018). The content of HMOs generally depends on maternal genetic factors, as they are divided into Secretors (Se+) and non-Sectors (Se-) according to the expression of the α-1-2-fucosyltransferase enzyme (Se gene encodes) in the mother. Metabolomics studies have shown a definite difference between the higher content of fucosylated oligosaccharides, 2α-fucosyl-lactose, lacto-difucotetraose, lactoN-fucopentaose, and lacto-N-difucosose and the BM of mothers Se+ and Se-. Therefore, newborns of mothers with the Se- gene may benefit from supplementation of specific HMOs to avoid NEC and other infections (Dessì et al., 2018). The first metabolomic study evaluating BM composition was conducted in 2012. While maltose was found in a higher concentration in formula milk (FM), the lactose concentration was higher in BM. Also, higher amounts of oleic and linoleic acids were detected in FM. A correlation with gestational age was highlighted, in which lactose increases during milk maturation, especially with regard to carbohydrates (Marincola et al., 2012). In one study, urine metabolomes in the first week of life were compared in groups of newborns classified as appropriate for gestational age (AGA), small for gestational age (SGA), and large for gestational age (LGA). With this study, the impact of early nutrition on neonatal metabolic pathways was emphasized. In conclusion, the urinary metabolome of the AGA group was found to be significantly different from LGA and SGA, and the urinary samples were mostly affected by nutrition (Dessì et al., 2016). Metabolites with the greatest variation are those related to energy metabolism, neuromodulation, antioxidant action, brain development, and surfactant synthesis. Variations in the HMO content and metabolites produced by the gut microbiome were also detected. These results highlight the effects of early feeding on neonatal development (Marincola et al., 2016).

Metabolomics and Sepsis

Sepsis caused by infectious pathogens is a common cause of morbidity and mortality in newborns and especially in premature infants. If it occurs in the first 72 hours of life, it is called early-onset sepsis, and sepsis that develops between 3-6 days is called late-onset sepsis. Although sepsis is a life-threatening condition, there is no clear early diagnosis marker yet. Metabolomics can reveal metabolic pathways related to sepsis, such as increased energy needs, hypoxia, and oxidative stress (Ng et al., 2018). In a study, urine samples collected from septic neonates were compared with healthy controls, highlighting effects on energy metabolites (including an increase in lactate, acetate, glucose, maltose, ketone products, and effects on antioxidants) (Fanos et al., 2014). In another study, attention was drawn to the urinary profile in a preterm neonate affected by fungal sepsis. As a result, increases in some amino acids were detected and the D-serine metabolite was seen as a good indicator of the antifungal treatment response by reducing itself during treatment (Dessì et al., 2014). Sarafidis et al., found that the urinary metabolic profile evaluated allowed a certain distinction to be made between septic and non-septic neonates by analyzing samples collected at the time of diagnosis and on the following days (days 3 and 10). Metabolite variations improved with the good conditions of the clinic, providing promising information for prognosis and treatment (Sarafidis et al., 2017). In another study in children with sepsis, an increase in lactate, glucose, creatinine, 2-oxoisocaproate, 2-hydroxysovalerate, and 2-hydroxybutyrate, and a decrease in threonine, acetate, 2-aminobutyrate, and adipate was found in the serum metabolomes of patients compared to healthy controls. According to the results of the studies, metabolomics can provide an early and accurate diagnosis of sepsis by showing disease progression, treatment efficacy, and toxicity in children (Dessì et al., 2014).

Metabolomics and Neuropsychiatry

Autism spectrum disorder (ASD) is a complex neurodevelopmental difference that is congenital or presents in the first years of life. Although it is not known what causes ASD, there is evidence that genetic, environmental factors, socioeconomic status, maternal and neonatal infections, formula feeding, and epigenetic components are effective. Although the incidence of ASD has increased in recent years, definitive biomarkers are not available for diagnosis. In recent years, metabolomics has emerged as promising for better knowledge of neuropsychiatric diseases as well, allowing for individualization, monitoring of biomarkers, and perhaps the delivery of innovative treatments. ASD-associated metabolites generally appear to be involved in amino acid metabolism, cholesterol metabolism, folate metabolism, antioxidants, nicotinic acid metabolism, and mitochondrial metabolism. Some metabolites produced in the gut microbiota may play a large role in shaping the behavior, metabolic patterns, and immune response of children with ADS, purine metabolism, amino acid biosynthesis such as phenylalanine, tryptophan, and tyrosine, vitamin B6 metabolism, and the TCA cycle (Fanos et al., 2018). When urine samples of patients with ASD were compared with their healthy siblings, differences were observed in nervous system-related amino acids such as catecholamine and serotonin. According to these results, diet may be considered a relevant epigenetic factor influencing the gut microbiome in the pathogenesis of ASD (Noto et al., 2014). Metabolic disorders associated with ASD can be detected in blood, urine, saliva, cortex, and cerebellum samples. Significant differences were found when many metabolites were compared in the prefrontal cortex of ASD patients and the healthy control group (Kurochkin et al., 2019). The study and application of metabolomics in neurological and psychiatric disorders is promising for the future. Specific biomarkers that have been present since the early stages of fetal life and that affect neuropsychiatric development from perinatal programming to adulthood should be identified (Faa et al., 2016).

Metabolomics and Some Organ Pathologies

Metabolomics studies have been carried out in systemic pathologies such as sudden idiopathic sensorineural hearing loss, nephrourological diseases, and cardiovascular diseases. The urinary metabolomes of patients with nephrological system diseases (vesicoureteral reflux, urinary tract infection, acute renal failure, renal dysplasia) and healthy children were evaluated. Metabolomics seems a promising, non-invasive tool in nephrourological disease (Atzori et al., 2010). Another study advocated the applicability of metabolomics to predict chronic kidney disease early in healthy adults born with extremely low birth weight (Atzori et al., 2011). Metabolomics can also help in detecting the risks of cardiovascular diseases early before clinical signs and can help prevent fatal outcomes (Dang et al., 2018). Metabolomics associated with cardiovascular risk is generally related to the gut; Trimethylamine N-oxide has recently been associated with an increased rate of atherosclerosis and thrombosis. Trimethylamine N-oxide levels appear to be associated with an increased risk of cardiovascular problems in stroke patients via increased proinflammatory cells (Jia et al., 2019). Metabolic studies have also been conducted on pathologies such as sudden idiopathic sensorineural hearing loss. Metabolomics can be used to predict clinical outcomes and to evaluate treatment responses to steroids. A study evaluated the urinary metabolome of patients with sudden idiopathic sensorineural hearing loss and analyzed it according to clinical outcomes after steroids. There were significant differences in urinary metabolomes (B-Alanine, 3-hydroxybutyrate and trimethylamine N-oxide, citrate, and creatinine) between responders and non-responders to steroid therapy (Carta et al., 2017).

Metabolomics and Inborn Errors of Metabolism

Although newborn screenings are important for public health, their content is not very diverse. Not all IEMs can be identified in routine newborn screening programs. Metabolic profiling can contribute significantly to expanding metabolic knowledge by obtaining an accurate diagnosis and discovering new IEMs. Recently, numerous metabolomic studies have been published focusing on IEMs. Metabolomics also seems promising in predicting the early recognition of metabolic diseases and the treatment and prognosis of inborn errors of metabolism. Metabolomics was first evaluated in the IEMs screening in maple syrup urine disease and phenylketonuria. There were significant differences between the metabolome of healthy children and the metabolome of children with maple syrup disease. Also, metabolomics has been used to differentiate phenylketonuria from maple syrup urine disease (Constantinou et al., 2004). Another study compared the urinary metabolomes of patients with IEM (argininosuccinic aciduria, homocystinuria, methylmalonic acidemia, maple syrup urine disease, phenylketonuria, and type II tyrosinemia) and healthy controls (Pan et al., 2007). According to the study, the urinary metabolic profile of each patient was significantly different from that of the controls, which appears promising for the use of metabolomics in the differential diagnosis of metabolic diseases. In a large study in Italy, metabolomics was used in newborn screening for the preclinical diagnosis of IEMs. In this study, it was aimed to identify newborns at risk, including organic acidemia, hyperammonemia, branched-chain amino acid deficiency, fatty acid oxidation disorders, and maternally acquired metabolic diseases. According to the results of the study, it was determined that metabolomics has an important place to improve clinical risk estimation with the presymptomatic diagnosis of IEMs (Scolamiero et al., 2015). Fabry disease is an X-linked complex, multisystemic lysosomal storage disease characterized by the accumulation of globotriaosylsphingosin (lyso-Gb3) and globotriaosylceramide (Gb3) in the body due to a deficiency of the α galactosidase A enzyme. Some studies have found different isoforms/ analogues of galabiosylceramide (Ga2) of Gb3 and Ga2 in the urine of untreated Fabry patients (Boutin and Auray-Blais, 2015). Detection of these isoforms has provided new insight into the pathophysiology and metabolic mechanisms of Fabry disease. Using metabolomes, amino acid pathologies, fatty acid oxidation disorders, and organic acidurias were also investigated (Sandlers, 2017). A study evaluated genetic metabolic disorders using metabolomics. In conclusion, this study demonstrated that targeted disorders are potentially useful as a screening tool for a large group of IEMs (Jacob et al., 2018).

Conclusion

Metabolomics is the study of metabolites in a sample and is the one that corresponds most closely to the function of the cell, tissue, or organism compared to the sciences of omics such as genomics, transcriptomics, or proteomics. Although the clinical efficacy and safety of metabolomics need to be formalized with large-scale randomized or multicenter studies for routine use in patients, metabolomics is promising for the future according to the results of the studies. In the near future, metabolomics appears to be extremely promising in the early diagnosis, monitoring, optimization of therapy, and disease progression of a variety of fetal, perinatal, and pediatric conditions through the detection of specific biomarkers.

References

Atzori, L., Antonucci, R., Barberini, L., Locci, E., Marincola, F. C., Scano, P., Cortesi, P., Agostiniani, R., Weljie, A., Lai, A., & Fanos, V. (2010). 1H NMR-based metabolic profiling of urine from children with nephrouropathies. *Frontiers in bioscience (Elite edition)*, *2*(2), 725–732. https://doi.org/10.2741/e132.

Atzori, L., Mussap, M., Noto, A., Barberini, L., Puddu, M., Coni, E., Murgia, F., Lussu, M., & Fanos, V. (2011). Clinical metabolomics and urinary NGAL for the early prediction of chronic kidney disease in healthy adults born ELBW. *The journal of maternal-fetal & neonatal medicine: the official journal of the European Association of Perinatal Medicine, the Federation of Asia and Oceania Perinatal Societies, the International Society of Perinatal Obstetricians*, *24 Suppl 2*, 40–43. https://doi.org/10.3109/14767058.2011.606678.

Boutin, M., & Auray-Blais, C. (2015). Metabolomic discovery of novel urinary galabiosylceramide analogs as Fabry disease biomarkers. *Journal of the American Society for Mass Spectrometry*, *26*(3), 499–510. https://doi.org/10.1007/s13361-014-1060-3.

Carta, F., Lussu, M., Bandino, F., Noto, A., Peppi, M., Chuchueva, N., Atzori, L., Fanos, V., & Puxeddu, R. (2017). Metabolomic analysis of urine with Nuclear Magnetic Resonance spectroscopy in patients with idiopathic sudden sensorineural hearing loss: A preliminary study. *Auris, nasus, larynx*, *44*(4), 381–389. https://doi.org/10.1016/j.anl.2016.10.003.

Constantinou, M. A., Papakonstantinou, E., Benaki, D., Spraul, M., Shulpis, K., Koupparis, M. A., Mikros, E. (2004). Application of nuclear magnetic resonance spectroscopy combined with principal component analysis in detecting inborn errors of metabolism using blood spots: a metabonomic approach. Anal Chim Acta, 511, 303-12. https://doi.org/10.1016/j.aca.2004.02.012.

Dang, V. T., Huang, A., & Werstuck, G. H. (2018). Untargeted Metabolomics in the Discovery of Novel Biomarkers and Therapeutic Targets for Atherosclerotic Cardiovascular Diseases. *Cardiovascular & hematological disorders drug targets*, *18*(3), 166–175. https://doi.org/10.2174/1871529X18666180420170108.

Debuf, M. J., Carkeek, K., & Piersigilli, F. (2021). A Metabolomic Approach in Search of Neurobiomarkers of Perinatal Asphyxia: A Review of the Current Literature. *Frontiers in pediatrics*, *9*, 674585. https://doi.org/10.3389/fped.2021.674585.

Dessì, A., Liori, B., Caboni, P., Corsello, G., Giuffrè, M., Noto, A., Serraino, F., Stronati, M., Zaffanello, M., & Fanos, V. (2014). Monitoring neonatal fungal infection with metabolomics. *The journal of maternal-fetal & neonatal medicine: the official journal of the European Association of Perinatal Medicine, the Federation of Asia and*

Oceania Perinatal Societies, the International Society of Perinatal Obstetricians, *27 Suppl 2*, 34–38. https://doi.org/10.3109/14767058.2014.954787.

Dessì, A., Murgia, A., Agostino, R., Pattumelli, M. G., Schirru, A., Scano, P., Fanos, V., & Caboni, P. (2016). Exploring the Role of Different Neonatal Nutrition Regimens during the First Week of Life by Urinary GC-MS Metabolomics. *International journal of molecular sciences*, *17*(2), 265. https://doi.org/10.3390/ijms17020265.

Dessì, A., Briana, D., Corbu, S., Gavrili, S., Marincola, F. C., Georgantzi, S., Pintus, R., Fanos, V., & Malamitsi-Puchner, A. (2018). Metabolomics of Breast Milk: The Importance of Phenotypes. *Metabolites*, *8*(4), 79. https://doi.org/10.3390/metabo8040079.

Dettmer, K., Aronov, P. A., & Hammock, B. D. (2007). Mass spectrometry-based metabolomics. *Mass spectrometry reviews*, *26*(1), 51–78. https://doi.org/10.1002/mas.20108.

Dobrzynski, W., Trafikowska, U., Trafikowska, A., Pilecki, A., Szymanski, W., & Zachara, B. A. (1998). Decreased selenium concentration in maternal and cord blood in preterm compared with term delivery. *The Analyst*, *123*(1), 93–97. https://doi.org/10.1039/a704884j.

Ergaz, Z., Avgil, M., & Ornoy, A. (2005). Intrauterine growth restriction-etiology and consequences: what do we know about the human situation and experimental animal models?. *Reproductive toxicology (Elmsford, N.Y.)*, *20*(3), 301–322. https://doi.org/10.1016/j.reprotox.2005.04.007.

Faa, G., Manchia, M., Pintus, R., Gerosa, C., Marcialis, M. A., & Fanos, V. (2016). Fetal programming of neuropsychiatric disorders. *Birth defects research. Part C, Embryo today: reviews*, *108*(3), 207–223. https://doi.org/10.1002/bdrc.21139.

Fanos, V., Caboni, P., Corsello, G., Stronati, M., Gazzolo, D., Noto, A., Lussu, M., Dessì, A., Giuffrè, M., Lacerenza, S., Serraino, F., Garofoli, F., Serpero, L. D., Liori, B., Carboni, R., & Atzori, L. (2014). Urinary (1)H-NMR and GC-MS metabolomics predicts early and late onset neonatal sepsis. *Early human development*, *90 Suppl 1*, S78–S83. https://doi.org/10.1016/S0378-3782(14)70024-6.

Fanos, V., Noto, A., Caboni, P., Pintus, M. C., Liori, B., Dessì, A., & Mussap, M. (2014). Urine metabolomic profiling in neonatal nephrology. *Clinical biochemistry*, *47*(9), 708–710. https://doi.org/10.1016/j.clinbiochem.2014.05.020.

Fanos, V., Noto, A., Mussap, M. (2018). The juniper bush of autism spectrum disorder (ASD): metabolomics, microbiomics, acetaminophen. What else? *J Pediatr Neonat Individual Med,7*, e070205.

Fanos, V., Reali, A., Marcialis, M A., Bardanzellu, F. (2018). What you have to know about human Milk oligosaccharides. *J Pediatr Neonat Individual Med, 7*, e070137.

Hofstee, P., McKeating, D. R., Perkins, A. V., & Cuffe, J. S. (2018). Placental adaptations to micronutrient dysregulation in the programming of chronic disease. *Clinical and experimental pharmacology & physiology*, *45*(8), 871–884. https://doi.org/10.1111/1440-1681.12954.

Horgan, R. P., Clancy, O. H., Myers, J. E., & Baker, P. N. (2009). An overview of proteomic and metabolomic technologies and their application to pregnancy research. *BJOG: an international journal of obstetrics and gynaecology*, *116*(2), 173–181. https://doi.org/10.1111/j.1471-0528.2008.01997.x.

Ismail, I. T., Showalter, M. R., & Fiehn, O. (2019). Inborn Errors of Metabolism in the Era of Untargeted Metabolomics and Lipidomics. *Metabolites*, *9*(10), 242. https://doi.org/10.3390/metabo9100242.

Jacob, M., Malkawi, A., Albast, N., Al Bougha, S., Lopata, A., Dasouki, M., & Abdel Rahman, A. M. (2018). A targeted metabolomics approach for clinical diagnosis of inborn errors of metabolism. *Analytica chimica acta*, *1025*, 141–153. https://doi.org/10.1016/j.aca.2018.03.058.

Jia, J., Dou, P., Gao, M., Kong, X., Li, C., Liu, Z., & Huang, T. (2019). Assessment of Causal Direction Between Gut Microbiota-Dependent Metabolites and Cardiometabolic Health: A Bidirectional Mendelian Randomization Analysis. *Diabetes*, *68*(9), 1747–1755. https://doi.org/10.2337/db19-0153.

Kaingade, P., Somasundaram, I., Nikam, A., Behera, P., Kulkarni, S., Patel, J. (2017). Breast milk cell components and its beneficial effects on neonates: need for breast milk cell banking. *JPNIM*,6,060115.

Kurochkin, I., Khrameeva, E., Tkachev, A., Stepanova, V., Vanyushkina, A., Stekolshchikova, E., Li, Q., Zubkov, D., Shichkova, P., Halene, T., Willmitzer, L., Giavalisco, P., Akbarian, S., & Khaitovich, P. (2019). Metabolome signature of autism in the human prefrontal cortex. *Communications biology*, *2*, 234. https://doi.org/10.1038/s42003-019-0485-4.

Liu, J., Litt, L., Segal, M. R., Kelly, M. J., Pelton, J. G., & Kim, M. (2011). Metabolomics of oxidative stress in recent studies of endogenous and exogenously administered intermediate metabolites. *International journal of molecular sciences*, *12*(10), 6469–6501. https://doi.org/10.3390/ijms12106469.

Locci, E., Noto, A., Puddu, M., Pomero, G., Demontis, R., Dalmazzo, C., Delogu, A., Fanos, V., d'Aloja, E., & Gancia, P. (2018). A longitudinal 1H-NMR metabolomics analysis of urine from newborns with hypoxic-ischemic encephalopathy undergoing hypothermia therapy. Clinical and medical legal insights. *PloS one*, *13*(4), e0194267. https://doi.org/10.1371/journal.pone.0194267.

Longini, M., Giglio, S., Perrone, S., Vivi, A., Tassini, M., Fanos, V., Sarafidis, K., & Buonocore, G. (2015). Proton nuclear magnetic resonance spectroscopy of urine samples in preterm asphyctic newborn: a metabolomic approach. *Clinica chimica acta; international journal of clinical chemistry*, *444*, 250–256. https://doi.org/10.1016/j.cca.2015.02.004.

Marincola, F. C., Noto, A., Caboni, P., Reali, A., Barberini, L., Lussu, M., Murgia, F., Santoru, M. L., Atzori, L., & Fanos, V. (2012). A metabolomic study of preterm human and formula milk by high resolution NMR and GC/MS analysis: preliminary results. *The journal of maternal-fetal & neonatal medicine: the official journal of the European Association of Perinatal Medicine, the Federation of Asia and Oceania Perinatal Societies, the International Society of Perinatal Obstetricians*, *25*(Suppl 5), 62–67. https://doi.org/10.3109/14767058.2012.715436.

Marincola, F. C., Corbu, S., Lussu, M., Noto, A., Dessì, A., Longo, S., Civardi, E., Garofoli, F., Grenci, B., Mongini, E., Budelli, A., Grinzato, A., Fasano, F., Fanos, V., & Stronati, M. (2016). Impact of Early Postnatal Nutrition on the NMR Urinary Metabolic Profile of Infant. *Journal of proteome research*, *15*(10), 3712–3723. https://doi.org/10.1021/acs.jproteome.6b00537.

Mazzone, P. J., Wang, X. F., Beukemann, M., Zhang, Q., Seeley, M., Mohney, R., Holt, T., & Pappan, K. L. (2016). Metabolite Profiles of the Serum of Patients with Non-Small Cell Carcinoma. *Journal of thoracic oncology: official publication of the International Association for the Study of Lung Cancer*, *11*(1), 72–78. https://doi.org/10.1016/j.jtho.2015.09.002.

Mussap, M., Antonucci, R., Noto, A., & Fanos, V. (2013). The role of metabolomics in neonatal and pediatric laboratory medicine. *Clinica chimica acta; international journal of clinical chemistry*, *426*, 127–138. https://doi.org/10.1016/j.cca.2013.08.020.

Ng, S., Strunk, T., Jiang, P., Muk, T., Sangild, P. T., & Currie, A. (2018). Precision Medicine for Neonatal Sepsis. *Frontiers in molecular biosciences*, *5*, 70. https://doi.org/10.3389/fmolb.2018.00070.

Noto, A., Fanos, V., Barberini, L., Grapov, D., Fattuoni, C., Zaffanello, M., Casanova, A., Fenu, G., De Giacomo, A., De Angelis, M., Moretti, C., Papoff, P., Ditonno, R., & Francavilla, R. (2014). The urinary metabolomics profile of an Italian autistic children population and their unaffected siblings. *The journal of maternal-fetal & neonatal medicine: the official journal of the European Association of Perinatal Medicine, the Federation of Asia and Oceania Perinatal Societies, the International Society of Perinatal Obstetricians*, *27 Suppl 2*, 46–52. https://doi.org/10.3109/14767058.2014.954784.

Pan, Z., Gu, H., Talaty, N., Chen, H., Shanaiah, N., Hainline, B. E., Cooks, R. G., & Raftery, D. (2007). Principal component analysis of urine metabolites detected by NMR and DESI-MS in patients with inborn errors of metabolism. *Analytical and bioanalytical chemistry*, *387*(2), 539–549. https://doi.org/10.1007/s00216-006-0546-7.

Rebouche, C. J. (2004). Kinetics, pharmacokinetics, and regulation of L-carnitine and acetyl-L-carnitine metabolism. *Annals of the New York Academy of Sciences*, *1033*, 30–41. https://doi.org/10.1196/annals.1320.003.

Saugstad, O. D. (1988). Hypoxanthine as an indicator of hypoxia: its role in health and disease through free radical production. *Pediatric research*, *23*(2), 143–150. https://doi.org/10.1203/00006450-198802000-00001.

Sandlers, Y. (2017). The future perspective: metabolomics in laboratory medicine for inborn errors of metabolism. *Translational research: the journal of laboratory and clinical medicine*, *189*, 65–75. https://doi.org/10.1016/j.trsl.2017.06.005.

Sarafidis, K., Chatziioannou, A. C., Thomaidou, A., Gika, H., Mikros, E., Benaki, D., Diamanti, E., Agakidis, C., Raikos, N., Drossou, V., & Theodoridis, G. (2017). Urine metabolomics in neonates with late-onset sepsis in a case-control study. *Scientific reports*, *7*, 45506. https://doi.org/10.1038/srep45506.

Scolamiero, E., Cozzolino, C., Albano, L., Ansalone, A., Caterino, M., Corbo, G., di Girolamo, M. G., Di Stefano, C., Durante, A., Franzese, G., Franzese, I., Gallo, G., Giliberti, P., Ingenito, L., Ippolito, G., Malamisura, B., Mazzeo, P., Norma, A., Ombrone, D., Parenti, G., Pellecchia, S., Pecce, R., Pierucci, I., Romanelli, R., Rossi, A., Siano, M., Stoduto, T., Villani, G.R., Andria, G., Salvatore, F., Frisso, G., & Ruoppolo, M. (2015). Targeted metabolomics in the expanded newborn screening for inborn errors of metabolism. *Molecular bioSystems*, *11*(6), 1525–1535. https://doi.org/10.1039/c4mb00729h.

Villar, J., Abdel-Aleem, H., Merialdi, M., Mathai, M., Ali, M. M., Zavaleta, N., Purwar, M., Hofmeyr, J., Nguyen, T. N., Campódonico, L., Landoulsi, S., Carroli, G., Lindheimer, M., & World Health Organization Calcium Supplementation for the Prevention of Preeclampsia Trial Group (2006). World Health Organization randomized trial of calcium supplementation among low calcium intake pregnant women. *American journal of obstetrics and gynecology*, *194*(3), 639–649. https://doi.org/10.1016/j.ajog.2006.01.068.

Wishart, D. S., Jewison, T., Guo, A. C., Wilson, M., Knox, C., Liu, Y., Djoumbou, Y., Mandal, R., Aziat, F., Dong, E., Bouatra, S., Sinelnikov, I., Arndt, D., Xia, J., Liu, P., Yallou, F., Bjorndahl, T., Perez-Pineiro, R., Eisner, R., Allen, F., Neveu, V., Greiner, R., & Scalbert, A. (2013). HMDB 3.0--The Human Metabolome Database in 2013. *Nucleic acids research*, *41*(Database issue), D801–D807. https://doi.org/ 10.1093/nar/gks1065.

Chapter 22

Metabolomic Profiles of Body Fluids in Preterm Births

Seda Yilmaz Semerci*, **MD**
and Adviye Cakil Saglik, MD
Department of Neonatology, Pediatrics, University of Health Sciences, Kanuni Sultan Suleyman Training and Research Hospital, Istanbul, Turkey

Abstract

Preterm birth is a multi-sided condition affecting more than 15 billion infants and women per year around the world. In the challenges of dealing with preterm birth and its accompanying morbidities, including respiratory and neurological disorders, increase the medical and pecuniary burden due to the increased survival of very preterm infants. Therefore, prevention and early detection of preterm birth associated mortality and/or morbidity is crucial to deal with these challenges. Metabolomics are promising ‘clue’ molecules of human metabolism. Maternal, fetal, and neonatal body fluids include many metabolomics that can be used as either early biomarkers or targeted therapeutic molecules of major preterm birth-related morbidities, including respiratory distress syndrome, pulmonary hypertension, and bronchopulmonary dysplasia. Given the wide range of prematurity associated disorders and human body fluid bioenvironment, more metabolomics are expected to be identified to improve quality of care. Thus, future research on body fluid metabolomics is expected to bring today’s individualized medicine closer to predict PTB by providing a better understanding of its underlying mechanisms.

* Corresponding Author’s Email: sedayilmazsemerci@gmail.com.

In: Metabolomics and Clinical Approach
Editors: Sevgi Durna Daştan and Taner Daştan
ISBN: 979-8-89113-095-1

Keywords: body fluids, metabolomics, newborn, perinatal medicine, precision medicine, preterm birth

Introduction

Preterm birth (<37 gestational weeks) (PTB) is a major obstetric condition resulting in prematurity-associated mortality and various morbidities, including respiratory distress syndrome, bronchopulmonary dysplasia, necrotizing enterocolitis, and neurologic disorders. Recent advances in obstetrics and newborn medicine are still inadequate to elucidate the exact mechanisms for the timing of birth due to it is multifactorial and complex nature. Thus, scientific effort focuses on preventing or predicting PTB by dredging for novel determinants including biomarkers, screening tools, or new scoring systems. At this point, biological fluids represent a suitable and dynamic bioenvironment representing the actual pathophysiological state of maternal and/or neonatal metabolism.

Metabolomics are micro products of the metabolism which provide a specific metabolic phenotype (metabotype) for each individual (Monni et al., 2022). The unique nature of metabolomics serves as novel biomarkers, disease predictors, and/or therapeutic agents in precision medicine. Since recent advances in newborn medicine provided an enhanced survival of even extremely preterm infants, the burden of PTB is increased. Therefore, anticipating the risk and accompanying neonatal disorders is particularly important in reducing the mortality and morbidity associated with PTB. Hence, the number of research on metabolomics has been increasing since the 1960s by the discovery of metabolites in maternal serum, amniotic fluid, umbilical cord blood, and placenta under various medical conditions (Fanos et al., 2013a). The risk of preterm premature rupture of membranes and placental abruption are some of the conditions that can be predicted by metabolomic analyses of maternal serum even in the first trimester (Gelaye et al., 2016). Therefore, the newborn metabotype in PTB can guide the physician in dealing with both PTB itself and common co-morbidities such as pulmonary hypertension as well as the rare ones including congenital abnormalities and inborn errors of metabolism (Gil & Duarte, 2018; Monni et al., 2021).

Biological fluids for metabolomic sampling can be classified as maternal plasma, urine, cervicovaginal secretions and postnatal breastmilk, fetal amniotic fluid (AF), placenta, umbilical cord blood, and neonatal plasma, urine, feces, and saliva (Table 1). Multiple methods including nuclear magnetic resonance spectroscopy (N-MRS), gas chromatography-mass spectrometry (GC-MS), and liquid chromatography-mass spectrometry (LC-MS) can be used in determining the metabolomics (Holmes et al., 2008). Furthermore, as more cost effective, practical, and non-invasive metabolomic analysis ways, near-infrared (NIR) and/or mid-infrared (MIR) spectroscopy are promising to overcome the technical issues with the other methods (Graça et al., 2013; Power et al., 2011). However, existing metabolomic studies using NIR and/or MIR are inadequate to reach a certain result due to their small sample size.

Table 1. The sources of body fluids for metabolomic analysis

	Prenatal	Postnatal
Maternal	• Blood • Urine • Cervicovaginal Secretions	• Blood • Breastmilk • Urine
Fetal	• Amniotic Fluid • Cord Blood • Placenta	• Umbilical Cord Blood • Saliva • Buccal swab • Tracheal aspirate • Bronchoalveolar lavage fluid • Urine • Meconium

Metabolomics in Predicting Preterm Birth

Accurate estimation of the gestational age is crucial for a better understanding of the PTB process, distinguishing the small for gestational age (SGA) infants and/or intra uterine growth restriction (IUGR) from preterm ones. Since common ways of estimating gestational age, including the last menstrual period, prenatal ultrasound, and birth weight, have a respectable potential for miscalculation, human cord blood metabolomics in combination with birth weight are thought to be more reliable tools in prediction of PTB prevalence (Jasper et al., 2022).

Preterm birth can be triggered by dysregulated maternal immune reactions through proinflammatory processes and/or fetal haematological disorganisation in fetal/placental angiogenesis or growth. Regardless of the etiopathology, all those processes include cell-to-cell interactions reverberate to metabolomics of biological fluids including amniotic fluid, maternal, and fetal plasma. Hence, Brou et al. demonstrated significant differences between the amniotic fluid, maternal and umbilical cord plasma metabolomics, in a race dependent manner, particularly those with inflammatory and haematological functioning ones including IL8, TNFα, IL1b, IL1RA in PTB (Brou et al., 2012). Herewith the race-dependent changes in biofluid compartment metabolomics, the impact of genetic structure manifests the multifactorial etiopathology of PTB. Given its complex configuration, multivariate adaptive regression splines analysis (MARS) based on a machine-learning algorithm is developed to define the biomarkers including the metabolomics of spontaneous PTB (Menon et al., 2014a). Although demographic and clinical data did not have a significant effect on this MARS model, racial variations and different levels of specific metabolomics including IL1RA, IL1b, TNFα, angiopoietin 2 between maternal-foetal biofluid compartments is caught. Moreover, a metabolomic analysis revealed that preterm labor is associated with a higher carbohydrate content than amino acids in the amniotic fluid, reflecting the catabolic state of the fetus, thus making it possible to determine the risk of preterm delivery (Romero et al., 2010). In contrast to the previous research, the metabolomic profiling of the mid-trimester amniotic fluid did not point to any relevance with PTB (Hallingström et al., 2022). Consequently, these findings can be attributable to the possible importance of timing and the cumulative effect of fetal and/or placental maturation level on the amniotic fluid bioenvironment, since the majority of AF metabolomics related to PTB are involved in inflammatory pathways and/or energy metabolism. Nevertheless, another second trimester AF metabolomic analysis found an increase in allantoin regarding in utero oxidative stress and a decrease in alanine, citrate and myoinositol due to the membrane phospholipid production and lung maturation (Graça et al., 2010). Untargeted metabolomic analysis of amniotic fluid at the time of delivery by Menon et al. revealed more than a hundred of metabolomics predominantly hepatic metabolites including xenobiotic detoxification, fatty acid, coenzyme A and histidine metabolism differed in PTB (Menon et al., 2014b). However, it is still controversial whether those different levels of metabolomics are the result or cause of the PTB. Presumptively, due to the enhanced fetal catabolism, reduced amino acids such as histidine, isoleucine/leucine, methionine, phenylalanine and valine with elevated hexoses are reported in second trimester AF despite concurrent maternal urine analysis that revealed no significant differences (Graça et al., 2012). Furthermore, in comparison with dysregulated lipid profile of the paired maternal blood, glutamine, glutamic acid and pyruvic acid changes in the second trimester AF indicating altered fetal energy metabolism are reported to be associated with PTB (Virgiliou et al., 2017). Thus, maternal circulating metabolomics is thought to be in a dynamic relationship with the fetal metabolism during the pregnancy which makes them probable markers to be used in predicting the maternal-fetal conditions including PTB. In terms of sample timing, while 28-32 gestational weeks' maternal serum serpin B7 levels were found to be higher in pregnancies ended by PTB, they were detected as normal for the same women at 19-24 weeks of gestation (Parry et al., 2014). Although a NIR spectroscopic analysis study revealed that the second trimester AF of pregnancies ended by term and PTB had significantly distinct metabotypes, providing the estimation of the PTB with a notable sensitivity, scientific evidence is yet inadequate for certain results due to the small sample size of this study (Power et al., 2011). Similarly, another study of MIR metabolic profiling unveiled potential metabolomics predicting PTB cases in second trimester AF, but these results should be re-evaluated with further research due to the limited number of participants (Graça et al., 2013). In addition to the increased risk of PTB in pregnant women with higher total cholesterol, triglycerides, and low-density lipoprotein cholesterol, the second trimester maternal plasma was also reported to have a predictive metabolic phospholipid profile for PTB (Mudd et al., 2012; Pinto et al., 2014). Additionally, Lizewska et al. defined distinct maternal plasma metabotypes that can be used to predict preterm birth (Lizewska et al., 2018). A recent report revealed higher plasma levels of diglycerides along with lower levels of some glycerophospholipids in PTB, indicating the possible descriptive role of maternal plasma lipidomic profile in the mechanism of PTB (Morillon et al., 2020). The predictive power of metabolomics can be enhanced by using the metabolomic analyses in combination with different clinical scoring systems, statistical analysis, and/or artificial intelligent-based methods. Therefore, PTB has been shown to be predicted in the second trimester by collating the results of serial maternal plasma metabolomic analyses with specific depression scale scores (Huang et al., 2021). Ultimately, a comprehensive study showed altered levels of various fatty acids along with decreased phosphocholines associated with PTB in 24-28 weeks of maternal plasma (Chen et al., 2022). Besides, a previous study suggested a model for metabolic processes proceeding PTB by using metabolomics with concurrent gene correlation network analysis and machine-learning strategies.

Maternal urine stands for a practical, non-invasive, and superior to plasma sample for metabolomic research. Nevertheless, the second trimester maternal urine choline and 2-hydroxibutirate levels were found to be associated with PTB (Diaz et al., 2011). The maternal urine ingredient in metabolomics, including histidine, hexose, phenylalanine, and methionine, was reported to differ between the term and PTB (Fanos et al., 2013b). Besides, PTB was reported to be in association with increased lysine and lower formate levels in maternal urine in the first trimester (Maitre et al., 2014). Interestingly, in the previous study, induced PTB was also shown to have a distinct metabolomic profile with higher levels of glycoprotein N-acetyl in maternal urine. Hence, the metabolomic reflection of maternal urine can be considered as a practical and time sensitive environment for the prediction and evaluation of PTB.

Several metabolomics were detected to have significantly different levels in PTB compared to normal controls by prenatal metabolomic analyses in maternal cervicovaginal secretions. A mass spectrometric study revealed that maternal cervicovaginal secretion sampling at 31-33 gestational weeks can be predictive of PTB (Auray-Blais et al., 2011). Alongside a detailed metabolomic analysis indicated that cervicovaginal secretions evolved dynamically during pregnancy with enhanced sialic acid, N-acetylneuraminate levels and reduced dipeptide levels in the third trimester samples (Ghartey et al., 2015). Given the well-defined role of amniotic microbial invasion due to maternal infection in PTB, cervicovaginal metabolomic changes are not surprising to indicate PTB. Therefore, Vicente-Muñoz et al. demonstrated elevated levels of hypoxanthine, proline, choline, and acetylcholine accompanied by lower phenylalanine, glutamine, isoleucine, leucine and glycerophosphocholine levels in PTB associated with amniotic infection (Vicente-Muñoz et al., 2020). In contrast to the existing data, Thomas et al. suggested that early pregnancy cervicovaginal metabolomics were not predictive of PTB (Thomas et al., 2015). However, these findings can be related to the importance of the timing of the biologic sample, the effect of the microbiota, racial or genetic factors, and technical methods of metabolomic analysis. Considering the role of race and micro flora on the cervical remodelling during pregnancy, Gerson et al. that indicated particular metabolomics included in dipeptide and amino acid metabolism were related to PTB in association with regional microbiota in non-Hispanic Black women (Gerson et al., 2021). Thus, a recent proteomic study determined specific metabolomics such as fibronectin-1, the precursor of the extracellular matrix protein 1 isoform 1, the laminin alpha 3 subunit isoform, the laminin A/C isoform 2, the calsyntenin 1 isoform 2 as potential biomarkers for PTB in cervicovaginal secretions by using both targeted and shotgun analysis techniques (Parry et al., 2020).

Elemental metabolomics is also a new research area for predicting and diagnosing PTB. In this context, elevated plasma levels of Ca, Cr, Ni, As, Sr, Mo, Sn, I, Au, and U were detected along with lower levels of Na, Mg, P, Mn, Pb, and Ba were detected in human cord blood (McKeating et al., 2020). In accordance with these data, maternal exposure to Cr before birth increased the risk of PTB as well as increased lead level in maternal urine is also linked to PTB (Pan et al., 2017; Zhang et al., 2015). Umbilical cord plasma ratios of Sn/Pb, Cr/Pb, and Pb/U have been shown to have considerable diagnostic power on PTB (McKeating et al., 2020).

Metabolomics in Preterm Morbidities

Accurate recognition of PTB is a must to prevent or mitigate disorders due to prematurity. Since today's medical advances are not yet able to prevent PTB, an individual metabolomic map for the preterm infant can guide the clinicians to provide a better neonatal care. Since prematurity alone is a major issue for the infant, it is extremely important to avoid additional stressors such as invasive laboratory tests or treatment modalities. Thus, metabolomic studies focused on postnatal biologic samples revealed promising metabolomics that foresee or facilitate the treatment of preterm morbidities. Maternal blood, breastmilk, urine, umbilical cord blood, amniotic fluid, neonatal saliva, urine, and meconium are the biofluids of interest for postnatal metabolomic research in PTB (Table 1).

The placenta states an active, complex, and dynamic bridge between the mother and newborn allowing perpetual metabolic interactions that are mirrored by biologic fluids including maternal-neonatal blood and urine. Therefore, several metabolomics including amino acids, carbohydrates, lipids and lipoprotein molecules are defined as predictive markers of preterm morbidities in prenatal and/or postnatal biofluid samples.

Necrotizing enterocolitis (NEC) is the most common gastrointestinal disease in preterm infants. Since specific diagnosis modalities for NEC cannot be defined yet, recent metabolomic research pointed to a variety of substantive metabolomics as predictors of NEC (Agakidou et al., 2020). Therefore, a lower level of IL1AR was determined as a potential predictor of NEC in buccal swab samples from preterm infants under 32 gestational weeks (Murgas Torrazza et al., 2013). Notable work revealed that NEC development showed a strong and time sensitive relation with the levels of alanine, phenylalanine, free carnitine, C16, arginine, C14:1/C16, and citrulline/phenylalanine levels in sequential dried blood samples from preterm infants under 32 gestational weeks (Sinclair et al., 2020). Fecal calprotectin, a specific metabotype of fecal volatile organic compounds, urinary serum amiloid A, intestinal fatty acid-binding protein, prostaglandin E2 major urinay metabolit are defined as non-invasive biomarkers for NEC (de Meij et al., 2015; Konishi et al., 2019; Moschino et al., 2022; Wang et al., 2019).

Bronchopulmonary dysplasia (BPD) is one of the probable long-term respiratory consequences of PTB. Although clinical and respiratory follow-up of the infant has some clues whether BPD develops in the future, only genetic and metabolomic analysis has the potential to make an accurate prediction of BPD early in the newborn period (Piersigilli & Bhandari, 2020). Therefore, AF, tracheal aspirate, bronchoalveolar lavage fluid, umbilical cord blood, and neonatal urine were analyzed for BPD predictive metabolomics (Baraldi et al., 2016a; la Frano et al., 2018; Piersigilli et al., 2019; Pintus et al., 2018). The first postnatal week tracheal aspirate of the ventilated newborns under 30 weeks of gestation was analyzed and the researchers evidenced that significant time dependent metabotypes were subject to foresee BPD development (Piersigilli et al., 2019). In the previous work, elevated histidine, citrulline, glycine, glutamic acid was detected along with higher isoleucine amino acids and C16-OH, C18:1-OH acylcarnitines particularly in more preterm ones. Since BPD incidence is in the reverse ratio of gestational age at birth those data are considered extremely noteworthy for further research on elucidating the ethiopathogenesis of BPD. A decent representative of integrative research revealed that multiple metabolomic changes together with concurrent altered respiratory tract microbiome associated with four pre-defined genes predictive for BPD in an experimental model (el Saie et al., 2022). Besides, disturbance in lipid metabolism allowed us to determine the severity of bronchopulmonary dysplasia and related pulmonary hypertension by detecting lower levels of phosphatidylcholine, sphingomyelin, along with a higher level of many oxylipins, including COX-derived prostaglandins, in preterm infants' umbilical cord blood (la Frano et al., 2018). Recent scientific evidence showed that increased levels of hydroxylated and oxidated fatty acids, fatty aldehydes, and amino acids were associated with both PTB and further development of BPD in the newborn infant pointing to the acute and long-lasting impact of in-utero fetal exposure to oxidative stress on the birth process and the neonate (Baraldi et al., 2016b). Meanwhile, a longitudinal study of metabolomics did not show a significant correlation between serum metabolomics and preterm morbidities, including BPD and retinopathy of prematurity, in extremely preterm infants (Nilsson et al., 2022). However, those findings can be related to the effect of genetic and racial factors, differences in postnatal environmental conditions, sample timing, and the choice of proper analysis and statistical methods.

Hemodynamically significant patent ductus arteriosus (hsPDA) is a common prematurity associated morbidity. The diagnosis of hsPDA requires an echocardiographic examination with a detailed clinical evaluation. As well as the other disorders of prematurity, hsPDA pathophysiology has not been elucidated yet. Therefore, early diagnosis and prediction is crucial to prevent ductus-related cardiac failure, renal and/or systemic hypoperfusion. Since echocardiographic evaluation cannot be continuously available for all settings, metabolomics is considered a practical way to treat hsPDA. As a non-invasive method within postnatal 12 hours neonatal urine showed to have higher levels of lactate and glucose along with lower betaine, glycylproline, 4-hydroxyproline, 3-methylxanthine, myoinositol, tryptophan, and trimethylamine-N-Oxide levels (Bardanzellu et al., 2020). Given the time advantage of early urinary metabolomic analysis for the diagnosis of hsPDA, a further supportive study can reduce the need for unnecessary echocardiologic screening of the preterm infants within the first 48-72 hours. Moreover, serum metabolomics was also studied for the early detection of hsPDA in several remarkable work, but the results did not point to specific ones neither and had controversy in terms of some amino acids, particularly for altered glutamate levels (Huizing et al., 2021; Oltman et al., 2021; Ryckman et al., 2013).

Preterm birth itself becomes a significant issue for long-term neurodevelopmental disabilities of the infant. Although it is more frequent in term birth, hypoxic ischemic encephalopathy (HIE) occurs in PTB and is still the most common cause of preventable neonatal mortality. Together with possible injury due to PTB, overlapped HIE can be detrimental for preterm infants. Given that the exact etiopathogenesis and underlying mechanisms of HIE are not completely defined to date, the unique evidence-based therapy is therapeutic hypothermia that is not an accurate solution. Hence, the preterm population benefits most from the detection of the metabolomics predicting and understanding of HIE development. Nevertheless, both clinical and experimental metabolomic research in HIE intensified at term births, revealing elevated acylcarnitine along with altered levels of several amino acids in umbilical cord plasma, distinct L-lysine, L-3-methylhistidine levels in neonatal urine (El-Farghali et al., 2018; Locci et al., 2020; Mikrogeorgiou et al., 2020; Rasineni et al., 2022; Valerio et al., 2022). Therefore, further scientific evidence is required to understand whether previously defined metabolomics also work for PTB; otherwise, novel metabolomic marker studies are urgently expected for HIE in PTB.

Intraventricular haemorrhage (IVH) is a devastating cause of brain damage associated with PTB. Actually, there is no accurate prevention strategy nor curative therapy for IVH, therefore serial targeted metabolomic analyses of neonatal urine samples revealed that a specific metabotype can be used to monitor the presence and the follow-up of IVH (Sarafidis et al., 2019).

Conclusion

Currently, a wealth of biofluid-derived metabolomics is studied in the pathophysiology of PTB. However, the metabolomics alone is not subject to predict or prevent PTB. Instead, risk scoring and early diagnosis algorithms based on the evaluation of the individual metabotype of maternofetal biofluids in combination with pathway analysis and clinical parameters can reduce global PTB related morbidity and mortality. Thus, metabolomics can be used as a fortune teller for PTB, as well as many other medical conditions. Therefore, further scientific collaborative effort is required to develop non-invasive novel diagnostic tools and targeted solutions for PTB by combining the benefit of metabolomics with computer technology.

References

Agakidou, E., Agakidis, C., Gika, H., & Sarafidis, K. (2020). Emerging Biomarkers for Prediction and Early Diagnosis of Necrotizing Enterocolitis in the Era of Metabolomics and Proteomics. *Frontiers in Pediatrics*, *8,* 1-17. https://doi.org/10.3389/fped.2020.602255.

Auray-Blais, C., Raiche, E., Gagnon, R., Berthiaume, M., & Pasquier, J.-C. (2011). Metabolomics and preterm birth: What biomarkers in cervicovaginal secretions are predictive of high-risk pregnant women? *International Journal of Mass Spectrometry*, *307*(1–3), 33–38. https://doi.org/10.1016/j.ijms.2011.02.009.

Baraldi, E., Giordano, G., Stocchero, M., Moschino, L., Zaramella, P., Tran, M. R., Carraro, S., Romero, R., & Gervasi, M. T. (2016a). Untargeted Metabolomic Analysis of Amniotic Fluid in the Prediction of Preterm Delivery and Bronchopulmonary Dysplasia. *PLOS ONE*, *11*(10), e0164211. https://doi.org/10.1371/journal.pone.0164211.

Baraldi, E., Giordano, G., Stocchero, M., Moschino, L., Zaramella, P., Tran, M. R., Carraro, S., Romero, R., & Gervasi, M. T. (2016b). Untargeted Metabolomic Analysis of Amniotic Fluid in the Prediction of Preterm Delivery and Bronchopulmonary

Dysplasia. *PLOS ONE*, *11*(10), e0164211. https://doi.org/10.1371/journal.pone.0164211.

Bardanzellu, F., Piras, C., Atzei, A., Neroni, P., & Fanos, V. (2020). Early Urinary Metabolomics in Patent Ductus Arteriosus Anticipates the Fate: Preliminary Data. *Frontiers in Pediatrics*, *8*, 1-18. https://doi.org/10.3389/fped.2020.613749.

Brou, L., Almli, L., Pearce, B., Bhat, G., Drobek, C., Fortunato, S., & Menon, R. (2012). Dysregulated biomarkers induce distinct pathways in preterm birth. *BJOG: An International Journal of Obstetrics & Gynaecology*, *119*(4), 458–473. https://doi.org/10.1111/j.1471-0528.2011.03266.x.

Chen, Y., He, B., Liu, Y., Aung, M. T., Rosario-Pabón, Z., Vélez-Vega, C. M., Alshawabkeh, A., Cordero, J. F., Meeker, J. D., & Garmire, L. X. (2022). Maternal plasma lipids are involved in the pathogenesis of preterm birth. *GigaScience*, *11*, 1-11. https://doi.org/10.1093/gigascience/giac004.

de Meij, T. G. J., van der Schee, M. P. C., Berkhout, D. J. C., van de Velde, M. E., Jansen, A. E., Kramer, B. W., van Weissenbruch, M. M., van Kaam, A. H., Andriessen, P., van Goudoever, J. B., Niemarkt, H. J., & de Boer, N. K. H. (2015). Early Detection of Necrotizing Enterocolitis by Fecal Volatile Organic Compounds Analysis. *The Journal of Pediatrics*, *167*(3), 562-567.e1. https://doi.org/10.1016/j.jpeds.2015.05.044.

Diaz, S. O., Pinto, J., Graça, G., Duarte, I. F., Barros, A. S., Galhano, E., Pita, C., Almeida, M. do C., Goodfellow, B. J., Carreira, I. M., & Gil, A. M. (2011). Metabolic Biomarkers of Prenatal Disorders: An Exploratory NMR Metabonomics Study of Second Trimester Maternal Urine and Blood Plasma. *Journal of Proteome Research*, *10*(8), 3732–3742. https://doi.org/10.1021/pr200352m.

el Saie, A., Fu, C., Grimm, S. L., Robertson, M. J., Hoffman, K., Putluri, V., Ambati, C. S. R., Putluri, N., Shivanna, B., Coarfa, C., & Pammi, M. (2022). Metabolome and microbiome multi-omics integration from a murine lung inflammation model of bronchopulmonary dysplasia. *Pediatric Research, 2022,* 1-10. https://doi.org/10.1038/s41390-022-02002-1.

El-Farghali, O. G., El-Chimi, M. S., El-Abd, H. S., & El-Desouky, E. (2018). Amino acid and acylcarnitine profiles in perinatal asphyxia: a case-control study. *The Journal of Maternal-Fetal & Neonatal Medicine*, *31*(11), 1462–1469. https://doi.org/10.1080/14767058.2017.1319354.

Fanos, V., Atzori, L., Makarenko, K., Melis, G. B., & Ferrazzi, E. (2013a). Metabolomics Application in Maternal-Fetal Medicine. *BioMed Research International*, *2013*, 1–9. https://doi.org/10.1155/2013/720514.

Fanos, V., Atzori, L., Makarenko, K., Melis, G. B., & Ferrazzi, E. (2013b). Metabolomics Application in Maternal-Fetal Medicine. *BioMed Research International*, *2013*, 1–9. https://doi.org/10.1155/2013/720514.

Gelaye, B., Sumner, S. J., McRitchie, S., Carlson, J. E., Ananth, C. V., Enquobahrie, D. A., Qiu, C., Sorensen, T. K., & Williams, M. A. (2016). Maternal Early Pregnancy Serum Metabolomics Profile and Abnormal Vaginal Bleeding as Predictors of Placental Abruption: A Prospective Study. *PLOS ONE*, *11*(6), e0156755. https://doi.org/10.1371/journal.pone.0156755.

Gerson, K. D., Liao, J., McCarthy, C., Burris, H. H., Korem, T., Levy, M., Ravel, J., & Elovitz, M. A. (2021). A non-optimal cervicovaginal microbiota in pregnancy is associated with a distinct metabolomic signature among non-Hispanic Black individuals. *Scientific Reports*, *11*(1), 22794. https://doi.org/10.1038/s41598-021-02304-0.

Ghartey, J., Bastek, J. A., Brown, A. G., Anglim, L., & Elovitz, M. A. (2015). Women with preterm birth have a distinct cervicovaginal metabolome. *American Journal of Obstetrics and Gynecology*, *212*(6), 776.e1-776.e12. https://doi.org/10.1016/j.ajog.2015.03.052.

Gil, A. M., & Duarte, D. (2018). Biofluid Metabolomics in Preterm Birth Research. *Reproductive Sciences*, *25*(7), 967–977. https://doi.org/10.1177/1933719118756748.

Graça, G., Duarte, I. F., Barros, A. S., Goodfellow, B. J., Diaz, S. O., Pinto, J., Carreira, I. M., Galhano, E., Pita, C., & Gil, A. M. (2010). Impact of Prenatal Disorders on the Metabolic Profile of Second Trimester Amniotic Fluid: A Nuclear Magnetic Resonance Metabonomic Study. *Journal of Proteome Research*, *9*(11), 6016–6024. https://doi.org/10.1021/pr100815q.

Graça, G., Goodfellow, B. J., Barros, A. S., Diaz, S., Duarte, I. F., Spagou, K., Veselkov, K., Want, E. J., Lindon, J. C., Carreira, I. M., Galhano, E., Pita, C., & Gil, A. M. (2012). UPLC-MS metabolic profiling of second trimester amniotic fluid and maternal urine and comparison with NMR spectral profiling for the identification of pregnancy disorder biomarkers. *Molecular BioSystems*, *8*(4), 1243. https://doi.org/10.1039/c2mb05424h.

Graça, G., Moreira, A. S., Correia, A. J. v., Goodfellow, B. J., Barros, A. S., Duarte, I. F., Carreira, I. M., Galhano, E., Pita, C., Almeida, M. do C., & Gil, A. M. (2013). Mid-infrared (MIR) metabolic fingerprinting of amniotic fluid: A possible avenue for early diagnosis of prenatal disorders? *Analytica Chimica Acta*, *764*, 24–31. https://doi.org/10.1016/j.aca.2012.12.023.

Hallingström, M., Barman, M., Savolainen, O., Viklund, F., Kacerovsky, M., Brunius, C., & Jacobsson, B. (2022). Metabolomic profiles of mid-trimester amniotic fluid are not associated with subsequent spontaneous preterm delivery or gestational duration at delivery. *The Journal of Maternal-Fetal & Neonatal Medicine*, *35*(11), 2054–2062. https://doi.org/10.1080/14767058.2020.1777271.

Holmes, E., Wilson, I. D., & Nicholson, J. K. (2008). Metabolic Phenotyping in Health and Disease. *Cell*, *134*(5), 714–717. https://doi.org/10.1016/j.cell.2008.08.026.

Huang, D., Liu, Z., Liu, X., Bai, Y., Wu, M., Luo, X., & Qi, H. (2021). Stress and Metabolomics for Prediction of Spontaneous Preterm Birth: A Prospective Nested Case-Control Study in a Tertiary Hospital. *Frontiers in Pediatrics*, *9*, 1-8. https://doi.org/10.3389/fped.2021.670382.

Huizing, M. J., Borges-Luján, M., Cavallaro, G., González-Luis, G. E., Raffaeli, G., Bas-Suárez, P., Bakker, J. A., Moonen, R. M., & Villamor, E. (2021). Plasma Amino Acid Concentrations at Birth and Patent Ductus Arteriosus in Very and Extremely Preterm Infants. *Frontiers in Pediatrics*, *9*, 1-7. https://doi.org/10.3389/fped.2021.647018.

Jasper, E. A., Oltman, S. P., Rogers, E. E., Dagle, J. M., Murray, J. C., Kamya, M., Kakuru, A., Kajubi, R., Ochieng, T., Adrama, H., Okitwi, M., Olwoch, P., Jagannathan, P.,

Clark, T. D., Dorsey, G., Ruel, T., Jelliffe-Pawlowski, L. L., & Ryckman, K. K. (2022). Targeted newborn metabolomics: prediction of gestational age from cord blood. *Journal of Perinatology*, *42*(2), 181–186. https://doi.org/10.1038/s41372-021-01253-w.

Konishi, K., Yoshida, M., Nakao, A., Tsuchiya, K., Tsurisawa, C., Ichiki, K., Takeda, T., Hisaeda, Y., Hirota, A., Amagata, S., Odashima, T., Yokomori, K., Ishida, K., Matsuura, M., Ito, S., Fujiwara, M., & Nakahara, S. (2019). Prostaglandin E-major urinary metabolite as a noninvasive surrogate marker for infantile necrotizing enterocolitis. *Journal of Pediatric Surgery*, *54*(8), 1584–1589. https://doi.org/10.1016/j.jpedsurg.2018.08.044.

la Frano, M. R., Fahrmann, J. F., Grapov, D., Pedersen, T. L., Newman, J. W., Fiehn, O., Underwood, M. A., Mestan, K., Steinhorn, R. H., & Wedgwood, S. (2018). Umbilical cord blood metabolomics reveal distinct signatures of dyslipidemia prior to bronchopulmonary dysplasia and pulmonary hypertension. *American Journal of Physiology-Lung Cellular and Molecular Physiology*, *315*(5), L870–L881. https://doi.org/10.1152/ajplung.00283.2017.

Lizewska, B., Teul, J., Kuc, P., Lemancewicz, A., Charkiewicz, K., Goscik, J., Kacerovsky, M., Menon, R., Miltyk, W., & Laudanski, P. (2018). Maternal Plasma Metabolomic Profiles in Spontaneous Preterm Birth: Preliminary Results. *Mediators of Inflammation*, *2018*, 1–13. https://doi.org/10.1155/2018/9362820.

Locci, E., Bazzano, G., Demontis, R., Chighine, A., Fanos, V., & d'Aloja, E. (2020). Exploring Perinatal Asphyxia by Metabolomics. *Metabolites*, *10*(4), 141. https://doi.org/10.3390/metabo10040141.

Maitre, L., Fthenou, E., Athersuch, T., Coen, M., Toledano, M. B., Holmes, E., Kogevinas, M., Chatzi, L., & Keun, H. C. (2014). Urinary metabolic profiles in early pregnancy are associated with preterm birth and fetal growth restriction in the Rhea mother–child cohort study. *BMC Medicine*, *12*(1), 110. https://doi.org/10.1186/1741-7015-12-110.

McKeating, D. R., Fisher, J. J., Zhang, P., Bennett, W. W., & Perkins, A. V. (2020). Elemental metabolomics in human cord blood: Method validation and trace element quantification. *Journal of Trace Elements in Medicine and Biology*, *59*, 126419. https://doi.org/10.1016/j.jtemb.2019.126419.

Menon, R., Bhat, G., Saade, G. R., & Spratt, H. (2014a). Multivariate adaptive regression splines analysis to predict biomarkers of spontaneous preterm birth. *Acta Obstetricia et Gynecologica Scandinavica*, *93*(4), 382–391. https://doi.org/10.1111/aogs.12344.

Menon, R., Jones, J., Gunst, P. R., Kacerovsky, M., Fortunato, S. J., Saade, G. R., & Basraon, S. (2014b). Amniotic Fluid Metabolomic Analysis in Spontaneous Preterm Birth. *Reproductive Sciences*, *21*(6), 791–803. https://doi.org/10.1177/1933719113518987.

Mikrogeorgiou, A., Chen, Y., Lee, B. S., Bok, R., Sheldon, R. A., Barkovich, A. J., Xu, D., & Ferriero, D. M. (2020). A Metabolomics Study of Hypoxia Ischemia during Mouse Brain Development Using Hyperpolarized ^{13}C. *Developmental Neuroscience*, *42*(1), 49–58. https://doi.org/10.1159/000506982.

Monni, G., Atzori, L., Corda, V., Dessolis, F., Iuculano, A., Hurt, K. J., & Murgia, F. (2021). Metabolomics in Prenatal Medicine: A Review. *Frontiers in Medicine*, *8*, 1-17. https://doi.org/10.3389/fmed.2021.645118.

Monni, G., Murgia, F., Corda, V., Iuculano, A., & Atzori, L. (2022). Metabolomics Application in Fetal Medicine. In *Perinatology* (pp. 537–548). Springer International Publishing. https://doi.org/10.1007/978-3-030-83434-0_30.

Morillon, A.-C., Yakkundi, S., Thomas, G., Gethings, L. A., Langridge, J. I., Baker, P. N., Kenny, L. C., English, J. A., & McCarthy, F. P. (2020). Association between phospholipid metabolism in plasma and spontaneous preterm birth: a discovery lipidomic analysis in the cork pregnancy cohort. *Metabolomics*, *16*(2), 19. https://doi.org/10.1007/s11306-020-1639-6.

Moschino, L., Verlato, G., Duci, M., Cavicchiolo, M. E., Guiducci, S., Stocchero, M., Giordano, G., Fascetti Leon, F., & Baraldi, E. (2022). The Metabolome and the Gut Microbiota for the Prediction of Necrotizing Enterocolitis and Spontaneous Intestinal Perforation: A Systematic Review. *Nutrients*, *14*(18), 3859. https://doi.org/10.3390/nu14183859.

Mudd, L. M., Holzman, C. B., Catov, J. M., Senagore, P. K., & Evans, R. W. (2012). Maternal lipids at mid-pregnancy and the risk of preterm delivery. *Acta Obstetricia et Gynecologica Scandinavica*, *91*(6), 726–735. https://doi.org/10.1111/j.1600-0412.2012.01391.x.

Murgas Torrazza, R., Li, N., Young, C., Kobeissy, F., Chow, M., Chen, S., Mai, V., Sharma, R., Hudak, M., Shuster, J., & Neu, J. (2013). Pilot Study Using Proteomics to Identify Predictive Biomarkers of Necrotizing Enterocolitis from Buccal Swabs in Very Low Birth Weight Infants. *Neonatology*, *104*(3), 234–242. https://doi.org/10.1159/000353721.

Nilsson, A. K., Tebani, A., Malmodin, D., Pedersen, A., Hellgren, G., Löfqvist, C., Hansen-Pupp, I., Uhlén, M., & Hellström, A. (2022). Longitudinal Serum Metabolomics in Extremely Premature Infants: Relationships with Gestational Age, Nutrition, and Morbidities. *Frontiers in Neuroscience*, *16*. https://doi.org/10.3389/fnins.2022.830884.

Oltman, S. P., Rogers, E. E., Baer, R. J., Jasper, E. A., Anderson, J. G., Steurer, M. A., Pantell, M. S., Petersen, M. A., Partridge, J. C., Karasek, D., Ross, K. M., Feuer, S. K., Franck, L. S., Rand, L., Dagle, J. M., Ryckman, K. K., & Jelliffe-Pawlowski, L. L. (2021). Newborn metabolic vulnerability profile identifies preterm infants at risk for mortality and morbidity. *Pediatric Research*, *89*(6), 1405–1413. https://doi.org/10.1038/s41390-020-01148-0.

Pan, X., Hu, J., Xia, W., Zhang, B., Liu, W., Zhang, C., Yang, J., Hu, C., Zhou, A., Chen, Z., Cao, J., Zhang, Y., Wang, Y., Huang, Z., Lv, B., Song, R., Zhang, J., Xu, S., & Li, Y. (2017). Prenatal chromium exposure and risk of preterm birth: a cohort study in Hubei, China. *Scientific Reports*, *7*(1), 3048. https://doi.org/10.1038/s41598-017-03106-z.

Parry, S., Leite, R., Esplin, M. S., Bukowski, R., Zhang, H., Varner, M., Andrews, W. W., Saade, G. R., Ilekis, J., Reddy, U. M., Huang, H., Sadovsky, Y., Blair, I. A., & Biggio, J. (2020). Cervicovaginal fluid proteomic analysis to identify potential biomarkers for preterm birth. *American Journal of Obstetrics and Gynecology*, *222*(5), 493.e1-493.e13. https://doi.org/10.1016/j.ajog.2019.11.1252.

Parry, S., Zhang, H., Biggio, J., Bukowski, R., Varner, M., Xu, Y., Andrews, W. W., Saade, G. R., Esplin, M. S., Leite, R., Ilekis, J., Reddy, U. M., Sadovsky, Y., & Blair, I. A.

(2014). Maternal serum serpin B7 is associated with early spontaneous preterm birth. *American Journal of Obstetrics and Gynecology*, *211*(6), 678.e1-678.e12. https://doi.org/10.1016/j.ajog.2014.06.035.

Piersigilli, F., & Bhandari, V. (2020). Metabolomics of bronchopulmonary dysplasia. *Clinica Chimica Acta*, *500*, 109–114. https://doi.org/10.1016/j.cca.2019.09.025.

Piersigilli, F., Lam, T. T., Vernocchi, P., Quagliariello, A., Putignani, L., Aghai, Z. H., & Bhandari, V. (2019). Identification of new biomarkers of bronchopulmonary dysplasia using metabolomics. *Metabolomics*, *15*(2), 20. https://doi.org/10.1007/s11306-019-1482-9.

Pinto, J., Maciel, E., Melo, T. S., Domingues, M. R. M., Galhano, E., Pita, C., Almeida, M. do C., Carreira, I. M., & Gil, A. M. (2014). Maternal plasma phospholipids are altered in trisomy 21 cases and prior to preeclampsia and preterm outcomes. *Rapid Communications in Mass Spectrometry*, *28*(14), 1635–1638. https://doi.org/10.1002/rcm.6941.

Pintus, M. C., Lussu, M., Dessì, A., Pintus, R., Noto, A., Masile, V., Marcialis, M. A., Puddu, M., Fanos, V., & Atzori, L. (2018). Urinary ^{1} H-NMR Metabolomics in the First Week of Life Can Anticipate BPD Diagnosis. *Oxidative Medicine and Cellular Longevity*, *2018*, 1–7. https://doi.org/10.1155/2018/7620671.

Power, K. M., Sanchez-Galan, J. E., Luskey, G. W., Koski, K. G., & Burns, D. H. (2011). Use of Near-Infrared Spectroscopic Analysis of Second Trimester Amniotic Fluid to Assess Preterm Births. *Journal of Pregnancy*, *2011*, 1–6. https://doi.org/10.1155/2011/980985.

Rasineni, G. K., Panigrahy, N., Rath, S. N., Chinnaboina, M., Konanki, R., Chirla, D. K., & Madduri, S. (2022). Diagnostic and Therapeutic Roles of the "Omics" in Hypoxic–Ischemic Encephalopathy in Neonates. *Bioengineering*, *9*(10), 498. https://doi.org/10.3390/bioengineering9100498.

Romero, R., Mazaki-Tovi, S., Vaisbuch, E., Kusanovic, J. P., Chaiworapongsa, T., Gomez, R., Nien, J. K., Yoon, B. H., Mazor, M., Luo, J., Banks, D., Ryals, J., & Beecher, C. (2010). Metabolomics in premature labor: a novel approach to identify patients at risk for preterm delivery. *The Journal of Maternal-Fetal & Neonatal Medicine*, *23*(12), 1344–1359. https://doi.org/10.3109/14767058.2010.482618.

Ryckman, K. K., Dagle, J. M., Shchelochkov, O. A., Ehinger, N., Poole, S. D., Berberich, S. L., Reese, J., & Murray, J. C. (2013). Association of amino acids with common complications of prematurity. *Pediatric Research*, *73*(6), 700–705. https://doi.org/10.1038/pr.2013.43.

Sarafidis, K., Begou, O., Deda, O., Gika, H., Agakidis, C., Efstathiou, N., & Theodoridis, G. (2019). Targeted urine metabolomics in preterm neonates with intraventricular hemorrhage. *Journal of Chromatography B*, *1104*, 240–248. https://doi.org/10.1016/j.jchromb.2018.11.024.

Sinclair, T. J., Ye, C., Chen, Y., Zhang, D., Li, T., Ling, X. B., Cohen, H. J., Shaw, G. M., Stevenson, D. K., Chace, D., Clark, R. H., & Sylvester, K. G. (2020). Progressive Metabolic Dysfunction and Nutritional Variability Precedes Necrotizing Enterocolitis. *Nutrients*, *12*(5), 1275. https://doi.org/10.3390/nu12051275.

Thomas, M., Sulek, K., McKenzie, E., Jones, B., Han, T.-L., Villas-Boas, S., Kenny, L., McCowan, L., & Baker, P. (2015). Metabolite Profile of Cervicovaginal Fluids from

Early Pregnancy Is Not Predictive of Spontaneous Preterm Birth. *International Journal of Molecular Sciences*, *16*(11), 27741–27748. https://doi.org/10.3390/ijms161126052.

Valerio, E., Mardegan, V., Stocchero, M., Cavicchiolo, M. E., Pirillo, P., Poloniato, G., D'Onofrio, G., Bonadies, L., Giordano, G., & Baraldi, E. (2022). Urinary metabotypes of newborns with perinatal asphyxia undergoing therapeutic hypothermia. *PLOS ONE*, *17*(8), e0273175. https://doi.org/10.1371/journal.pone.0273175.

Vicente-Muñoz, S., Cobo, T., Puchades-Carrasco, L., Sánchez-García, A. B., Agustí, N., Palacio, M., Pineda-Lucena, A., & Gratacós, E. (2020). Vaginal metabolome: towards a minimally invasive diagnosis of microbial invasion of the amniotic cavity in women with preterm labor. *Scientific Reports*, *10*(1), 5465. https://doi.org/10.1038/s41598-020-62542-6.

Virgiliou, C., Gika, H. G., Witting, M., Bletsou, A. A., Athanasiadis, A., Zafrakas, M., Thomaidis, N. S., Raikos, N., Makrydimas, G., & Theodoridis, G. A. (2017). Amniotic Fluid and Maternal Serum Metabolic Signatures in the Second Trimester Associated with Preterm Delivery. *Journal of Proteome Research*, *16*(2), 898–910. https://doi.org/10.1021/acs.jproteome.6b00845.

Wang, K., Tao, G., Sun, Z., & Sylvester, K. G. (2019). Recent Potential Noninvasive Biomarkers in Necrotizing Enterocolitis. *Gastroenterology Research and Practice*, *2019*, 1–9. https://doi.org/10.1155/2019/8413698.

Zhang, B., Xia, W., Li, Y., Bassig, B. A., Zhou, A., Wang, Y., Li, Z., Yao, Y., Hu, J., Du, X., Zhou, Y., Liu, J., Xue, W., Ma, Y., Pan, X., Peng, Y., Zheng, T., & Xu, S. (2015). Prenatal exposure to lead in relation to risk of preterm low birth weight: A matched case–control study in China. *Reproductive Toxicology*, *57*, 190–195. https://doi.org/10.1016/j.reprotox.2015.06.051.

Chapter 23

The Use of Metabolomics in Diagnosing and Evaluating Inborn Metabolism Errors

Adviye Cakil Saglik*, MD
Department of Neonatology, Pediatrics, University of Health Sciences,
Kanuni Sultan Suleyman Training and Research Hospital, Istanbul, Turkey

Abstract

Metabolites are small molecules that are the end products of enzymatic processes in the human body. Inborn errors of metabolism (IEM) are inherited, known to have a poor prognosis, generally and luckily rarely diseases. More than 1000 diseases were defined about metabolite deficiency, enzymatic dysfunction, or absence (Ferreira & van Karnebeek, 2019). The first studies on inborn errors of metabolism started in the 1900s with most popular diseases including albinisim, cystinuria, and alkaptonuria (Vangala & Tonelli, 2007). From those years, with the help of new technology, new studies are performed with a few drops of blood and provided to check more than 20 metabolic diseases with one sample. More than 100 years before, diagnosed metabolic diseases numbers were smaller, but for now the diagnostic ratio of IEM increased 5 times much more than those years. Thus, an early diagnosis can be possible with screening all newborns, not only probable patients or newborns with a family history. So, in many countries it becomes a part of the routine neonatal screening programme to diagnose in early newborn period before symptoms occur. By the help of technological systems, the new study area of the point is metabolomics and the analysing of the metabolite profiles of the biological system to understand genes' effects in many metabolic inherited diseases.

---

* Corresponding Author's Email: adviye_mtf@yahoo.com.

In: Metabolomics and Clinical Approach
Editors: Sevgi Durna Daştan and Taner Daştan
ISBN: 979-8-89113-095-1

Keywords: inborn error of metabolism, metabolomics, metabolic diseases, newborn

Introduction

Inborn errors of metabolism (IEM) are inherited diseases seen rarely and the caused by different enzyme defects in the newborn period and result in several progressive diseases. These enzymes contribute to different systems of the organism. In the carbohydrate, fatty acids, amino acids, nucleic acids, and urea cycle system, enzyme defects disturb the metabolism of substrates and cause accumulation of the toxins (Baumgartner & Baumgartner, 2006). By the blockage of system at any stage, clinical symptoms start and lead to death. It was first named in 1908 by a British physician, and first diagnosed diseases were alkaptonuria, albinism, and cystinuria (Mussap et al., 2018). More than a century of studies continue to focus on IEM. For today IEM prevalence is known as 1 in 1000 people all over the world (Coene et al., 2018). IEM are generally rare diseases and their prevalence change from disease to disease. For example, congenital hypothyroidism is seen approximately 60 times much more than branched chain ketoaciduria, which are both IEM (Baumgartner & Baumgartner, 2006). If any disease seems to have such high incidence in a society, it is much more important to diagnose it earlier. Symptoms and signs of IEM differ in a wide range. Neurological signs are hypotonia, myopathy, ataxia, convulsions, myelopathy, encephalopathy, movement disorders, intellectual problems. Gastrointestinal signs are food intolerance, hepatomegaly, and hepatic failure, splenomegaly, and jaundice. As cardiac signs, cardiomyopathy is the most seen. In the skeletal system, joints easily dislocated, short or tall heights are possible, osteochondrosis and osteopenia can be seen. Also, eye problems such as lens dislocation, cataract or retinopathy, and hearing loss can occur. And the metabolic problems are dysregulation of blood glucose level, hiper or hypoketosis, hypocalcemia, adrenal failure, and failure to thrive (Mordaunt et al., 2020).

In this view, newborn screening tests become more important by years. Nowadays it is possible to check the IEM with a small blood sample as dry blood spots (DBS) in developed and low-income countries. Early diagnosis is essential to provide treatment or a better quality of life and a longer life. But when delayed in diagnosis, it may result in metabolic decompensation, progressive neuromotor disturbance, severe complications, and early death.

Metabolomics in the Diagnosis of IEM

'Omics' are new molecules that are used to understand biological systems. It can be checked proteins, lipids, carbohydrates, metabolites. As one of them is metabolomics, they are small molecules in metabolic pathways and fingerprints of the metabolic processes of the organism. The term of 'metabolomics' was first defined in 2002 (Fiehn, 2002). In metabolic pathways, the process is affected both by genetic factors and non-genetic environmental factors. Laboratory tests for metabolomics can be categorised in four groups which are general metabolic screening tests, specific metabolic tests, enzymatic studies, and nucleic acid analysis. By this technology we can now diagnose more than 50 congenital metabolic diseases such as aminoacidopathies, organic acidemias, fatty acid oxidations, and lysosomal storage diseases. For specific diagnosis amino acid profiles, urine organic acid profiles, enzyme activity assays, plasma acylcarnitine profiles, free fatty acid profiles, oligosaccharides, mucopolysaccharides and mutational analyses (Baumgartner & Baumgartner, 2006).

Nuclear Magnetic Resonance (NMR) spectroscopy and Tandem mass spectrometry (MS) are reference methods to analyse complex metabolites objectively. NMR spectroscopy measures the intrinsic magnetic speciality of atomic nucleus (Beckonert et al., 2007). One dimensional proton NMR spectroscopy is the most preferred method to study metabolomics due to its advantages of no preanalytic stage needs, no manipulation to sample and no destruction to the products occur and it analyses fast and highly reproducible (Markley et al., 2017). Aygen et al., in 2014 in Turkey studied 989 newborns urine samples by NMR and for outliers analyses checked 65 metabolites to diagnose IEM (Aygen et al., 2014). By this NMR technology, they can diagnose those with IEM in addition to the other newborns who have statistical outliers. Maybe in the future, it will be a combined diagnosis method for asymptomatic but suspected IME in newborns. Another method which is reliable, cheaper and more suitable for complex metabolites is Tandem mass spectrometry (TMS) (González-Domínguez et al., 2017). It first started to be used in the 1980s and became one of the most important diagnostic methods in IEM. Since it can be studied with a little DBS like general screening tests, it is a practical method to check all newborns. There are two pathways to analyse in TMS. One is direct infusion mode, in which the sample is infused directly to the mass spectrometer, and the other method is conjunction with high resolution separation such as liquid or gas chromatography (LC-MS or GC-MS) or capillary electrophoresis (CE-MS) (Begou et al., 2017). The direct infusion method is used to separate metabolites from complex compounds. LC-MS is the most commonly chosen method for polar and non-polar products, GC-MS is used to analyse volatile compounds, and CE-MS is generally used for polar metabolites (Begou et al., 2017). New technological methods are ultra-performance liquid chromatography (UP-LC) and supercritical liquid chromatography (SLC). However, any of the methods is the sole and perfect for all metabolomes. Therefore, combined methods are considered to be more preferable.

Metabolic Screening Tests in Neonates

Metabolic screening tests for newborn infants were first started in the 1960s in the United States of America for Phenylketonuria (PKU) (Maccready & Hussey, 1964). In 1968 newborn metabolic screening tests became World Health Organization (WHO) standards for newborn infants (Wilson et al., 1968). Standard screening tests for diseases that are important to public health, are easily detectable, early treatment is beneficial, and it must be cost effective (Arnold, 2018). With a single DBS, at least 50 and more metabolic diseases should be checked.

Early diagnosis to start treatment in some IEM diseases improves life quality and extends life in patients. Thus, we see that neonatal screening becomes more important by the years, in particular for developing countries. Although not all IEM can be detected with these tests, the chance of finding as many as possible, plays an important role in public health. In the Human Metabolome Data Base (HMDB), 247 metabolites are defined and 147 of them are associated with IEM. This project named as multinational named Human Metabolome Project (HMP) to facilitate diagnosis and find associated genes of IEM (Lee et al., 2009; Ninomiya et al., 2020). Therefore, it is possible to diagnose diseases with whole exome sequence analysis (Yu et al., 2013).

Metabolomic Tests Diversity

Metabolomic tests in diseases of metabolism can be classified as targeted or untargeted. Untargeted tests have many limitations, such as expensive instruments and special methods which need expensive instruments (Dhiman et al., 2011; Koelmel et al., 2017). Apart from the other omics, metabolomics is affected by gender, diet, or other physiological factors (Zhang et al., 2013). For example, age is one of the most significant factors including both gestational age and chronological age (Courraud et al., 2021). As environmental factors, temperature and humidity affect the sample preparation and the results of metabolic profiles (Biagini et al., 2019). Complex analysis takes more time to perform, however, timely accurate diagnosis and correlation with clinical outcomes are extremely important in IEM (Beebe & Kennedy, 2016). For metabolic diseases, ethnicity also has a crucial role, and many variations can be seen in different regions around the world. Therefore, studies for metabolomics must be variated for ethnicity differences (Rosenfeld et al., 2012). Up to now, by the analysing systems improved, in the most popular database -Human Metabolome Database (HMDB)- metabolite numbers have doubled (Wishart et al., 2022).

In different organ-specific diseases and sample types, distinct metabolomic profiles need to be analyzed. However, the sensitivity of untargeted metabolomics is lower than the targeted metabolomics (Hertzog et al., 2022). Almontashiri et al., controlled the trueness of the untargeted metabolomic analysis in 87 known IEMs patients and found that its sensitivity is as high as 86% (Almontashiri et al., 2020). Besides, Steinbusch et al., found a similar sensitivity rate as 87% (Steinbusch et al., 2021).

For targeted tests on specific metabolites studies, many studies focus on targeted tests. Both targeted and untargeted metabolomic studies are done for a wide range of disease-associated metabolites (Vécsei et al., 2013). By DBS more than 400 metabolites can be detected, such as lipids, organic acids, carbohydrates, bile acids, and acylcarnitines. Galactosemia can be diagnosed by detecting hexose metabolomes. A study carried out in Italy between 2007 and 2014, to detect IEM in the newborn period. They performed with LC-MS/GC-MS for fatal diseases such as fatty acid oxidation, organic acidemia, and hyperammonemia (Scolamiero et al., 2015). As the result, it is understood that metabolomics can be used for diagnosis before symptoms occur. Phenylketonuria and maple syrup urine disease (MSUD) are the most important metabolic diseases for screening metabolomics (Constantinou et al., 2004).

As an example, diagnose of an IEM for a clinician starts with the first suspect. There are many factors that affect the decision. In some countries or in some of regions some diseases are seen much more because of genetic factors, or somewhere environmental factors affect the composition of DNA. Physical signs are the main suspicious factors for an IEM, such as facial signs, finger numbers and configurations, other abdominal or cardiac problems, neurologic impairments, and psychiatric problems help to make the decision. If any screening test has been performed in the newborn period, it helps to rule out some of the diseases, but of course not all. So, the clinician can start with untargeted tests to tend a smaller disease group. Targeted tests can help directly to the specific disease for restrict diagnosis.

Neuropsychiatric Symptoms of IEM

Generally, diagnosis of any suspected IEM is made if a family history is known or in neonatal screening it is detected or after any physical symptom occurs. But, of course, some IEM diseases have neuropsychiatric symptoms such as cognitive dysfunctions, emotional stress disturbance, mental deficiency, developmental delay. These symptoms may be seen in hormonal change periods such as childbirth (for example, ornithine transcarbamylase, urea cycle disorders) or in puberty (Fassier et al., 2011; Peterson, 2003; Sedel et al., 2007). If it is a milder form of disease, it takes so long years to diagnose, may be after adolescence or in adulthood years. So if we can diagnose more early IEM with neuropsychiatric symptoms, may be in the following years new parameters can be added in neonatal screening tests for more severe or atypical neuropsychiatric diseases (Naylor et al., 1987).

Conclusion

IEM are genetically transmitted familial diseases. They are rarely seen and increased in some regions with high-incidence marriages with relatives. Sometimes the underlying reason is a gene defect, or sometimes an enzyme deficiency or absence is the source of the disease. Any standard or sole classification for IEM could not be done yet. However, several classifications according to pathophysiology, clinical features, enzyme defects, accumulated toxins, and many more exist. The most used one is divided into 3 groups as follows; intoxication, energy deficiency, and complex molecules (Saudubray, 2001).

Metabolomics is at the core of IEM studies. Early diagnosis is important because treatment costs are highly expensive. Targeted and untargeted metabolomics with a combination of genomics improve early diagnosis and start treatment of IEM, decrease morbidity and mortality and finally better prognosis. The role of epigenetics must be continued to study to better understand the mechanisms underlying complex processes in the occurrence of IEM. It is possible that every newborn who has and does not familial risk factors of IEM, should be controlled with DBS for early diagnosis and to increase quality of life.

References

Almontashiri, N. A. M., Zha, L., Young, K., Law, T., Kellogg, M. D., Bodamer, O. A., & Peake, R. W. A. (2020). Clinical Validation of Targeted and Untargeted Metabolomics Testing for Genetic Disorders: A 3 Year Comparative Study. *Scientific Reports*, *10*(1), 9382. https://doi.org/10.1038/s41598-020-66401-2.

Arnold, G. L. (2018). Inborn errors of metabolism in the 21st century: past to present. *Annals of Translational Medicine*, *6*(24), 467. https://doi.org/10.21037/atm.2018.11.36.

Aygen, S., Dürr, U., Hegele, P., Kunig, J., Spraul, M., Schäfer, H., Krings, D., Cannet, C., Fang, F., Schütz, B., Bülbül, S. F. H., Aydin, H. I., Sarıcı, S. U., Yalaz, M., Ors, R., Atalan, R., & Tuncer, O. (2014). NMR-Based Screening for Inborn Errors of Metabolism: Initial Results from a Study on Turkish Neonates. *JIMD Reports*, *16*, 101–111. https://doi.org/10.1007/8904_2014_326.

Baumgartner, C., & Baumgartner, D. (2006). Biomarker Discovery, Disease Classification, and Similarity Query Processing on High-Throughput MS/MS Data of Inborn Errors of Metabolism. *SLAS Discovery*, *11*(1), 90–99. https://doi.org/10.1177/1087057105280518.

Beckonert, O., Keun, H. C., Ebbels, T. M. D., Bundy, J., Holmes, E., Lindon, J. C., & Nicholson, J. K. (2007). Metabolic profiling, metabolomic and metabonomic procedures for NMR spectroscopy of urine, plasma, serum and tissue extracts. *Nature Protocols*, *2*(11), 2692–2703. https://doi.org/10.1038/nprot.2007.376.

Beebe, K., & Kennedy, A. D. (2016). Sharpening Precision Medicine by a Thorough Interrogation of Metabolic Individuality. *Computational and Structural Biotechnology Journal*, *14*, 97–105. https://doi.org/10.1016/j.csbj.2016.01.001.

Begou, O., Gika, H. G., Wilson, I. D., & Theodoridis, G. (2017). Hyphenated MS-based targeted approaches in metabolomics. *The Analyst*, *142*(17), 3079–3100. https://doi.org/10.1039/c7an00812k.

Biagini, D., Lomonaco, T., Ghimenti, S., Onor, M., Bellagambi, F. G., Salvo, P., di Francesco, F., & Fuoco, R. (2019). Using labelled internal standards to improve needle trap micro-extraction technique prior to gas chromatography/mass spectrometry. *Talanta*, *200*, 145–155. https://doi.org/10.1016/j.talanta.2019.03.046.

Coene, K. L. M., Kluijtmans, L. A. J., van der Heeft, E., Engelke, U. F. H., de Boer, S., Hoegen, B., Kwast, H. J. T., van de Vorst, M., Huigen, M. C. D. G., Keularts, I. M. L. W., Schreuder, M. F., van Karnebeek, C. D. M., Wortmann, S. B., de Vries, M. C., Janssen, M. C. H., Gilissen, C., Engel, J., & Wevers, R. A. (2018). Next-generation metabolic screening: targeted and untargeted metabolomics for the diagnosis of inborn errors of metabolism in individual patients. *Journal of Inherited Metabolic Disease*, *41*(3), 337–353. https://doi.org/10.1007/s10545-017-0131-6.

Constantinou, M. A., Papakonstantinou, E., Benaki, D., Spraul, M., Shulpis, K., Koupparis, M. A., & Mikros, E. (2004). Application of nuclear magnetic resonance spectroscopy combined with principal component analysis in detecting inborn errors of metabolism using blood spots: a metabonomic approach. *Analytica Chimica Acta*, *512*(2), 303–312.

Courraud, J., Ernst, M., Svane Laursen, S., Hougaard, D. M., & Cohen, A. S. (2021). Studying Autism Using Untargeted Metabolomics in Newborn Screening Samples. *Journal of Molecular Neuroscience : MN*, *71*(7), 1378–1393. https://doi.org/10.1007/s12031-020-01787-2.

Dhiman, N., Hall, L., Wohlfiel, S. L., Buckwalter, S. P., & Wengenack, N. L. (2011). Performance and cost analysis of matrix-assisted laser desorption ionization-time of flight mass spectrometry for routine identification of yeast. *Journal of Clinical Microbiology*, *49*(4), 1614–1616. https://doi.org/10.1128/JCM.02381-10.

Fassier, T., Guffon, N., Acquaviva, C., D'Amato, T., Durand, D. V., & Domenech, P. (2011). Misdiagnosed postpartum psychosis revealing a late-onset urea cycle disorder. *The American Journal of Psychiatry*, *168*(6), 576–580. https://doi.org/10.1176/appi.ajp.2010.10071032.

Ferreira, C. R., & van Karnebeek, C. D. M. (2019). *Inborn errors of metabolism* (pp. 449–481). https://doi.org/10.1016/B978-0-444-64029-1.00022-9.

Fiehn, O. (2002). Metabolomics--the link between genotypes and phenotypes. *Plant Molecular Biology*, *48*(1–2), 155–171.

González-Domínguez, R., Sayago, A., & Fernández-Recamales, Á. (2017). Direct infusion mass spectrometry for metabolomic phenotyping of diseases. *Bioanalysis*, *9*(1), 131–148. https://doi.org/10.4155/bio-2016-0202.

Hertzog, A., Selvanathan, A., Devanapalli, B., Ho, G., Bhattacharya, K., & Tolun, A. A. (2022). A narrative review of metabolomics in the era of "-omics": integration into clinical practice for inborn errors of metabolism. *Translational Pediatrics*, *11*(10), 1704–1716. https://doi.org/10.21037/tp-22-105.

Koelmel, J. P., Ulmer, C. Z., Jones, C. M., Yost, R. A., & Bowden, J. A. (2017). Common cases of improper lipid annotation using high-resolution tandem mass spectrometry data and corresponding limitations in biological interpretation. *Biochimica et Biophysica Acta. Molecular and Cell Biology of Lipids*, *1862*(8), 766–770. https://doi.org/10.1016/j.bbalip.2017.02.016.

Lee, M. N., Ha, S. H., Kim, J., Koh, A., Lee, C. S., Kim, J. H., Jeon, H., Kim, D.-H., Suh, P.-G., & Ryu, S. H. (2009). Glycolytic flux signals to mTOR through glyceraldehyde-3-phosphate dehydrogenase-mediated regulation of Rheb. *Molecular and Cellular Biology*, *29*(14), 3991–4001. https://doi.org/10.1128/MCB.00165-09.

Maccready, R. A., & Hussey, M. G. (1964). Newborn Phenylketonuria Detection Program In Massachusetts. *American Journal of Public Health and the Nation's Health*, *54*(12), 2075–2081. https://doi.org/10.2105/ajph.54.12.2075.

Markley, J. L., Brüschweiler, R., Edison, A. S., Eghbalnia, H. R., Powers, R., Raftery, D., & Wishart, D. S. (2017). The future of NMR-based metabolomics. *Current Opinion in Biotechnology*, *43*, 34–40. https://doi.org/10.1016/j.copbio.2016.08.001.

Mordaunt, D., Cox, D., & Fuller, M. (2020). Metabolomics to Improve the Diagnostic Efficiency of Inborn Errors of Metabolism. *International Journal of Molecular Sciences*, *21*(4), 1195. https://doi.org/10.3390/ijms21041195.

Mussap, M., Zaffanello, M., & Fanos, V. (2018). Metabolomics: a challenge for detecting and monitoring inborn errors of metabolism. *Annals of Translational Medicine*, *6*(17), 338–338. https://doi.org/10.21037/atm.2018.09.18.

Naylor, E. W., Ennis, D., Davidson, A. G., Wong, L. T., Applegarth, D. A., & Niederwieser, A. (1987). Guanosine triphosphate cyclohydrolase I deficiency: early diagnosis by routine urine pteridine screening. *Pediatrics*, *79*(3), 374–378. https://doi.org/10.1542/peds.79.3.374.

Ninomiya, S., Nakamura, N., Nakamura, H., Mizutani, T., Kaneda, Y., Yamaguchi, K., Matsumoto, T., Kitagawa, J., Kanemura, N., Shiraki, M., Hara, T., Shimizu, M., & Tsurumi, H. (2020). Low Levels of Serum Tryptophan Underlie Skeletal Muscle Atrophy. *Nutrients*, *12*(4), 978. https://doi.org/10.3390/nu12040978.

Peterson, D. E. (2003). Acute postpartum mental status change and coma caused by previously undiagnosed ornithine transcarbamylase deficiency. *Obstetrics and Gynecology*, *102*(5 Pt 2), 1212–1215. https://doi.org/10.1016/s0029-7844(03)00165-0.

Rosenfeld, J. A., Mason, C. E., & Smith, T. M. (2012). Limitations of the human reference genome for personalized genomics. *PloS One*, *7*(7), e40294. https://doi.org/10.1371/journal.pone.0040294.

Saudubray, J.-M. (2001). Clinical phenotypes: diagnosis/algorithms. In *The Metabolic and Molecular Bases of Inherited Disease* (pp. 1327–1403). McGraw-Hill.

Scolamiero, E., Cozzolino, C., Albano, L., Ansalone, A., Caterino, M., Corbo, G., di Girolamo, M. G., di Stefano, C., Durante, A., Franzese, G., Franzese, I., Gallo, G., Giliberti, P., Ingenito, L., Ippolito, G., Malamisura, B., Mazzeo, P., Norma, A., Ombrone, D., Parenti, G., Pellecchia, S., Pecce, R., Pierucci, I., Romanelli, R., Rossi, A., Siano, M., Stoduto, T., Villani, G. R., Andria, G., Salvatore, F., Frisso, G., & Ruoppolo, M. (2015). Targeted metabolomics in the expanded newborn screening for inborn errors of metabolism. *Molecular BioSystems*, *11*(6), 1525–1535. https://doi.org/10.1039/c4mb00729h.

Sedel, F., Baumann, N., Turpin, J.-C., Lyon-Caen, O., Saudubray, J.-M., & Cohen, D. (2007). Psychiatric manifestations revealing inborn errors of metabolism in adolescents and adults. *Journal of Inherited Metabolic Disease*, *30*(5), 631–641. https://doi.org/10.1007/s10545-007-0661-4.

Steinbusch, L. K. M., Wang, P., Waterval, H. W. A. H., Stassen, F. A. P. M., Coene, K. L. M., Engelke, U. F. H., Habets, D. D. J., Bierau, J., & Körver-Keularts, I. M. L. W. (2021). Targeted urine metabolomics with a graphical reporting tool for rapid diagnosis of inborn errors of metabolism. *Journal of Inherited Metabolic Disease*, *44*(5), 1113–1123. https://doi.org/10.1002/jimd.12385.

Vangala, S., & Tonelli, A. (2007). Biomarkers, metabonomics, and drug development: Can inborn errors of metabolism help in understanding drug toxicity? *The AAPS Journal*, *9*(3), E284–E297. https://doi.org/10.1208/aapsj0903031.

Vécsei, L., Szalárdy, L., Fülöp, F., & Toldi, J. (2013). Kynurenines in the CNS: recent advances and new questions. *Nature Reviews. Drug Discovery*, *12*(1), 64–82. https://doi.org/10.1038/nrd3793.

Wilson J, Jungner G, & WHO. (1968). Principles and practice of screening for disease. Retrieved from http://www.who.int/iris/handle/10665/37650.

Wishart, D. S., Guo, A., Oler, E., Wang, F., Anjum, A., Peters, H., Dizon, R., Sayeeda, Z., Tian, S., Lee, B. L., Berjanskii, M., Mah, R., Yamamoto, M., Jovel, J., Torres-Calzada, C., Hiebert-Giesbrecht, M., Lui, V. W., Varshavi, D., Varshavi, D., Allen, D., Arndt, D., Khetarpal, N., Sivakumaran, A., Harford, K., Sanford, S., Yee, K., Cao, X., Budinski, Z., Liigand, J., Zhang, L., Zheng, J., Mandal, R., Karu, N., Dambrova, M., Schiöth, H. B., Greiner, R., & Gautam, V. (2022). HMDB 5.0: the Human Metabolome Database for 2022. *Nucleic Acids Research*, *50*(D1), D622–D631. https://doi.org/10.1093/nar/gkab1062.

Yu, H.-C., Sloan, J. L., Scharer, G., Brebner, A., Quintana, A. M., Achilly, N. P., Manoli, I., Coughlin, C. R., Geiger, E. A., Schneck, U., Watkins, D., Suormala, T., van Hove, J. L. K., Fowler, B., Baumgartner, M. R., Rosenblatt, D. S., Venditti, C. P., & Shaikh, T. H. (2013). An X-linked cobalamin disorder caused by mutations in transcriptional coregulator HCFC1. *American Journal of Human Genetics*, *93*(3), 506–514. https://doi.org/10.1016/j.ajhg.2013.07.022.

Zhang, A., Sun, H., Xu, H., Qiu, S., & Wang, X. (2013). Cell Metabolomics. *OMICS: A Journal of Integrative Biology*, *17*(10), 495–501. https://doi.org/10.1089/omi.2012.0090.

Chapter 24

Metabolomics in Biomarker Identification for Cardiovascular Diseases

Mesude Avci[*], PhD
Department of Chemical Engineering, Sivas Cumhuriyet University, Sivas, Turkey

Abstract

Metabolomics is the systematic analysis of the particular chemical fingerprints of small molecules or metabolite profiles which are associated with a different cellular metabolic process in a cell, organ, or organism. Events in a cell are not described completely by messenger RNA gene expression data and proteomic analyses, but metabolic profiling supplies direct and indirect physiological insights, which can possibly be measurable in a broad range of biospecimens. Even though not specific to cardiac conditions, identification, confirmation, clinical validation, and bedside tests are a biomarker exploration path to translate metabolomics into cardiovascular biomarkers. Technological progress in metabolomic tools (such as nuclear magnetic resonance spectroscopy and mass spectrometry) and more complicated bioinformatics and analytical techniques help to evaluate low- molecular-weight metabolites in biospecimens and ultimately supply a unique insight into determined and novel metabolic pathways. Systematic metabolomics can provide physiological knowledge of cardiovascular disease states in addition to traditional profiling and can include the definition of metabolic reactions of an individual or population to therapeutic interventions or environmental exposures.

---

[*] Corresponding Author's E-mail: mesude@cumhuriyet.edu.tr.

In: Metabolomics and Clinical Approach
Editors: Sevgi Durna Daştan and Taner Daştan
ISBN: 979-8-89113-095-1

Keywords: metabolomics, cardiovascular diseases (CVDs), heart failure, atherosclerosis, biomarker, metabolites

Introduction

A severe popular health challenge and the main cause of death has been cardiovascular diseases (CVDs) (D'Agostino et al., 2000; Kordalewska & Markuszewski, 2015). According to the World Health Organization, CVD is responsible for 17.9 million deaths in 2019 which is 32% of global deaths (World Health Organization (WHO), 2009). Future predictions show that CVDs could reach 23.3 million deaths in 2030 (Mathers & Loncar, 2006). For the European Union, the estimated number of the costs per year is 196 billion euros which include 54% direct healthcare, 24% performance deficits and 22% casual nursing of patients with CVD (Nichols et al., 2012).

Complications of the blood vessels and heart, which is a result of atherosclerosis, cause CVDs and are mostly diagnosed in old age in both men and women. These groups of diseases contain infarction, cardiogenic shock, and myocardial ischemia, atherosclerosis, anthracycline-induced cardiotoxicity, atrial fibrillation heart failure, ischemic cardiomyopathy, non-ischemic cardiomyopathy, coronary artery disease (CAD). Early diagnosis and intervention procedure will decrease the prevalence of CVD.

While many risk factors are responsible for CVDs, such as smoking, gender, renal failure, lack of nutritious dietary, overweight as a result of less body movements, cholesterol, increased blood pressure, and hyperglycemia, the pathological mechanism fundamental to most CVDs are still not fully known (Hackam & Anand, 2003; Kordalewska & Markuszewski, 2015; Libby, 2002; P. W. Wilson et al., 1998; P. W. F. Wilson, 2008). Moreover, in addition to popular risk factors for CVD, it is mostly expected that a patient with CVD could have another CVD as time progresses (Hunt et al., 2013; World Health Organization (WHO), 2007). Furthermore, one of the major problems for CVD patients is that signs of the diseases do not appear early in the progression of the disease. Actually, plaque formation will be formed during asymptomatic processes, which will build up silent but growing tissue damage (Barderas et al., 2011). When atheroma plaques subsequently tear, an atherothrombotic event arises due to the discharge of highly thrombogenic material (Barderas et al., 2011). When the metabolism is considered, the heart is a very significant part of the human being. Therefore, complications in the cardiac energy metabolism cause many cardiovascular diseases (Müller et al.,

2021; van Bilsen et al., 2009). Moreover, cardiac function and myocardial metabolism can be affected by the pathogenesis of cardiovascular disease. Cardiovascular diseases also induce changes in substrate metabolism that result in distinct changes in the patient's metabolic profile (Nascimben et al., 1996; Smith et al., 2006).

Depending on these events, clinical intervention and early diagnosis of CVDs require the discovery of original and practically important biomarkers, which are used alone or together with existing ones (Barderas et al., 2011). When evaluating particular responses to determine standard risk factors, a mixture of existing biomarkers will only contribute slightly (T. J. Wang et al., 2006). Thus, there is considerable interest in exploring and operating new biomarkers, which will help decide the most useful from the current list and diagnosing people with the potential to be caught in CVDs (Barderas et al., 2011). Especially, if the used biomarkers predict the risk of rupture, it will help patients receive pharmacological treatment in time and will create a protective lifestyle. The investigation and innovation of biomarkers for developments in outpatient and inpatient care adds a new dimension to the landscape of CVD. The improvements in "-omics" technologies (genomics, transcriptomics, proteomics, and metabolomics), which have fast, sensitive and robust tools, have made it easier to examine these small molecules in cardiovascular diseases.

Metabolomics Technologies

Tiny particles, which are responsible for common responses related to metabolism and which are necessary to continue the sustenance, advancement, and regular action of a cell, are called metabolites. Moreover, metabolome, derived from the word genomics, is defined as the entire group of metabolites, which can be found in a living thing and its organs (Fiehn et al., 2000; Oliver et al., 1998) or the whole metabolites in a cell (Tweeddale et al., 1998). Thus, usage regarding investigative procedures on determining and measuring whole metabolites in the body, along with observing the differences in the metabolome of the cell cultivation, tissue model, or a biofluid as a result of perturbation are called as metabolomics and metabonomics (Fiehn et al., 2000; Nicholson et al., 1999).

Cardiovascular diseases cause pathophysiological molecular, cellular and functional changes, which can be better understood with the help of new "omics" tools (genomics, transcriptomics, proteomics, and metabolomics)

(Roberts & Gerszten, 2013). The excessive number of these small molecules in liquid body substances (saliva, urine, blood) and breathing exhalation can be measured by the use of modern metabolomics technologies (Müller et al., 2021; Shah et al., 2012). This information might be used as predictive and characteristic tools to analyze early specific alterations during the beginning and progression of cardiovascular disease (Müller et al., 2021). For that reason, metabolomics is projected as a valuable means of providing additional insight into pathologic physiology in CVDs along with increasing practitioners' knowledge of pathogenesis of CVDs (Müller et al., 2021).

One of the interesting characteristics in the area of metabolites is that the number of metabolites in the body is slightly small (≈7000) when compared to the approximate number of transcripts (100000), genes (25000), and proteins (1000000) (Shah et al., 2012). Nonetheless, concentration ranges of metabolites are very wide, and metabolites display significant chemical diversity. Therefore, it is impossible to measure the metabolites in the human metabolome with the use of currently available instruments in an individual analysis (Shah et al., 2012). Alternatively, metabolome analysis can be performed with several analytical strategies (Dunn et al., 2005), such as nuclear magnetic resonance (NMR) (Nicholson & Wilson, 2003), mass spectrometry (MS), Fourier transformation infrared spectroscopy (FT-IR) (Harrigan et al., 2004; Johnson et al., 2004), along with analysis methods for example capillary electrophoresis (CE), gas chromatography (GC), or high performance liquid chromatography (HPLC) (Barderas et al., 2011). The metabolomics study includes various research approaches such as metabolic fingerprinting, metabolic profiling, and metabolic foot printing (Kordalewska & Markuszewski, 2015). Metabolic profiling is an illustration of the targeted approach and in this technique metabolites, which have similar physical characteristics such as carbohydrates, amino acids, grouped in a specific biological approach such as purine metabolism and glycolysis are discovered. A specific section of the metabolome composition can be learned better qualitatively and quantitatively with the help of the data, which is gathered with this strategy (Kordalewska & Markuszewski, 2015; Patti et al., 2012). In the case of the metabolic fingerprinting method, which is an example of an untargeted approach, metabolites are investigated without previous information. Therefore, the whole metabolome might be discovered. Metabolites' levels vary under precise systems' conditions by showing a specific pattern, which can be described by this method. The metabolic footprinting approach is used mostly in molecular biology and microbiological studies. Metabolites, which are secreted into the culture medium by cells and microorganisms, could be recognized in these experiments (Kordalewska & Markuszewski, 2015; Patti et al., 2012).

Metabolomics in Cardiovascular Diseases (CVDs)

Metabolomics is being performed to examine various forms of causes of CVDs such as diabetes mellitus, fatness, and metabolic syndrome (Dumas et al., 2006; Faber et al., 2007; T. J. Wang et al., 2011). Mostly, it has focused on analyzing markers and explaining the natural history linked with various common pathologies in CVDs. These have extended markers for cardiogenic shock (Nicholls et al., 2007), myocardial ischemia (Lewis et al., 2008, 2010; Sabatine et al., 2005), risk of developing atherosclerosis or future cardiovascular events (Tang et al., 2009; Z. Wang et al., 2009b, 2011), atrial fibrillation (Mayr et al., 2008), risk of developing diabetes mellitus (T. J. Wang et al., 2011), chemotherapy-induced cardiotoxicity (Andreadou et al., 2009) and pulmonary hypertension related to advanced heart failure (Shao et al., 2012). These are some of the examples of cardiovascular events showing that metabolomic data metabolomic data have a wide application in the control of CVDs (Senn et al., 2012).

Metabolomics in Myocardial Ischemia, Cardiogenic Shock, and Infarction

The possible discovery of metabolic imbalance, which may occur during or after myocardial ischemia, can become an encouraging diagnostic instrument. In the work of Sabatine et al., (Sabatine et al., 2005), LC-MS (Liquid chromatography mass spectrometry), an untargeted approach, was used to examine metabolic profiling of myocardial ischemia. In their work, specimens of patients with and without myocardial ischemia were collected to test the difference of workout in patients. Therefore, differences in small molecules (metabolite) before and after to stress examination helped them determine the possible signs (biomarkers) of coronary ischemia. The levels of 6 metabolites changed and were recognized as inducible ischemia with a validated risk score. γ-aminobutyric acid, citric acid, uric acid, and several more metabolites were determined at an abnormal level. It was concluded that studies in metabolomics will be helpful in diagnostic studies and eventually will analyze new goals for therapeutic intervention. Apparently, cardiovascular metabolic changes, which can be discovered with serial blood sampling, occur after exercise (Senn et al., 2012).

To continue further ischemia, Lewis et al., (Lewis et al., 2008) worked on an artificial infarction design with environment of a septal ablation for obstructive hypertrophic cardiomyopathy to determine the momentary diversities metabolomic profiling throughout the progression of myocardial infarction. The interesting results of their work showed that the plasma marker of threonine, aconitic acid, hypoxanthine, and trimethylamine-N-oxide (TMAO) discriminated among with infarcted and with coronary angiography patients.

The array of disorders in the body can also help to understand the level of the disease. Intense heart attack (acute myocardial infarction (AMI)), which is made difficult by cardiogenic shock, causes serious morbidity and mortality rates in spite of tough therapy techniques such as revascularization (Hochman et al., 1999; Hochman et al., 2001). Nitric oxide (NO) has useful impacts containing coronary vasodilation and additional resting in the bed. Moreover, NO has various harmful effects, such as, lowering the ability of heart to contract, thus it can perform an essential duty in the hypotension and reduced heart functionality, which describe cardiogenic shock. It has been hypothesized that NO may participate in the pathogenesis of shocks in the heart, depending on the idea that stimulation in the inflammatory cells may cause isoforms of NO synthesize (Hochman, 2003). People with and without coronary artery disease are studied in the work of Nicholls et al., (Nicholls et al., 2007), and comparisons of metabolic profiles were made. Thus, patients after AMI are complicated by cardiogenic shock. In their results, it was found that the increased amount of the NO synthesize blockage, asymmetric dimethylarginine (ADMA) presents to be a free predictor of death. On the other hand, a future study of that group could not find a death advantage with inhibition of therapeutic NO synthase by L-NG-monomethyl arginine (TRIUMPH Investigators et al., 2007).

Metabolomics in Atherosclerosis

The metabolic profile that occurred during atherosclerosis should be examined because approximately all CVDs have atherosclerosis as an underlying process. The Multi-Ethnic Study of Atherosclerosis was started in 2000 in the US and that project also included the metabolomics approach (Bild et al.,

2002; MESA, 2022). In one of the studies, the relation between inflammation in the immune system caused by fat having a dangerous effect on atherosclerosis and plasma phospholipid polyunsaturated fatty acids degrees of was examined (Steffen et al., 2012).

Another broad investigation was occurred in 2012 to improve the identification of atherosclerosis before the infirmary stage. Tyrosine, glutamine, and docosahexaenoic acid were found to be a possible indicator of atherosclerosis growth as a result of serum metabolic profile analysis by using the NMR technique (Vorkas et al., 2015). Chen et al., (Chen et al., 2010) the used GC–MS method along progressive bioinformatics devices and 1-monolinoleoylglycerol, stearate, and palmitate were found as a possible plasma biomarkers of the disease.

The metabolic phenotype of the atherosclerotic plaque was examined and a comparison of the metabolome arrangement of the intima tissue along with atherosclerotic plaque tissue of people with carotid or femoral endarterectomy was obtained. UHPLC–MS (Ultra-high performance liquid chromatography-Mass spectrometer) method was applied to analyze tissue extracts. The degrees of acylcarnitines were different, which demonstrated changes in β-oxidation operation in the atherosclerotic plaque tissue. Also, phosphatidylethanoleamine-ceramides were recommended to be possible biomarkers of atherosclerosis pathogenesis (Vorkas et al., 2015).

Metabolomics in Heart Failure

Zhang et al., (Zhang et al., 2009) analyzed the sequence of myocardial infarction caused by isoproterenol in rats in metabolism. They performed UHPLC–TOF/MS (ultra-high performance liquid chromatography time-of-flight/ mass spectrometry) examination and found differences in the degrees of 13 plasma lipids (phospholipids and fatty acids) in rats with activated myocardial infarction (heart attack) as distinguished from healthy people.

Another study on heart attack was performed in pigs and in the control zone, the "at-risk" regions and the necrotic districts of the hearts were imposed on resection. As a result of the NMR-based metabolic fingerprinting approach, the quantity of small metabolites decreased and the lipid signs were found in necrotic cells (Barba et al., 2007).

The operation of the GC–TOF/MS (Gas Chromatography–Time-of-Flight/Mass Spectrometry) method showed the existence of possible serum biomarkers in the diagnosis of heart failure. As a result of the comparison between patients and healthy individuals, 2-hydroxy 2-methylpropanoicacid, pseudouridine, 2-oxoglutarate, 2,4,6- trihydroxypyrimidine and erythritol were different (Dunn et al., 2007).

The application of the LC–QqQ/MS (liquid chromatographic-triple quadrupole tandem mass spectrometry) technique was used to perform metabolomic analyses in plasma and it was found that asymmetrical dimethylarginine, N-mono-methylarginine, and symmetrical dimethylarginine were possible dangerous predictors of incident cardiac occurrences (Z. Wang et al., 2009a).

The molecular process of acute coronary syndrome was analyzed using the GC–MS technique with the help of plasma metabolic fingerprinting. Comparison was made between the metabolic characterization of 9 samples from acute coronary syndrome patients, ten examples of constant atherosclerosis patients, and ten examples of patients in good health. As a result of the comparison between acute coronary syndrome and healthy individuals, aspartic acid, 4-hydroxyproline, citric acid, and fructose levels decreased while glucose, urea, lactate, and valine amounts enhanced. The partial least squares discriminant examination (PLS-DA) was performed to discover the changes in metabolome composition and, as a result, the groups were classified as excellent. The categorization error was 5.3% for sick people with acute coronary syndrome and 0% for controls and patients with stable atherosclerosis (Vallejo et al., 2009).

Conclusion

The scientific community has a growing interest in the metabolomics, which is one of the most commonly used omic-related sciences, over the last decade. A mixture of different sensitive analytical techniques and advanced chemometric tools are needed to be used in metabolomics analyses. The molecular processes underlying different diseases can be explained and understood better with the help of metabolomics application. As a result of acquired knowledge, determining the reasons behind diseases, optimizing the cure, and choosing particular characteristic biomarkers can be explained easily. When diseases progress asymptomatically or without particular diagnostic biomarkers, the operation of metabolomics approach becomes more important. These metabolomics analyses have a difficulty of excluding the several effects, for example, age, dietary, used pharmacotherapy and additional environmental aspects influencing differences in the metabolome.

The composition of the metabolites should change as a result of the development of disease particularly. In the case of untargeted analysis, knowledge on organisms' metabolome structure is provided. Nevertheless, confirmation of possible disease markers can only be provided by the quantitatively targeting the analysis of selected metabolites. These compounds will gain a diagnostic and prognostic power by the measurement of them in a large-scale population along with parallel validation. To summarize, the operation of metabolomics in biomedical research can develop the advancement in pharmaceutical studies. The work reviewed in this chapter demonstrated that there has been an increasing concern about the use of metabolomics in CVDs. The likelihood of utilizing various example classes such as urine, tissue, blood, and breath with a concurrent operation of particular analytic methods may supply the inclusion of all metabolites exist in the body. The above cited works presents cases in which the metabolomic path is becoming more developed into an effective instrument in the CVDs analysis.

References

Andreadou, I., Papaefthimiou, M., Zira, A., Constantinou, M., Sigala, F., Skaltsounis, A.-L., Tsantili-Kakoulidou, A., Iliodromitis, E. K., Kremastinos, D. T., & Mikros, E. (2009). Metabonomic identification of novel biomarkers in doxorubicin cardiotoxicity and protective effect of the natural antioxidant oleuropein. *NMR in Biomedicine*, *22*(6), 585–592. https://doi.org/10.1002/nbm.1370.

Barba, I., Jaimez-Auguets, E., Rodriguez-Sinovas, A., & Garcia-Dorado, D. (2007). 1H NMR-based metabolomic identification of at-risk areas after myocardial infarction in swine. *Magma (New York, N.Y.)*, *20*(5–6), 265–271. https://doi.org/10.1007/s10334-007-0097-8.

Barderas, M. G., Laborde, C. M., Posada, M., de la Cuesta, F., Zubiri, I., Vivanco, F., & Alvarez-Llamas, G. (2011). Metabolomic profiling for identification of novel potential biomarkers in cardiovascular diseases. *Journal of Biomedicine & Biotechnology*, *2011*, 790132. https://doi.org/10.1155/2011/790132.

Bild, D. E., Bluemke, D. A., Burke, G. L., Detrano, R., Diez Roux, A. V, Folsom, A. R., Greenland, P., Jacob, D. R. J., Kronmal, R., Liu, K., Nelson, J. C., O'Leary, D., Saad, M. F., Shea, S., Szklo, M., & Tracy, R. P. (2002). Multi-Ethnic Study of Atherosclerosis: objectives and design. *American Journal of Epidemiology*, *156*(9), 871–881. https://doi.org/10.1093/aje/kwf113.

Chen, X., Liu, L., Palacios, G., Gao, J., Zhang, N., Li, G., Lu, J., Song, T., Zhang, Y., & Lv, H. (2010). Plasma metabolomics reveals biomarkers of the atherosclerosis. *Journal of Separation Science*, *33*(17–18), 2776–2783. https://doi.org/10.1002/jssc.201000395.

D'Agostino, R. B., Russell, M. W., Huse, D. M., Ellison, R. C., Silbershatz, H., Wilson, P. W., & Hartz, S. C. (2000). Primary and subsequent coronary risk appraisal: new results from the Framingham study. *American Heart Journal*, *139*(2 Pt 1), 272–281. https://doi.org/10.1067/mhj.2000.96469.

Dumas, M.-E., Barton, R. H., Toye, A., Cloarec, O., Blancher, C., Rothwell, A., Fearnside, J., Tatoud, R., Blanc, V., Lindon, J. C., Mitchell, S. C., Holmes, E., McCarthy, M. I., Scott, J., Gauguier, D., & Nicholson, J. K. (2006). Metabolic profiling reveals a contribution of gut microbiota to fatty liver phenotype in insulin-resistant mice. *Proceedings of the National Academy of Sciences of the United States of America*, *103*(33), 12511–12516. https://doi.org/10.1073/pnas.0601056103.

Dunn, W. B., Bailey, N. J. C., & Johnson, H. E. (2005). Measuring the metabolome: current analytical technologies. *The Analyst*, *130*(5), 606–625. https://doi.org/10.1039/b418288j.

Dunn, W. B., Broadhurst, D. I., Deepak, S. M., Buch, M. H., & McDowell, G. (2007). Serum metabolomics reveals many novel metabolic markers of heart failure, including pseudouridine and 2-oxoglutarate. *Metabolomics*, *3*(413–426).

Faber, J. H., Malmodin, D., Toft, H., Maher, A. D., Crockford, D., Holmes, E., Nicholson, J. K., Dumas, M. E., & Baunsgaard, D. (2007). Metabonomics in diabetes research. *Journal of Diabetes Science and Technology*, *1*(4), 549–557. https://doi.org/10.1177/193229680700100413.

Fiehn, O., Kopka, J., Dörmann, P., Altmann, T., Trethewey, R. N., & Willmitzer, L. (2000). Metabolite profiling for plant functional genomics. *Nature Biotechnology*, *18*(11), 1157–1161. https://doi.org/10.1038/81137.

Hackam, D. G., & Anand, S. S. (2003). Emerging Risk Factors for Atherosclerotic Vascular DiseaseA Critical Review of the Evidence. *JAMA*, *290*(7), 932–940. https://doi.org/10.1001/jama.290.7.932.

Harrigan, G. G., LaPlante, R. H., Cosma, G. N., Cockerell, G., Goodacre, R., Maddox, J. F., Luyendyk, J. P., Ganey, P. E., & Roth, R. A. (2004). Application of high-throughput Fourier-transform infrared spectroscopy in toxicology studies: contribution to a study on the development of an animal model for idiosyncratic toxicity. *Toxicology Letters*, *146*(3), 197–205. https://doi.org/10.1016/j.toxlet.2003.09.011.

Hochman, J. S., Sleeper, L. A., Webb, J. G., Sanborn, T. A., White, H. D., Talley, J. D., Buller, C. E., Jacobs, A. K., Slater, J. N., Col, J., McKinlay, S. M., & LeJemtel, T. H. (1999). Early revascularization in acute myocardial infarction complicated by cardiogenic shock. SHOCK Investigators. Should We Emergently Revascularize Occluded Coronaries for Cardiogenic Shock. *The New England Journal of Medicine*, *341*(9), 625–634. https://doi.org/10.1056/NEJM199908263410901.

Hochman, J. S. (2003). Cardiogenic shock complicating acute myocardial infarction: expanding the paradigm. *Circulation*, *107*(24), 2998–3002. https://doi.org/10.1161/01.CIR.0000075927.67673.F2.

Hochman, J. S, Sleeper, L. A., White, H. D., Dzavik, V., Wong, S. C., Menon, V., Webb, J. G., Steingart, R., Picard, M. H., Menegus, M. A., Boland, J., Sanborn, T., Buller, C. E., Modur, S., Forman, R., Desvigne-Nickens, P., Jacobs, A. K., Slater, J. N., LeJemtel, T. H., & Investigators, for the S. (2001). One-Year Survival Following

Early Revascularization for Cardiogenic Shock. *JAMA*, *285*(2), 190–192. https://doi.org/10.1001/jama.285.2.190.

Hunt, J., Nicholson, D., & Selbie, D. (2013). *Cardiovascular Disease Outcomes Strategy Improving outcomes for people with or at risk of cardiovascular disease.* DH Department of Health, Cardiovascular Disease Outcomes Strategy "Improving Outcomes for People with or at Risk of Cardiovascular Disease." https://assets.publishing.service.gov.uk/government/uploads/system/uploads/attachment_data/file/214895/9387-2900853-CVD-Outcomes_web1.pdf%0A https://assets.publishing.service.gov.uk/government/uploads/system/uploads/attachment_data/file/217118/9387-2900853.

Johnson, H. E., Broadhurst, D., Kell, D. B., Theodorou, M. K., Merry, R. J., & Griffith, G. W. (2004). High-throughput metabolic fingerprinting of legume silage fermentations via Fourier transform infrared spectroscopy and chemometrics. *Applied and Environmental Microbiology*, *70*(3), 1583–1592. https://doi.org/10.1128/AEM.70.3.1583-1592.2004.

Kordalewska, M., & Markuszewski, M. J. (2015). Metabolomics in cardiovascular diseases. *Journal of Pharmaceutical and Biomedical Analysis*, *113*, 121–136. https://doi.org/10.1016/j.jpba.2015.04.021.

Lewis, G. D., Farrell, L., Wood, M. J., Martinovic, M., Arany, Z., Rowe, G. C., Souza, A., Cheng, S., McCabe, E. L., Yang, E., Shi, X., Deo, R., Roth, F. P., Asnani, A., Rhee, E. P., Systrom, D. M., Semigran, M. J., Vasan, R. S., Carr, S. A., Wang, T. J., Sabatine, M. S., Clish, C. B., & Gerszten, R. E. (2010). Metabolic signatures of exercise in human plasma. *Science Translational Medicine*, *2*(33), 33ra37. https://doi.org/10.1126/scitranslmed.3001006.

Lewis, G. D., Wei, R., Liu, E., Yang, E., Shi, X., Martinovic, M., Farrell, L., Asnani, A., Cyrille, M., Ramanathan, A., Shaham, O., Berriz, G., Lowry, P. A., Palacios, I. F., Taşan, M., Roth, F. P., Min, J., Baumgartner, C., Keshishian, H., Addona, T., Mootha, V. K., Rosenzweig, A., Carr, S. A., Fifer, M. A., Sabatine, M. S., & Gerszten, R. E. (2008). Metabolite profiling of blood from individuals undergoing planned myocardial infarction reveals early markers of myocardial injury. *The Journal of Clinical Investigation*, *118*(10), 3503–3512. https://doi.org/10.1172/JCI35111.

Libby, P. (2002). Inflammation in atherosclerosis. *Nature*, *420*. 868–874. https://doi.org/10.1038/nature01323.

Mathers, C. D., & Loncar, D. (2006). Projections of Global Mortality and Burden of Disease from 2002 to 2030. *PLOS Medicine*, *3*(11), e442. https://doi.org/10.1371/journal.pmed.0030442.

Mayr, M., Yusuf, S., Weir, G., Chung, Y.-L., Mayr, U., Yin, X., Ladroue, C., Madhu, B., Roberts, N., De Souza, A., Fredericks, S., Stubbs, M., Griffiths, J. R., Jahangiri, M., Xu, Q., & Camm, A. J. (2008). Combined metabolomic and proteomic analysis of human atrial fibrillation. *Journal of the American College of Cardiology*, *51*(5), 585–594. https://doi.org/10.1016/j.jacc.2007.09.055.

MESA. (2022). The Multi-Ethnic Study of Atherosclerosis (MESA). Retrieved December 3, 2022 from *http://www.mesa-nhlbi.org/.*

Müller, J., Bertsch, T., Volke, J., Schmid, A., Klingbeil, R., Metodiev, Y., Karaca, B., Kim, S.-H., Lindner, S., Schupp, T., Kittel, M., Poschet, G., Akin, I., & Behnes, M. (2021). Narrative review of metabolomics in cardiovascular disease. *Journal of Thoracic Disease*, *13*(4), 2532–2550. https://doi.org/10.21037/jtd-21-22.

Nascimben, L., Ingwall, J. S., Pauletto, P., Friedrich, J., Gwathmey, J. K., Saks, V., Pessina, A. C., & Allen, P. D. (1996). Creatine kinase system in failing and nonfailing human myocardium. *Circulation*, *94*(8), 1894–1901. https://doi.org/ 10.1161/01.cir.94.8.1894.

Nicholls, S. J., Wang, Z., Koeth, R., Levison, B., DelFraino, B., Dzavik, V., Griffith, O. W., Hathaway, D., Panza, J. A., Nissen, S. E., Hochman, J. S., & Hazen, S. L. (2007). Metabolic Profiling of Arginine and Nitric Oxide Pathways Predicts Hemodynamic Abnormalities and Mortality in Patients With Cardiogenic Shock After Acute Myocardial Infarction. *Circulation*, *116*(20), 2315–2324. https://doi.org/10.1161/CIRCULATIONAHA.107.693986.

Nichols, M., Townsend, N., Luengo-Fernandez, R., Leal, J., Gray, A., Scarborough, P., & Rayner, M. (2012). European CardiovascularDisease Statistics. *European Heart Network and European Society of Cardiology*.

Nicholson, J. K., Lindon, J. C., & Holmes, E. (1999). "Metabonomics": understanding the metabolic responses of living systems to pathophysiological stimuli via multivariate statistical analysis of biological NMR spectroscopic data. *Xenobiotica; the Fate of Foreign Compounds in Biological Systems*, *29*(11), 1181–1189. https://doi.org/10.1080/004982599238047.

Nicholson, J. K., & Wilson, I. D. (2003). Opinion: understanding "global" systems biology: metabonomics and the continuum of metabolism. *Nature reviews. Drug discovery*, *2*(8), 668–676. https://doi.org/10.1038/nrd1157.

Oliver, S. G., Winson, M. K., Kell, D. B., & Baganz, F. (1998). Systematic functional analysis of the yeast genome. *Trends in Biotechnology*, *16*(9), 373–378. https://doi.org/10.1016/s0167-7799(98)01214-1.

Patti, G. J., Yanes, O., & Siuzdak, G. (2012). Metabolomics: the apogee of the omics trilogy. *Nature Reviews Molecular Cell Biology*, *13*(4), 263–269. https://doi.org/10.1038/nrm3314.

Roberts, L. D., & Gerszten, R. E. (2013). Toward new biomarkers of cardiometabolic diseases. *Cell Metabolism*, *18*(1), 43–50. https://doi.org/10.1016/j.cmet.2013.05.009.

Sabatine, M. S., Liu, E., Morrow, D. A., Heller, E., McCarroll, R., Wiegand, R., Berriz, G. F., Roth, F. P., & Gerszten, R. E. (2005). Metabolomic identification of novel biomarkers of myocardial ischemia. *Circulation*, *112*(25), 3868–3875. https://doi.org/10.1161/CIRCULATIONAHA.105.569137.

Senn, T., Hazen, S. L., & Tang, W. H. W. (2012). Translating metabolomics to cardiovascular biomarkers. *Progress in Cardiovascular Diseases*, *55*(1), 70–76. https://doi.org/10.1016/j.pcad.2012.06.004.

Shah, S. H., Kraus, W. E., & Newgard, C. B. (2012). Metabolomic profiling for the identification of novel biomarkers and mechanisms related to common cardiovascular diseases: form and function. *Circulation*, *126*(9), 1110–1120. https://doi.org/10.1161/CIRCULATIONAHA.111.060368.

Shao, Z., Wang, Z., Shrestha, K., Thakur, A., Borowski, A. G., Sweet, W., Thomas, J. D., Moravec, C. S., Hazen, S. L., & Tang, W. H. W. (2012). Pulmonary hypertension associated with advanced systolic heart failure: dysregulated arginine metabolism and importance of compensatory dimethylarginine dimethylaminohydrolase-1. *Journal of the American College of Cardiology*, *59*(13), 1150–1158. https://doi.org/10.1016/j.jacc.2011.12.022.

Smith, C. S., Bottomley, P. A., Schulman, S. P., Gerstenblith, G., & Weiss, R. G. (2006). Altered creatine kinase adenosine triphosphate kinetics in failing hypertrophied human myocardium. *Circulation*, *114*(11), 1151–1158. https://doi.org/10.1161/CIRCULATIONAHA.106.613646.

Steffen, B. T., Steffen, L. M., Tracy, R., Siscovick, D., Hanson, N. Q., Nettleton, J., & Tsai, M. Y. (2012). Obesity modifies the association between plasma phospholipid polyunsaturated fatty acids and markers of inflammation: the Multi-Ethnic Study of Atherosclerosis. *International Journal of Obesity (2005)*, *36*(6), 797–804. https://doi.org/10.1038/ijo.2011.157.

Tang, W. H. W., Wang, Z., Cho, L., Brennan, D. M., & Hazen, S. L. (2009). Diminished global arginine bioavailability and increased arginine catabolism as metabolic profile of increased cardiovascular risk. *Journal of the American College of Cardiology*, *53*(22), 2061–2067. https://doi.org/10.1016/j.jacc.2009.02.036.

TRIUMPH Investigators, Alexander, J. H., Reynolds, H. R., Stebbins, A.L., Dzavik, V., Harrington, R. A., Van de Werf, F., Hochman, J. S. (2007). Effect of Tilarginine Acetate in Patients With Acute Myocardial Infarction and Cardiogenic ShockThe TRIUMPH Randomized Controlled Trial. *JAMA*, *297*(15), 1657–1666. https://doi.org/10.1001/jama.297.15.joc70035.

Tweeddale, H., Notley-McRobb, L., & Ferenci, T. (1998). Effect of slow growth on metabolism of Escherichia coli, as revealed by global metabolite pool ("metabolome") analysis. *Journal of Bacteriology*, *180*(19), 5109–5116. https://doi.org/10.1128/JB.180.19.5109-5116.1998.

Vallejo, M., García, A., Tuñón, J., García-Martínez, D., Angulo, S., Martin-Ventura, J. L., Blanco-Colio, L. M., Almeida, P., Egido, J., & Barbas, C. (2009). Plasma fingerprinting with GC-MS in acute coronary syndrome. *Analytical and Bioanalytical Chemistry*, *394*(6), 1517–1524. https://doi.org/10.1007/s00216-009-2610-6.

van Bilsen, M., van Nieuwenhoven, F. A., & van der Vusse, G. J. (2009). Metabolic remodelling of the failing heart: beneficial or detrimental? *Cardiovascular Research*, *81*(3), 420–428. https://doi.org/10.1093/cvr/cvn282.

Vorkas, P. A., Shalhoub, J., Isaac, G., Want, E. J., Nicholson, J. K., Holmes, E., & Davies, A. H. (2015). Metabolic Phenotyping of Atherosclerotic Plaques Reveals Latent Associations between Free Cholesterol and Ceramide Metabolism in Atherogenesis. *Journal of Proteome Research*, *14*(3), 1389–1399. https://doi.org/10.1021/pr5009898.

Wang, T. J., Gona, P., Larson, M. G., Tofler, G. H., Levy, D., Newton-Cheh, C., Jacques, P. F., Rifai, N., Selhub, J., Robins, S. J., Benjamin, E. J., D'Agostino, R. B., & Vasan, R. S. (2006). Multiple Biomarkers for the Prediction of First Major Cardiovascular Events and Death. *New England Journal of Medicine*, *355*(25), 2631–2639. https://doi.org/10.1056/NEJMoa055373.

Wang, T. J., Larson, M. G., Vasan, R. S., Cheng, S., Rhee, E. P., McCabe, E., Lewis, G. D., Fox, C. S., Jacques, P. F., Fernandez, C., O'Donnell, C. J., Carr, S. A., Mootha, V. K., Florez, J. C., Souza, A., Melander, O., Clish, C. B., & Gerszten, R. E. (2011). Metabolite profiles and the risk of developing diabetes. *Nature Medicine*, *17*(4), 448–453. https://doi.org/10.1038/nm.2307.

Wang, Z., Klipfell, E., Bennett, B. J., Koeth, R., Levison, B. S., Dugar, B., Feldstein, A. E., Britt, E. B., Fu, X., Chung, Y.-M., Wu, Y., Schauer, P., Smith, J. D., Allayee, H., Tang, W. H. W., DiDonato, J. A., Lusis, A. J., & Hazen, S. L. (2011). Gut flora metabolism of phosphatidylcholine promotes cardiovascular disease. *Nature*, *472*(7341), 57–63. https://doi.org/10.1038/nature09922.

Wang, Z., Tang, W. H. W., Cho, L., Brennan, D. M., & Hazen, S. L. (2009a). Targeted metabolomic evaluation of arginine methylation and cardiovascular risks: potential mechanisms beyond nitric oxide synthase inhibition. *Arteriosclerosis, Thrombosis, and Vascular Biology*, *29*(9), 1383–1391. https://doi.org/10.1161/ATVBAHA.109.185645.

Wang, Z., Tang, W. H. W., Cho, L., Brennan, D. M., & Hazen, S. L. (2009b). Targeted Metabolomic Evaluation of Arginine Methylation and Cardiovascular Risks. *Arteriosclerosis, Thrombosis, and Vascular Biology*, *29*(9), 1383–1391. https://doi.org/10.1161/ATVBAHA.109.185645.

Wilson, P. W., D'Agostino, R. B., Levy, D., Belanger, A. M., Silbershatz, H., & Kannel, W. B. (1998). Prediction of coronary heart disease using risk factor categories. *Circulation*, *97*(18), 1837–1847. https://doi.org/10.1161/01.cir.97.18.1837.

Wilson, P. W. F. (2008). Progressing From Risk Factors to Omics. *Circulation: Cardiovascular Genetics*, *1*(2), 141–146. https://doi.org/10.1161/CIRCGENETICS.108.815605.

World Health Organization (WHO) (2007). *Prevention of cardiovascular disease : guidelines for assessment and management of total cardiovascular risk* (pp. vi, 86 p, with CD-ROM.). World Health Organization.

World Health Organization (WHO). (2009). *World Health Organization*. Eastern Mediterranean Health Journal = La Revue de Santé de La Méditerranée Orientale = Al-Majallah Al-Ihhīyah Li-Sharq Al-Mutawassi. https://doi.org/10.1093/yiel/yvs044.

Zhang, H., Chen, X., Hu, P., Liang, Q., Liang, X., Wang, Y., & Luo, G. (2009). Metabolomic profiling of rat serum associated with isoproterenol-induced myocardial infarction using ultra-performance liquid chromatography/time-of-flight mass spectrometry and multivariate analysis. *Talanta*, *79*(2), 254–259. https://doi.org/10.1016/j.talanta.2009.03.045.

Index

L

M

N

O

P

S

T

U

V